Drug dictionary
for dentistry

Dose schedules are being continually revised and new side effects recognized. Oxford University Press makes no representation, express or implied, that the drug dosages in this book are correct. For these reasons the reader is strongly urged to consult the pharmaceutical company's printed instructions before administering any of the drugs recommended in this book.

Drug dictionary
for dentistry

J.G. Meechan

and

R.A. Seymour

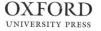

OXFORD
UNIVERSITY PRESS

Great Clarendon Street, Oxford OX2 6DP

Oxford University Press is a department of the University of Oxford.
It furthers the University's objective of excellence in research,
scholarship, and education by publishing worldwide in

Oxford New York

Auckland Bangkok Buenos Aires Cape Town Chennai
Dar es Salaam Delhi Hong Kong Istanbul Karachi
Kolkata Kuala Lumpur Madrid Melbourne Mexico City
Mumbai Nairobi São Paulo Shanghai Singapore Taipei
Tokyo Toronto

with an associated company in Berlin

Oxford is a registered trade mark of Oxford University Press
in the UK and in certain other countries

Published in the United States
by Oxford University Press Inc., New York

A catalogue record for this title is available from the British Library

Library of Congress Cataloging in Publication Data
Meechan, J. G.
Drug dictionary for dentistry/J. G. Meechan, R. A. Seymour.
p. cm.
1. Dental pharmacology–Dictionaries.   2. Dental therapeutics–
Dictionaries. I. Seymour, R. A. II. Title.
RK701.M442002   617.6'061'03–dc21   2001052052
ISBN 0 19 263274 4

10 9 8 7 6 5 4 3 2 1

Typeset by Newgen Imaging Systems (P) Ltd., Chennai, India
Printed in Great Britain on acid-free paper by
The Bath Press, Avon

This book is dedicated to:
The memory of my father (JGM)
Gayle, Tom and Oliver (RAS)

Preface

Drug therapy has an effect on the management of patients in dentistry. Many drugs produce oro-dental problems; in addition concurrent medication can interact with drugs which the dentist may prescribe. The aim of this dictionary is to draw together the effects of drugs on the teeth, oral and perioral structures and highlight drug interactions which impact on dental treatment. Drugs taken by out-patients which may be encountered in general dental practice and interactions with drugs contained in the *Dental Practitioners Formulary* have been included. Interactions which may occur with medication prescribed by dentists working in the hospital service have also been covered. Drugs which the dentist may prescribe have been annotated in greater detail to include any significant interactions that have been recorded. Drugs have been listed alphabetically by their Recommended Non-proprietary Name (rINN) rather than their British Approved Name (BAN). In those cases where it is still recommended that both the BAN and rINN should appear then drugs commonly found in dental out-patients are listed under both names.

It is hoped that this pocket-sized volume will act as a ready reference source for those dealing with dental patients taking medication.

J.G. Meechan
R.A. Seymour

October, 2001

How to use this dictionary

The drugs are listed in alphabetical order by their approved name in this dictionary. An alphabetical list of trade-names is provided in the Appendix in order to cross-reference to the approved name used in the dictionary.

Acknowledgement

The authors are pleased to acknowledge the assistance of Mrs Renata Taylor in the compilation of this dictionary.

Abacavir (Ziagen)

Description
A nucleoside reverse transcriptase inhibitor.

Indications
Used in the management of HIV infection.

Effects on oral and dental structures
This drug may produce oral ulceration.

Effects on patient management
Sensitive handling of the underlying disease state is essential. Excellent preventive dentistry and regular examinations are important in patients suffering from HIV, as dental infections are best avoided. HIV will interfere with postoperative healing and antibiotic prophylaxis prior to oral surgery may be advisable.

Drug interactions
None of importance in dentistry.

Acamprosate calcium (Campral EC)

Description
An anti-dependence drug.

Indications
Used in the management of alcohol dependence.

Effects on oral and dental structures
None known.

Effects on patient management
A history of alcohol dependence may cause bleeding disorders and affect drug metabolism.

Drug interactions
None relevant.

Acarbose (Glucobay)

Description
An inhibitor of intestinal alpha glucosidases.

Indications
Diabetes mellitus inadequately controlled by diet or by diet and oral hypoglycaemic agents.

Effects on oral and dental structures
None reported.

Effects on patient management
Hypoglycaemia can be a problem in patients taking acarbose, especially if they are also on insulin. Before commencing dental treatment, it is important to check that patients have had their normal food intake. If there is any doubt, give the patient a glucose drink. As with any diabetic patient try and treat in the first half of the morning and ensure that patients can eat after dental treatment. If a patient on acarbose requires a general anaesthetic then refer to hospital.

Drug interactions
Systemic corticosteroids antagonize the hypoglycaemic actions of acarbose. If these drugs are required, then consult the patient's physician before prescribing.

Acebutolol (Sectral)

Description
A beta-adrenoceptor blocking drug. Also combined with a diuretic, hydrochlorothiazide (Secadrex).

Indications
Hypertension.

Effects on oral and dental structures
Xerostomia and lichenoid eruptions can be produced.

Effects on patient management
Xerostomia will make the dentate patient more susceptible to dental caries (especially root caries) and will cause problems with denture retention. Postural hypotension may occur, and patients may feel dizzy when the dental chair is returned to the upright position after they have been treated in the supine position.

Drug interactions
NSAIDs such as ibuprofen may antagonize hypotensive action of acebutolol; possible interaction between epinephrine and acebutolol which may cause a slight increase in blood pressure. Do not exceed

more than 3 cartridges of epinephrine containing local anaesthetic solution per adult patient.

Aceclofenac (Preservex)

Description
A peripherally acting, non-steroidal anti-inflammatory analgesic.

Indications
Pain and inflammation associated with musculoskeletal disorders, e.g. rheumatoid arthritis, osteoarthritis, and ankylosing spondylitis.

Effects on oral and dental structures
Patients on long-term NSAIDs such as aceclofenac may be afforded some degree of protection against periodontal breakdown. This arises from the drug's inhibitory action on prostaglandin synthesis. The latter is an important inflammatory mediator in the pathogenesis of periodontal breakdown.

Effects on patient management
Rare unwanted effects of aceclofenac include angioedema and thrombocytopenia. If the platelet count is low (<100,000) then the socket should be packed and sutured. Persistent bleeding may require a platelet transfusion. The latter may cause an increased bleeding tendency following any dental surgical procedure.

Drug interactions
Ibuprofen, aspirin and diflunisal should be avoided in patients taking aceclofenac due to an increase in unwanted effects, especially gastrointestinal ulceration, renal and liver damage. Systemic corticosteroids also increase the risk of peptic ulceration and gastrointestinal bleeding.

Acemetacin (Emflex)

Description
A peripherally acting, non-steroidal anti-inflammatory analgesic.

Indications
Pain and inflammation associated with musculoskeletal disorders, e.g. rheumatoid arthritis, osteoarthritis, and ankylosing spondylitis. Postoperative analgesia.

Effects on oral and dental structures
Patients on long-term NSAIDs such as acemetacin may be afforded some degree of protection against periodontal breakdown. This arises from the drug's inhibitory action on prostaglandin synthesis. The latter is an important inflammatory mediator in the pathogenesis of

periodontal breakdown. Acemetacin has also been implicated for inducing oral lichenoid eruptions and oral ulceration. The drug does have a higher incidence of bone marrow suppression when compared to other NSAIDs. This can cause agranulocytosis, leucopenia, aplastic anaemia, and/or thrombocytopenia. Such depression of bone marrow function will affect the oral mucosa (high risk of ulceration), the periodontal tissue (high risk of gingival bleeding and periodontal breakdown) and healing after any dental surgical procedure.

Effects on patient management
The risk of thrombocytopenia will cause an increased bleeding tendency following dental surgical procedures. If the platelet count is low (<100,000) then the socket should be packed and sutured. Persistent bleeding may require a platelet transfusion.

Drug interactions
Ibuprofen, aspirin and diflunisal should be avoided in patients taking acemetacin due to an increase in unwanted effects, especially gastrointestinal ulceration, renal, and liver damage. Systemic corticosteroids increase the risk of peptic ulceration and gastrointestinal bleeding.

Acetazolamide

Description
A carbonic anhydrase inhibitor.

Indications
Used to treat glaucoma, as a prophylaxis against mountain sickness, as an add-on drug in epilepsy and in the emergency management of retrobulbar haemorrhage. Although it is a diuretic it is not used for that purpose.

Effects on oral and dental structures
Xerostomia, taste disturbance (metallic taste), paraesthesia, and Stevens–Johnson syndrome may occur.

Effects on patient management
Acetazolamide increases the toxicity of the local anaesthetic procaine, however this local anaesthetic agent is rarely used in modern dentistry. Acetazolamide can cause both thrombocytopenia and anaemia. Thrombocytopenia may cause postoperative bleeding. If the platelet count is low (<100,000) then the socket should be packed and sutured. Persistent bleeding may require a platelet transfusion. Anaemia may result in poor healing. Any anaemia will need correction prior to elective general anaesthesia and sedation.

Avoid high dose aspirin for postoperative pain control as a serious metabolic acidosis may occur. If the patient is receiving the drug for epilepsy control then fits are possible, especially if the pateint is stressed, therefore sympathetic handling and perhaps sedation should be considered for stressful procedures. Emergency anticonvulsant medication (diazepam or midazolam) must be available.

Drug interactions

The interactions with aspirin and procaine were mentioned above. Acetazolamide increases the plasma concentration of carbamazepine and increases the chances of osteomalacia when combined with phenytoin and phenobarbitone. It also increases the toxicity of ephedrine. Combined therapy with corticosteroids increases the chances of hypokalaemia.

Acetylsalicylic acid (Aspirin)

Description
A peripherally acting, non-steroidal analgesic.

Indications
Pain with a significant inflammatory component (e.g. postoperative pain after dental surgical procedures). Also used in the management of musculoskeletal pain, headache, and dysmenorrhoea, as an antipyretic, and for its antiplatelet actions in the prophylaxis for cerebrovascular disease or myocardial infarctions.

Presentations
(i) A 300 mg tablet.

(ii) Dispersible aspirin 300 mg.

(iii) A 75 mg tablet used for antiplatelet action.

Dose
Analgesia and antipyresis 300–900 mg every 4–6 hours.
Antiplatelet action 75–300 mg per day.

Contraindications
Cannot be prescribed to asthmatics (can precipitate bronchoconstriction), children under 12 years (risk of Reye's syndrome), patients with a history of peptic ulceration (aspirin is ulcerogenic), uncontrolled hypertension, patients suffering from gout (aspirin is uricosuric), patients with disorders of haemostasis (aspirin reduces platelet aggregation, therefore increases bleeding time), or patients with known hypersensitivity to the drug.

Precautions
Pregnancy and breastfeeding mothers.

Unwanted effects

Aspirin is ulcerogenic to the gastric mucosa and can cause the so-called 'aspirin burn' if a tablet is held against the oral mucosa. The effect of the drug on platelets can lead to an increase in bleeding time and possible problems with haemostasis. Local measures usually resolve an aspirin-induced bleed, but if these fail, the patient will need a platelet transfusion. High doses of aspirin can cause tinnitus due to a raise in labyrinthine pressure. Reducing the dose usually resolves the problem. The drug is also uricosuric and can precipitate an attack of gout.

Drug interactions

Aspirin should not be prescribed to patients taking anticoagulants since there is an increased risk of impaired haemostasis. Aspirin also enhances the effect of the antiepileptic drugs phenytoin and sodium valproate. Both aspirin and corticosteroids are ulcerogenic and should thus be avoided, especially in patients with a history of peptic ulceration. Aspirin reduces the renal excretion of the cytotoxic drug methotrexate and thus increases the unwanted effects of this drug. The diuretic actions of spironolactone and acetazolamide are reduced by aspirin. Metaclopramide and domperidone increase the rate of aspirin absorption by their actions on gastric emptying. The uricosuric effects of aspirin will reduce the actions of probenecid and sulfinpyrazone. Can produce hypoglycaemia, combined use with oral hypoglycaemic agents should be avoided.

Aciclovir [Acyclovir] (Zovirax)

Description
An antiviral drug.

Indications
Used in the treatment of herpes simplex and varicella-zoster infections.

Presentations
(i) 200 mg, 400 mg and 800 mg tablets.

(ii) 200 mg, 400 mg and 800 mg dispersible tablets.

(iii) Oral suspensions of 200 mg/5 mL and 400 mg/5 mL.

(iv) A 5% cream.

(v) 250 mg powder for reconstitution for intravenous infusion.

Dose
Adults: 200–400 mg 5 times daily (or topical application to lesion 5 times daily).

Children under 2 years: half adult dose.

Contraindications
Hypersensitivity.

Precautions
Renal disease, pregnancy, and breastfeeding. Maintenance of adequate fluid intake is required with high doses.

Unwanted effects
Stinging sensation at site of application, altered taste, gastrointestinal upset, renal failure, bone marrow depression, tremors and convulsions, lichenoid reactions, rash and urticaria.

Drug interactions
Aciclovir may reduce the effectiveness of the anticonvulsant drugs phenytoin and sodium valproate. Aciclovir may increase the toxicity of pethidine. Probenicid increases the plasma concentration of aciclovir.

Aclarubicin

Description
A cytotoxic antibiotic.

Indications
Acute non-lymphocytic leukaemia.

Effects on oral and dental structures
Aclarubicin causes bone marrow suppression with an accompanying thrombocytopenia and agranulocytosis. Bone marrow suppression can lead to troublesome oral ulceration, exacerbation of an existing periodontal condition and rapid spread of any residual (e.g. periapical) infections.

Effects on patient management
The effect of aclarubicin on the bone marrow is transient and routine dental treatment is best avoided until the white blood cells and platelet counts start to recover. If emergency dental treatment such as an extraction is required then antibiotic cover may be necessary, depending on the degree of myelosuppression. If the platelet count is low (<100,000) then the socket should be packed and sutured. Persistent bleeding may require a platelet transfusion.

Patients on chemotherapeutic agents such as aclarubicin often neglect their oral hygiene and thus there could be an increase in both caries and periodontal disease. If time permits, patients about to go on chemotherapy should have a dental check up and any potential areas of infection should be treated. Similarly, to reduce the mucosal irritation (sensitivity) that often accompanies chemotherapy, it is advisable to remove any ill-fitting dentures and smooth over rough cusps or restorations.

Drug interactions
None of any dental significance.

Acrivastine (Benadryl allergy relief, Semprex)

Description
An antihistamine.

Indications
Used in the treatment of allergies such as hay fever.

Effects on oral and dental structures
May produce xerostomia, but this is less common compared to older antihistamines.

Effects on patient management
The patient may be drowsy which may interfere with co-operation. Xerostomia may increase caries incidence and thus a preventive regimen is important. If the xerostomia is severe artificial saliva may be indicated.

Drug interactions
An enhanced sedative effect occurs with anxiolytic and hypnotic drugs. Tricyclic and monoamine oxidase inhibitor antidepressants increase antimuscarinic effects such as xerostomia.

Adrenaline (Epinephrine)

Description
A catecholamine sympathomimetic agent.

Indications
Used in dental local anaesthetic solutions to increase efficacy and duration and to aid in haemostasis.

Presentations
Epinephrine is contained in local anaesthetic solutions in concentrations of 1 : 80,000 (12.5 µg/mL), 1 : 100,000 (10 µg/mL) and 1 : 200,000 (5 µg/mL).

Dose
The *maximum* recommended dose over one visit in dental local anaesthetic solutions is 200 µg.

Contraindications
Severe cardiac disease such as uncontrolled arrhythmias and unstable angina are contraindications to the use of epinephrine. The

unusual catecholamine-secreting tumour of the adrenal gland known as phaeochromocytoma and thyroid storm (an acute hyperthyroid episode), are other contraindications to epinephrine in dental local anaesthesia.

Precautions
Dose reduction is wise when cardiac disease exists (see also drug interactions below).

Unwanted effects
Excessive dosage or inadvertent intravascular injection will produce symptoms of fear and anxiety such as tachycardia and tremors. Systolic blood pressure can rise and diastolic blood pressure may fall. Epinephrine, even at doses used in dentistry, can produce a hypokalaemia (reduction in plasma potassium) and this can lead to cardiac arrhythmias.

Drug interactions
Many drug interactions with epinephrine are theoretical; however some have been shown to produce effects that are clinically important. Tricyclic antidepressant drugs increase the pressor effects of epinephrine twofold; as the pressor effects are negligible at the doses used in dental local anaesthetics simple dose reduction is all that is required.

Adrenergic beta-blocking drugs such as propranolol can lead to unopposed increases in systolic blood pressure and dose reduction of epinephrine-containing local anaesthetics is advised. Non-potassium sparing diuretics exacerbate the hypokalaemia produced by epinephrine and this is apparent at the doses used in dental local anaesthesia; thus for patients receiving such diuretic therapy epinephrine dose reduction is advised. The volatile anaesthetics such as halothane increase cardiac sensitivity to the effects of epinephrine and a 50% dose reduction in the amount of catecholamine used is advised. Any agent with sympathomimetic properties has the potential to increase the toxicity of epinephrine and among these agents are drugs of abuse such as cocaine, cannabis, and amphetamines.

Albendazole (Eskazole)

Description
An antihelminthic drug.

Indications
Used in the management of tapeworms.

Effects on oral and dental structures
Xerostomia may occur.

Effects on patient management

Xerostomia may increase caries incidence and thus a preventive regimen is important. If the xerostomia is severe artificial saliva may be indicated. The drug can cause a leucopenia which may affect healing adversely; if severe, prophylactic antibiotics should be prescribed to cover surgical procedures.

Drug interactions

Serum levels of albendazole are raised by concurrent therapy with dexamethasone. Carbamazepine may accelerate the metabolism of albendazole.

Alendronic acid (Fosamax)

Description

A bisphosphonate.

Indications

Postmenopausal osteoporosis.

Effects on oral and dental structures

Alendronic acid has been cited as a cause of angioedema. Whilst this unwanted effect is rare, when it does occur, it often involves the lips, the tongue and the floor of the mouth. Drug-induced angioedema is difficult to predict and can be precipitated by dental treatment.

Effects on patient management

Since alendronic acid can cause angioedema, it is always advisable to check whether patients have experienced any problems with breathing or swallowing.

Drug interactions

NSAIDs such as ibuprofen should not be prescribed to patients taking alendronic acid, since both drugs are ulcerogenic to the gastrointestinal tract.

Alginates (Algicon, Gastrocote, Gaviscon, Peptac, Topal)

Description

Used to counteract gastro-oesophageal reflux, usually in combination with antacids.

Indications

Used in the management of dyspepsia and gastro-oesophageal reflux.

Effects on oral and dental structures
Patients may complain of a chalky taste. The underlying condition of reflux can lead to erosion of the teeth, especially the palatal surfaces.

Effects on patient management
The patient may not be comfortable in the fully supine position due to gastric reflux. Combinations which include an antacid will interact with the drugs listed below, and such drugs should be taken a few hours in advance of antacid dose.

Drug interactions
Combinations of alginates and antacids reduce absorption of phenytoin, tetracyclines, the non-steroidal analgesic diflunisal and the antifungal drugs ketoconazole and itraconazole. Antacids can increase the excretion of aspirin and reduce plasma concentration to nontherapeutic levels.

Alimemazine tartrate/Trimeprazine tartrate (Vallergan)

Description
An antihistamine.

Indications
Used in the treatment urticaria and pruritis and as a sedative.

Effects on oral and dental structures
Can produce xerostomia.

Effects on patient management
The patient may be drowsy which may interfere with co-operation. Xerostomia may increase caries incidence and thus a preventive regimen is important. If the xerostomia is severe artificial saliva may be indicated. This drug may cause thrombocytopenia, agranulocytosis, and anaemia. Thrombocytopenia may cause postoperative bleeding. If the platelet count is low (<100,000) then the socket should be packed and sutured. Persistent bleeding may require a platelet transfusion. Agranulocytosis may affect healing adversely. Anaemia may result in poor healing. Any anaemia will need correction prior to elective general anaesthesia and sedation.

Drug interactions
There is an enhanced sedative effect with anxiolytic and hypnotic drugs and increased CNS depression with opioid analgesics. Tricyclic and monoamine oxidase inhibitor antidepressants increase antimuscarinic effects such as xerostomia.

Allopurinol (Zyloric)

Description
A xanthine-oxidase inhibitor.

Indications
Prophylaxis of gout and to prevent uric acid and calcium oxalate renal stones.

Effects on oral and dental structures
Allopurinol can cause taste disturbances and paraesthesia. It is a rare cause of erythema multiforme and bone marrow suppression.

Effects on patient management
Allopurinol-induced bone marrow suppression can cause an increased risk of oral infections, especially after dental surgical procedures. The accompanying thrombocytopenia increases the risk of haemorrhage.

Drug interactions
None of any dental significance.

Alprazolam (Xanax)

Description
A benzodiazepine anxiolytic.

Indications
Used in the short term management of anxiety.

Effects on oral and dental structures
Xerostomia may occur.

Effects on patient management
Xerostomia may increase caries incidence and thus a preventive regimen is important. If the xerostomia is severe artificial saliva may be indicated. Patients on alprazolam are anxious individuals and may be subject to mood swings; thus they require gentle, sympathetic handling. The concurrent prescription of CNS inhibitors should be avoided.

Drug interactions
As with all benzodiazepines, there is enhancement of other CNS inhibitors. Serum alprazolam levels are reduced by combined therapy with carbamazepine. Erythromycin and ketoconazole and paroxetine inhibit the metabolism of alprazolam. Alprazolam increases serum imipramine levels.

Aluminium hydroxide (Algicon, Alu-cap, Gastrocote, Gaviscon Maalox, Maalox TC, Mucogel, Topal)

Description
An antacid.

Indications
Used to treat dyspepsia and hyperphosphataemia.

Effects on oral and dental structures
Patients may complain of a chalky taste. Excessive use of aluminium hydroxide can lead to hypophosphataemia which may cause bone pains. The underlying condition of reflux can lead to erosion of the teeth, especially the palatal surfaces.

Effects on patient management
The patient may not be comfortable in the fully supine position due to gastric reflux. Any fluoride supplementation should be taken a few hours in advance of antacid dose (the same applies to tetracyclines).

Drug interactions
Reduced absorption of fluoride, phenytoin, metronidazole, tetracyclines, the non-steroidal analgesic diflunisal, the corticosteroids prednisone and prednisolone, and the antifungal drugs ketoconazole and itraconazole occurs. Concurrent therapy with aluminium hydroxide causes some delay in the absorption of diazepam but this is clinically unimportant. Aluminium hydroxide can increase the excretion of aspirin and reduce plasma concentration to non-therapeutic levels.

Alverine citrate (Alvercol)

Description
An antispasmodic drug.

Indications
Used for symptomatic relief in gastrointestinal disorders such as dyspepsia, diverticular disease and irritable bowel syndrome. Also used in dysmenorrhoea.

Effects on oral and dental structures
None specific.

Effects on patient management
The patient may not be comfortable in fully supine position due to the underlying gastrointestinal disorder.

Drug interactions
None of importance in dentistry.

Amantadine hydrochloride (Symmetrel)

Description
A dopaminergic drug.

Indications
Used in the management of Parkinsonism and as an antiviral agent against herpes zoster.

Effects on oral and dental structures
Xerostomia and occasionally glossitis can occur.

Effects on patient management
Xerostomia may increase caries incidence and thus a preventive regimen is important. If the xerostomia is severe artificial saliva may be indicated. This drug may cause postural hypotension, thus the patient should not be changed from the supine to the standing position too rapidly. If the drug is being used to treat Parkinsonism the underlying disease can lead to management problems as the patient may have uncontrollable movement. Short appointments are recommended.

Drug interactions
None of importance in dentistry.

Amethocaine [tetracaine] (Ametop)

Description
An ester local anaesthetic for topical use.

Indications
Used for topical anaesthesia of the skin prior to venepuncture.

Presentations
A 4% gel.

Dose
1.5 g applied to skin surface.

Contraindications
Allergy to ester local anaesthetics and parabens. Should not be used in infants less than one year old.

Precautions
Care must be employed in patients with liver disease as absorption is rapid and toxicity may occur. Similarly, it should not be used

on traumatized or damaged tissue or highly vascularized mucous membranes.

Unwanted effects
Allergic reactions can occur. Amethocaine is more toxic than other ester local anaesthetics because of slower metabolism, thus it is no longer used as an injectable agent.

Drug interactions
Increased systemic toxicity when administered in combination with other local anaesthetics.

Amfebutamone [Bupropion] (Zyban)

Description
An anti-dependence drug.

Indications
Used in the management of smoking cessation.

Effects on oral and dental structures
Xerostomia and Stevens–Johnson syndrome may occur.

Effects on patient management
Xerostomia may increase caries incidence and thus a preventive regimen is important. If the xerostomia is severe artificial saliva may be indicated. Occasionally patients experience postural hypotension, thus sudden movements of the dental chair should be avoided.

Drug interactions
Carbamazepine reduces the plasma concentration of amfebutamone. Concurrent use with monoamine oxidase inhibitors should be avoided.

Amikacin (Amikin)

Description
An aminoglycoside antibiotic.

Indications
Use to treat serious Gram-negative infections resistant to gentamicin.

Effects on oral and dental structures
None specific.

Effects on patient management
This drug can produce disturbances of hearing and balance; rapid movements of the dental chair should be avoided and care taken when the patient leaves the chair.

Drug interactions
The ototoxic effect of this drug is exacerbated by vancomycin. Nephrotoxicity is increased when used in combination with amphotericin B and clindamycin. The risk of hypocalcaemia produced by bisphosphonates, which are used in the management of Paget's disease of bone, is increased by amikacin.

Amiloride

Description
A potassium-sparing diuretic.

Indications
Oedema, potassium conservation with thiazide, and loop diuretics.

Effects on oral and dental structures
Xerostomia leading to increased risk of root caries, candidal infections, and poor denture retention. If the xerostomia is severe, dentate patients should receive topical fluoride and be offered an artificial saliva.

Effect on patient management
Postural hypotension can occur.

Drug interactions
NSAIDs can enhance amiloride-induced hyperkalaemia.

Aminophylline (Phyllocontin Continus)

Description
A bronchodilator.

Indications
Used in the management of asthma and reversible airway obstruction.

Effects on oral and dental structures
Xerostomia and taste disturbance may be produced.

Effects on patient management
Patients may not be comfortable in the supine position if they have respiratory problems. If the patient suffers from asthma then aspirin-like compounds should not be prescribed as many asthmatic patients are allergic to these analgesics. Similarly, sulphite-containing compounds (such as preservatives in epinephrine-containing local anaesthetics) can produce allergy in asthmatic patients. Xerostomia may increase caries incidence and thus a preventive regimen is important. If the xerostomia is severe artificial saliva may be indicated. The use of a rubber dam in patients with obstructive airway disease may

further embarrass the airway. If a rubber dam is essential then supplemental oxygen via a nasal cannula may be required. (See drug interactions below.)

Drug interactions

There is an increased chance of dysrhythmia with halogenated general anaesthetic agents during combined therapy. Aminophylline decreases the sedative and anxiolytic effects of some benzodiazepines, including diazepam. Plasma aminophylline levels are reduced by carbamazepine and phenytoin. Plasma aminophylline concentration is increased by ciprofloxacin, clarithromycin, erythromycin, fluconazole and ketoconazole and tetracyclines. Aminophylline decreases the plasma concentration of erythromycin. Aminophylline levels may be affected by corticosteroids; hydrocortisone and methylprednisolone have been shown to both increase and decrease aminophylline levels. Concurrent therapy with quinolone antibacterials such as ciprofloxacin may lead to convulsions.

Amiodarone (Cordarone)

Description
A class III antidysrhythmic drug.

Indications
Cardiac arrhythmias.

Effects on oral and dental structures
Metallic taste may be produced.

Effects on patient management
Very rarely cause thrombocytopenia. If the platelet count is low (<100,000) then the socket should be packed and sutured. Persistent bleeding may require a platelet transfusion.

Drug indications
None of any dental significance.

Amisulpride (Solian)

Description
An atypical antipsychotic drug.

Indications
Used in the treatment of schizophrenia.

Effects on oral and dental structures
Xerostomia and uncontrollable oro-facial muscle activity (tardive dyskenesia) may be produced.

Effects on patient management

Xerostomia may increase caries incidence and thus a preventive regimen is important. If the xerostomia is severe artificial saliva may be indicated. Uncontrollable muscle movement of jaws and tongue as well as the underlying psychotic condition may interfere with management as satisfactory co-operation may not be achieved readily. There may be problems with denture retention and certain stages of denture construction (e.g. jaw registration) can be difficult. Postural hypotension can occur with this drug, therefore rapid changes in patient position should be avoided.

Drug interactions

There is increased sedation when used in combination with CNS depressant drugs such as alcohol, opioid analgesics, and sedatives. Combined therapy with tricyclic antidepressants increases the chances of cardiac arrythmias, and exacerbates antimuscarinic effects such as xerostomia.

Amitriptyline hydrochloride (Lentizol, Triptaphen, Tryptizol)

Description

A tricyclic antidepressant.

Indications

Used in the management of depressive illness and for the treatment of nocturnal enuresis in children.

Effects on oral and dental structures

Xerostomia, taste disturbance, stomatitis, oro-facial dysaesthesia, and pain in the salivary glands may occur.

Effects on patient management

Xerostomia may increase caries incidence and thus a preventive regimen is important. If the xerostomia is severe artificial saliva may be indicated. Postural hypotension and fainting may occur with this drug, therefore rapid changes in patient position should be avoided. This drug may cause thrombocytopenia, agranulocytosis, and leucopenia. Thrombocytopenia may cause postoperative bleeding. If the platelet count is low (<100,000) then the socket should be packed and sutured. Persistent bleeding may require a platelet transfusion. Agranulocytosis and leucopenia may affect healing adversely.

Drug interactions

Increased sedation occurs with alcohol and sedative drugs such as benzodiazepines. This drug may antagonize the action of anticonvulsants such as carbamazepine and phenytoin. This drug increases the pressor effects of epinephrine. Nevertheless, the use of epinephrine-containing local anaesthetics is not contraindicated; however, epinephrine dose limitation is recommended. Normal anticoagulant control by warfarin may be upset, both increases and decreases in INR have been noted during combined therapy with tricyclic antidepressants.

Combined therapy with other antidepressant should be avoided and if prescribing another class of antidepressant a period of one to two weeks should elapse between changeover. Antimuscarinic effects such as xerostomia are increased when used in combination with other anticholinergic drugs such as antipsychotics.

Amlodipine besylate (Istin)

Description
A calcium-channel blocker.

Indications
Hypertension and angina prophylaxis.

Effects on oral and dental structures
Amlodipine can cause gingival overgrowth, especially in the anterior part of the mouth. It also causes taste disturbances by inhibiting calcium-channel activity necessary for normal function of taste and smell receptors.

Effects on patient management
None of any significance.

Drug interactions
None of any dental significance.

Amobarbital (Amylobarbitone) [Amytal]

Description
A barbiturate hypnotic.

Indications
Only used in treatment of intractable insomnia in those already taking barbiturates.

Effects on oral and dental structures
Barbiturates may cause xerostomia and fixed drug eruptions.

Effects on patient management
The patient may be drowsy and confused. As respiratory depression is produced by this drug other medication which produces such depression, e.g. sedatives, must be avoided in general practice. Long term

treatment with this drug may produce anaemia, agranulocytosis and thrombocytopenia. Thrombocytopenia may cause postoperative bleeding. If the platelet count is low (<100,000) then the socket should be packed and sutured. Persistent bleeding may require a platelet transfusion. Anaemia and agranulocytosis may result in poor healing. Any anaemia will need correction prior to elective general anaesthesia and sedation.

Drug interactions

All barbiturates are enzyme-inducers and thus can increase the metabolism of concurrent medication. Drugs which are metabolized more rapidly in the presence of barbiturates include warfarin, carbamazepine, doxicycline, and tricyclic antidepressants. The effects of other CNS depressants, including alcohol, are increased in the presence of barbiturates.

Amoxapine (Asendis)

Description
A tricyclic antidepressant.

Indications
Used in the management of depressive illness.

Effects on oral and dental structures
Xerostomia and stomatitis may occur. Uncontrollable oro-facial movements (tardive dyskenesia) may be produced.

Effects on patient management
Xerostomia may increase caries incidence and thus a preventive regimen is important. If the xerostomia is severe artificial saliva may be indicated. Postural hypotension and fainting may occur with this drug, therefore rapid changes in patient position should be avoided. Tardive dyskenesia may make co-operation for treatment difficult. There may be problems with denture retention and certain stages of denture construction (e.g. jaw registration) can be difficult. This drug may cause thrombocytopenia, agranulocytosis and leucopenia. Thrombocytopenia may cause postoperative bleeding. If the platelet count is low (<100,000) then the socket should be packed and sutured. Persistent bleeding may require a platelet transfusion. Agranulocytosis and leucopenia may affect healing adversely.

Drug interactions
Increased sedation occurs with alcohol and sedative drugs such as benzodiazepines. This drug may antagonize the action of anticonvulsants such as carbamazepine and phenytoin. This drug increases the pressor effects of epinephrine. Nevertheless, the use of epinephrine-containing

local anaesthetics is not contraindicated; however, epinephrine dose limitation is recommended.

Normal anticoagulant control by warfarin may be upset, both increases and decreases in INR have been noted during combined therapy with tricyclic antidepressants. Combined therapy with other antidepressants should be avoided and if prescribing another class of antidepressant a period of one to two weeks should elapse between changeover. Antimuscarinic effects such as xerostomia are increased when used in combination with other anticholinergic drugs such as antipsychotics.

Amoxicillin (Amoxil)

Description
A broad spectrum beta-lactam antibacterial.

Indications
Used to treat bacterial infection such as a dental abscess. Used prophylactically in the prevention of infective endocarditis.

Presentations
 (i) Capsules of 250 mg and 500 mg.
 (ii) 500 mg dispersible tablets.
 (iii) Oral suspensions of 125 mg/5 mL and 250 mg/5 mL.
 (iv) Powder for reconstitution for oral administration 750 mg and 3 g.
 (v) 250 mg and 500 mg vials for reconstitution for injection.

Dose
(1) For management of dental infections
250–500 mg orally three times daily for out-patient treatment.
500–1000 mg intravenously four times daily for severe infections.
Child under 10 years: 50% adult dose.
(2) For prophylaxis of infective endocarditis.
3 g orally one hour preoperatively for prophylaxis when treatment under local anaesthesia. Under general anaesthesia 1 g intravenously or intramuscularly at induction followed by 500 mg 6 hours later: or 3 g orally 4 hours preoperatively followed by 3 g orally as soon as practicable after surgery.
Child under 5 years: 25% adult dose.
Child 5–10 years 50% adult dose.

Contraindications
Hypersensitivity.

Precautions
Renal disease.
Glandular fever.

Chronic lymphatic leukaemia.
HIV.

Unwanted effects
Glossitis and tongue discolouration.
Candidiasis.
Hypersensitivity.
Gastrointestinal upset.
Pseudomembranous colitis.
Hypokalaemia.

Drug interactions
Amoxicillin reduces the excretion of the cytotoxic drug methotrexate, leading to increased toxicity of the latter drug which may cause death. There may be a reduced efficacy of oral contraceptives and other methods of contraception are advised during antibiotic therapy. Amoxicillin activity is decreased by tetracyclines. Amoxicillin rarely increases the prothrombin time when given to patients receiving warfarin. Probenecid significantly increases the half-life of amoxicillin. Nifedipine increases amoxicillin absorption but this is of little clinical importance. Amiloride decreases the absorption of amoxicillin but this is probably of little significance. The production of rashes is increased during concomitant treatment with allopurinol.

Amphotericin (Fungilin, Fungizone)

Description
A polyene antifungal.

Indications
Used to treat candidal infections.

Presentations
(i) 100 mg tablets.
(ii) 10 mg lozenges.
(iii) 100 mg/mL oral suspension.
(iv) A 50 mg powder for reconstitution for intravenous infusion.

Dose
For oral infection suck one lozenge four times a day or place 1 mL of the oral suspension over the lesion four times daily for up to 14 days.

Contraindications
Other than allergy there are no contraindications to topical use.

Precautions
None for topical use but parenteral administration requires close monitoring and a test dose. Combined therapy with cyclosporin and cardiac glycosides (such as digoxin) should be avoided.

Unwanted effects
Gastrointestinal disturbances.
Renal damage.
Hypokalaemia.
Myopathy and neuropathy.

Drug interactions
Antifungal action is decreased during combined therapy with fluconazole, ketoconazole, and miconazole. Parenterally administered amphotericin has increased nephrotoxicity when administered with aminoglycoside antibiotics (e.g. gentamycin, vancomycin, and cyclosporin). Amphotericin can produce potassium loss (hypokalaemia) and this is exacerbated during concurrent treatment with corticosteroids. Similarly, the risk of hypokalaemia is increased during combined therapy with non-potassium sparing diuretics. Combined therapy with pentamidine, which is a drug used to treat pneumocystis pneumonia in AIDS patients, can lead to acute renal failure. Similarly the antiviral agent zalcitabine, which is used in the management of HIV, has increased toxicity when given concurrently with amphotericin.

Ampicillin (Penbritin)

Description
A broad spectrum beta-lactam antibacterial.

Indications
Used to treat bacterial infection such as a dental abscess.

Presentations
  (i) 250 mg and 500 mg capsules.
 (ii) Syrup with 125 mg/5 mL and 250 mg/5 mL.
(iii) Oral suspensions of 125 mg/1.25 mL, 125 mg/5 mL and 250 mg/5 mL.
 (iv) 250 mg and 500 mg vials for reconstitution for injection.
  (v) Also available in combination with cloxacillin as Ampiclox.

Dose
250–1000 mg four times daily.
Child under 10 years: 50% adult dose.

Contraindications
Hypersensitivity.

Precautions
Renal disease.
Glandular fever.
Chronic lymphatic leukaemia.
HIV.

Unwanted effects
Glossitis and tongue discolouration.
Candidiasis.
Hypersensitivity.
Stevens–Johnson syndrome.
Gastrointestinal upset.
Hypokalaemia.
Pseudomembranous colitis.

Drug interactions
Ampicillin reduces the excretion of the cytotoxic drug methotrexate, leading to increased toxicity of the latter drug which may cause death. There may be a reduced efficacy of oral contraceptives and other methods of contraception are advised during antibiotic therapy. Ampicillin activity is decreased by tetracyclines. Antagonism also occurs with chloramphenicol and the neurological side effects of the latter drug (e.g. deafness) are increased during combined therapy. Chloroquine reduces the absorption of ampicillin. Ampicillin rarely increases the prothrombin time when given to patients receiving warfarin. Ampicillin can increase the muscle weakness of patients with myasthenia gravis who are receiving anti-cholinergic drugs. Ampicillin reduces the efficacy of sulphasalazine which is used in the treatment of Crohn's disease.

Probenecid significantly increases the half-life of ampicillin. Nifedipine increases ampicillin absorption but this is of little clinical importance. Amiloride decreases the absorption of ampicillin but this is probably of little significance. The production of rashes is increased during concomitant treatment with allopurinol. Large single doses of ampicillin (1 g) decrease the serum levels of the anti-hypertensive drug atenolol by half.

Anastrozole (Arimidex)

Description
A non-steroidal aromatase inhibitor.

Indications
Advanced postmenopausal breast cancer.

Effects on oral and dental structures
Nothing reported.

Effects on patient management
Nothing of any significance.

Drug interactions
None of any dental significance.

Apomorphine hydrochloride (Britaject)

Description
A dopaminergic drug.

Indications
Used under specialist supervision for the management of refractory Parkinsonism.

Effects on oral and dental structures
Local administration can lead to swelling of the lips, oral ulceration, and stomatitis.

Effects on patient management
Parkinsonism can lead to management problems as the patient may have uncontrollable movement. Short appointments are recommended.

Drug interactions
None of importance in dentistry.

Articaine (Septanenst)

Description
An amide local anaesthetic.

Indications
Used to provide intra-oral anaesthesia by injection.

Presentations
In dental local anaesthetic cartridges of 1.7 mL containing 4% articaine (68 mg) with 1 : 100,000 (17 μg) or 1 : 200,000 (8.5 μg) epinephrine (adrenaline).

Dose
The maximum recommended dose is 7.0 mg/kg.

Contraindications
Allergy to the amide group of local anaesthetics is a contraindication. Articaine is unusual as an amide local anaesthetic in that it contains a sulphur component, thus allergy to sulphites contraindicates use (some asthmatic patients have sulphite allergies). The manufacturers do not recommend use in children under 12 years of age.

Precautions

Reduce the dose in hepatic disease. Epinephrine-containing solutions have additional precautions (see epinephrine).

Unwanted effects

Articaine has been implicated in the production of non-surgical paraesthesias after intra-oral injection.

Drug interactions

None known.

Atenolol (Tenorminx)

Description

A beta$_1$-adrenergic blocker, whose action is primarily targeted against the beta$_1$-adrenergic receptors in the heart. Although used in hypertension, its mode of action is uncertain. Atenolol is also combined with a diuretic, chlortalidone (Co-Tenidone) and with a calcium-channel blocker, nifedipine (Beta-Adalat).

Indications

Hypertension, angina pectoris, cardiac arrhythmias, early management of myocardial infarction.

Effects on oral and dental structures

Atenolol can cause dry mouth, lichenoid eruption, inhibition of calculus formation and tooth demineralization. The mechanism of the latter is uncertain and does not appear to be related to the reduction in salivary flow or change in salivary calcium or phosphate ion concentrations. It is thought that atenolol, along with other beta-adrenergic blockers, alters the physiochemical properties of saliva, which in turn makes tooth tissue more susceptible to demineralization.

Effects on patient management

The dry mouth and the other actions of atenolol on saliva will make the dentate patient more susceptible to dental caries, especially root surface caries. Regular topical fluoride treatment and dietary advice (e.g. sugar free chewing gum) will reduce the caries risk. Postural hypotension may occur and patients may feel dizzy when the dental chair is returned to upright after they have been treated in the supine position.

Dental Drug interactions

Possible interaction between epinephrine and atenolol may cause a slight increase in systolic blood pressure. The effect would be related to the dose of epinephrine used in either gingival retraction cord or in local anaesthetic solutions. Use of NSAIDs may decrease the hypotensive actions of atenolol.

Atorvastatin (Lipitor)

Description
A cholesterol lowering drug.

Indications
To reduce coronary events by lowering LDL cholesterol.

Effects on oral and dental structures
None reported.

Effects on patient management
None of any significance.

Drug interactions
None of any dental significance.

Atovaquone (Wellvone)

Description
An antiprotozoal drug.

Indications
Used to treat pneumonia caused by Pneumocystis carinii.

Effects on oral and dental structures
Altered taste and candidal infection can occur.

Effects on patient management
Opportunistic infection such as candida should be suspected and treated early. The drug can cause anaemia, and leucopenia which will interfere with general anaesthesia, sedation, and postoperative healing.

Drug interactions
Tetracycline reduces plasma levels of atovaquone which may lead to failure in therapy. There is a theoretical possibility that atovaquone increases the anticoagulant effect of warfarin.

Atropine sulphate

Description
An antimuscarinic drug.

Indications
Used in gastrointestinal disorders such as dyspepsia, diverticular disease, and irritable bowel syndrome. Used as a premedication and in ophthalmology.

Effects on oral and dental structures
Xerostomia may occur.

Effects on patient management
Usually atropine is used as an acute medication and thus xerostomia is a transient effect. However in prolonged use, as in management of gastrointestinal disorders, xerostomia may increase caries incidence and thus a preventive regimen is important. If the xerostomia is severe artificial saliva may be indicated.

Patients may not be comfortable in fully supine condition due to underlying gastrointestinal disorder.

Drug interactions
Absorption of ketoconazole is decreased, but this is only of concern with prolonged use of the antimuscarinic drug. Side effects are increased during concurrent medication with tricyclic and monoamine oxidase inhibitor antidepressants.

Auranofin (Ridaura)

Description
A gold salt.

Indications
Active progressive rheumatoid arthritis, juvenile arthritis.

Effects on oral and dental structures
Administration of gold salts is associated with oral lichenoid eruptions, oral ulceration and discolouration of the oral mucosa. Auranofin does suppress bone marrow activity and the accompanying thrombocytopenia will enhance gingival bleeding. Likewise, auranofin-induced oral ulceration may be secondary to bone marrow suppression.

Effects on patient management
Auranofin-induced bone marrow suppression can cause an increased risk of oral infection, especially after dental surgical procedures. The accompanying thrombocytopenia increases the risk of haemorrhage. If

the platelet count is low (<100,000) then the socket should be packed and sutured. Persistent bleeding may require a platelet transfusion.

Drug interactions
None of any dental significance.

Azapropazone (Rheumox)

Description
A peripherally acting, non-steroidal anti-inflammatory analgesic.

Indications
For use in rheumatoid arthritis, ankylosing spondylitis, and acute gout when all other NSAIDs have failed.

Effects on oral and dental structures
Patients on long-term NSAIDs such as azapropazone may be afforded some degree of protection against periodontal breakdown. This arises from the drug's inhibitory action on prostaglandin synthesis. The latter is an important inflammatory mediator in the pathogenesis of periodontal breakdown. Azapropazone has a high prevalence of photosensitivity reactions, which can cause a sunburn-type reaction affecting the lips and circumoral skin. Patients on this drug should always apply a sunblock cream to the skin and lips when exposed to sunlight.

Effects on patient management
Rare unwanted effects of azapropazone include angioedema and thrombocytopenia. The latter may cause an increased bleeding tendency following any dental surgical procedure. If the platelet count is low (<100,000) then the socket should be packed and sutured. Persistent bleeding may require a platelet transfusion.

Drug interactions
Ibuprofen, aspirin and diflunisal should be avoided in patients taking azapropazone due to an increase in unwanted effects, especially gastrointestinal ulceration, renal, and liver damage. Systemic corticosteroids increase the risk of peptic ulceration and gastrointestinal bleeding.

Azatadine maleate (Optimine)

Description
An antihistamine.

Indications
Used in the treatment of allergies such as hay fever and urticaria.

Effects on oral and dental structures
Can produce xerostomia.

Effects on patient management
The patient may be drowsy which may interfere with cooperation. Xerostomia may increase caries incidence and thus a preventive regimen is important. If the xerostomia is severe artificial saliva may be indicated. This drug may cause thrombocytopenia, agranulocytosis and anaemia. Thrombocytopenia may cause postoperative bleeding. If the platelet count is low (<100,000) then the socket should be packed and sutured. Persistent bleeding may require platelet transfusion. Agranulocytosis may affect healing adversely. Anaemia may result in poor healing. Any anaemia will need correction prior to elective general anaesthesia and sedation.

Drug interactions
Enhanced sedative effects occur with anxiolytic and hypnotic drugs. Tricyclic and monoamine oxidase inhibitor antidepressants increase antimuscarinic effects such as xerostomia.

Azathioprine (Imuran)

Description
An immunosuppressant.

Indications
To prevent graft rejection in organ transplant patients; used in the management of autoimmune and collagen diseases.

Effects on oral and dental structures
The immunosuppressant properties of azathioprine could impact upon expression of periodontal disease (reduce breakdown), cause delayed healing, and make the patient more susceptible to opportunist oral infections such as candida or herpetic infections. Organ transplant patients on azathioprine are more prone to malignancy and lesions which can affect the mouth, including Kaposi's sarcoma and lip cancer. Hairy leukoplakia can also develop in these patients and again this is attributed to the immunosuppressant properties of azathioprine.

Effects on patient management
All patients on immunosuppressant therapy should receive a regular oral screening because of their increased propensity to 'oral' and lip malignancies. Any suspicious lesion must be biopsied. Likewise any signs of opportunistic oral infections must be treated promptly to avoid systemic complications. The delayed healing and increased susceptibility to infection does not warrant the use of prophylactic antibiotic cover before specific dental procedures.

Drug interactions
None of any dental significance.

Azithromycin (Zithromax)

Description
A macrolide antibiotic.

Indications
Used to treat respiratory and soft tissue infections, otitis media, and genital chlamydial infections.

Effects on oral and dental structures
Taste disturbance, stomatitis, candidiasis, and Stevens–Johnson syndrome may occur.

Effects on patient management
Local treatment for stomatitis and candidiasis may be required.

Drug interactions
None of importance in dentistry.

Azlocillin (Securopen)

Description
A beta-lactam antibiotic.

Indications
Used in the treatment of infections caused by *Pseudomonas aeruginosa*.

Effects on oral and dental structures
Oral candidiasis may result from the use of this broad spectrum agent.

Effects on patient management
This drug may cause thrombocytopenia, neutropenia, and anaemia. Thrombocytopenia may cause postoperative bleeding. If the platelet count is low (<100,000) then the socket should be packed and sutured. Persistent bleeding may require platelet transfusion. Neutropenia and anaemia may result in poor healing. Any anaemia will need correction prior to elective general anaesthesia and sedation.

Drug interactions
Tetracyclines reduce the effectiveness of penicillins. This drug inactivates gentamicin if they are mixed together in the same infusion and this should be avoided.

Aztreonam (Azactam)

Description
A beta-lactam antibiotic.

Indications
Used to treat Gram-negative infections.

Effects on oral and dental structures
This drug may produce oral ulceration and taste disturbance.

Effects on patient management
Oral ulcers may require local therapy. This drug may cause thrombocytopenia and neutropenia Thrombocytopenia may cause postoperative bleeding. If the platelet count is low (<100,000) then the socket should be packed and sutured. Persistent bleeding may require platelet transfusion. Neutropenia may affect healing adversely.

Drug interactions
Aztreonam probably increases the anticoagulant effects of warfarin and nicoumalone.

Balsalazide sodium (Colazide)

Description
An aminosalicylate.

Indications
Used to treat ulcerative colitis.

Effects on oral and dental structures
May produce lupus erythematosus.

Effects on patient management
Due to the underlying condition non-steroidal inflammatory drugs are best avoided. In order to avoid pseudomembranous ulcerative colitis discussion with the supervising physician is advised prior to prescription of an antibiotic.

The aminosalicylates can produce blood dyscrasias including anaemia, leucopenia and thrombocytopenia. Anaemia may result in poor healing. Any anaemia will need correction prior to elective general anaesthesia and sedation. Leucopenia will affect healing adversely and if severe prophylactic antibiotics should be prescribed to cover surgical procedures. Thrombocytopenia may cause postoperative bleeding. If the platelet count is low (<100,000) then the socket should be packed and sutured. Persistent bleeding may require platelet transfusion. Patients may be receiving steroids in addition to aminosalicylates and thus the occurrence of adrenal crisis should be borne in mind.

Drug interactions

No drug interactions of importance in dentistry but see comments above related to non-steroidals and antibiotics.

Bambuterol hydrochloride (Bambec)

Description

A beta$_2$-adrenoceptor stimulant.

Indications

Used in the management of asthma and obstructive airway disease.

Effects on oral and dental structures

Xerostomia and taste alteration may occur.

Effects on patient management

Patients may not be comfortable in the supine position if they have respiratory problems. Aspirin-like compounds should not be prescribed as many asthmatic patients are allergic to these analgesics. Similarly, sulphite-containing compounds (such as preservatives in epinephrine-containing local anaesthetics) can produce allergy in asthmatic patients. Xerostomia may increase caries incidence and thus a preventive regimen is important. If the xerostomia is severe artificial saliva may be indicated. The use of a rubber dam in patients with obstructive airway disease may further embarrass the airway. If a rubber dam is essential then supplemental oxygen via a nasal cannula may be required.

Drug interactions

The hypokalaemia which may result from large doses of salbutamol may be exacerbated by a reduction in potassium produced by high doses of steroids and by epinephrine in dental local anaesthetics.

Beclometasone dipropionate (AeroBec, AsmaBec, Becloforte, Becodisks, Beconase, Becotide, Ventide, Propaderm, Qvar)

Description

A corticosteroid.

Indications

Used in the prophylaxis of asthma, in allergic rhinitis, and inflammatory skin disorders such as eczema.

Effects on oral and dental structures

The inhalational forms may produce xerostomia and candidiasis.

Effects on patient management

The patient may be at risk of adrenal crisis under stress. This is due to adrenal suppression. Whilst such suppression does occur physiologically, its clinical significance does appear to be overstated. As far as dentistry is concerned, there is increasing evidence that supplementary corticosteroids are not required. This would apply to all restorative procedures, periodontal surgery, and the uncomplicated dental extraction. For more complicated dentoalveolar surgery, each case must be judged on its merits. An apprehensive patient may well require cover. It is important to monitor the patient's blood pressure before, during and for 30 minutes after the procedure. If diastolic pressure drops by more than 25%, then hydrocortisone 100 mg IV should be administered and the patient's blood pressure should continue to be monitored.

Patients may not be comfortable in the supine position if they have respiratory problems. If the patient suffers from asthma then aspirin-like compounds should not be prescribed as many asthmatic patients are allergic to these analgesics. Similarly, sulphite-containing compounds (such as preservatives in epinephrine-containing local anaesthetics) can produce allergy in asthmatic patients. Xerostomia may increase caries incidence and thus a preventive regimen is important. If the xerostomia is severe artificial saliva may be indicated.

Drug interactions

When used topically, including by inhalation, drug interactions of relevance to dentistry are not a concern.

Bendrofluazide/Bendroflumethiazide

Description

A thiazide diuretic.

Indications

Heart failure, hypertension, and oedema.

Effects on oral and dental structures

Thiazide diuretics can cause lichenoid eruptions in the mouth, and taste disturbances due to hyperzincuria and xerostomia.

Effect on patient management

Postural hypertension and rarely blood disorders, including agranulocytosis, neutropenia, and thrombocytopenia can occur. The latter may have an effect on haemostasis after various dental surgical procedures. High doses of bendrofluazide can cause hypokalaemia which can be exacerbated by epinephrine local anaesthetic solutions (no more than 3 cartridges per adult patient).

Drug interactions

Epinephrine containing local anaesthetic solutions and systemic amphotericin may exacerbate a bendrofluazide hypokalaemia. Bendrofluazide may increase the nephrotoxicity of NSAIDs.

Benperidol (Anquil)

Description

A butyrophenone antipsychotic medication.

Indications

Used in the treatment of antisocial deviant sexual conditions.

Effects on oral and dental structures

Xerostomia and uncontrollable oro-facial muscle activity (tardive dyskenesia) may be produced.

Effects on patient management

Xerostomia may increase caries incidence and thus a preventive regimen is important. If the xerostomia is severe artificial saliva may be indicated. Uncontrollable muscle movement of jaws and tongue as well as the underlying psychotic condition may interfere with management as satisfactory co-operation may not be achieved readily. There may be problems with denture retention and certain stages of denture construction (e.g. jaw registration) can be difficult. Postural hypotension may occur with this drug, therefore rapid changes in patient position should be avoided.

Drug interactions

There is increased sedation when used in combination with CNS depressant drugs such as alcohol, opioid analgesics, and sedatives. Combined therapy with tricyclic antidepressants increases the chances of cardiac arrhythmias and exacerbates antimuscarinic effects such as xerostomia. The photosensitive effect of tetracyclines may be increased during combined therapy. There is a theoretical risk of hypotension being exacerbated by the epinephrine in dental local anaesthetics.

Benzatropine mesilate (Cogentin)

Description

An antimuscarinic drug.

Indications

Used in the management of Parkinsonism.

Effects on oral and dental structures

Xerostomia and glossitis can occur.

Effects on patient management
Xerostomia may increase caries incidence and thus a preventive regimen is important. If the xerostomia is severe artificial saliva may be indicated. Parkinsonism can lead to management problems as the patient may have uncontrollable movement. Short appointments are recommended.

Drug interactions
Absorption of ketoconazole is decreased. Side effects increase with concurrent medication with tricyclic antidepressants, mono-amine oxidase inhibitors and selective serotonin reuptake inhibitor antidepressants.

Benzhexol hydrochloride/Trihexyphenidyl hydrochloride (Broflex)

Description
An antimuscarinic drug.

Indications
Used in the management of Parkinsonism.

Effects on oral and dental structures
Xerostomia and glossitis can occur.

Effects on patient management
Xerostomia may increase caries incidence and thus a preventive regimen is important. If the xerostomia is severe artificial saliva may be indicated. Parkinsonism can lead to management problems as the patient may have uncontrollable movement. Short appointments are recommended.

Drug interactions
Absorption of ketoconazole is decreased. Side effects increase with concurrent medication with tricyclic and monoamine oxidase inhibitor antidepressants.

Benzocaine

Description
An ester local anaesthetic.

Indications
Used to provide intra-oral topical anaesthesia.

Presentations
Topical preparations in concentrations from 6% to 20%.

Dose

Due to its poor solubility and poor absorption, toxic reactions to benzocaine are rare. Dosage recommendations for the various preparations are provided by the manufacturer.

Contraindications

Allergy to the ester group of local anaesthetics and allergy to parabens are contraindications.

Precautions

Avoid excessive use in the mouth as loss of sensation in the tongue and pharynx can reduce protection of the airway.

Unwanted effects

Allergic reactions to the ester anaesthetics are more common than to the amides such as lidocaine. Benzocaine can produce methaemoglobinaemia at high dose or as an idiosyncratic reaction. Methaemoglobinaemia presents as cyanosis and is caused by the iron in haemoglobin being present as the ferric, rather than the ferrous form that reduces oxygen carriage.

Drug interactions

Benzocaine can antagonize the activity of the sulfonamide antibacterials.

Benzyl penicillin (Penicillin G, Crystapen)

Description

A beta-lactam antibacterial drug.

Indications

Used to treat bacterial infections such as dental abscesses.

Presentations

600 mg and 1.2 g vials of powder for reconstitution for intramuscular or intravenous administration (Penicillin G).

Dose

Adult: 600 mg–1.2 g four times a day.
Child: 1–12 years 100–300 mg/kg daily in 4–6 doses.

Contraindications

Hypersensitivity.

Precautions

Renal disease.

Unwanted effects

Hypersensitivity reactions.
Gastrointestinal upset.

Drug interactions

Penicillin reduces the excretion of the cytotoxic drug methotrexate, leading to increased toxicity of the latter drug which may cause death. There may be a reduced efficacy of oral contraceptives and other methods of contraception are advised during antibiotic therapy. Penicillin activity is decreased by tetracyclines. Penicillin G rarely increases the prothrombin time when given to patients receiving warfarin. Probenecid, phenylbutazone, sulphaphenazole, sulphinpyrazone, and the anti-inflammatory drugs aspirin and indomethacin significantly increase the half-life of penicillin G.

Betahistine dihydrochloride (Serc)

Description
A drug specific for Ménière's disease.

Indications
Used in the treatment of Ménière's disease.

Effects on oral and dental structures
None specific to this drug.

Effects on patient management
Due to the underlying condition rapid changes in patient position should be avoided.

Drug interactions
None of importance in dentistry.

Betamethasone (Betnesol)

Description
A corticosteroid.

Indications
Suppression of inflammation and allergic disorders. Used in the management of inflammatory bowel diseases, asthma, immunosuppression, and in various rheumatic diseases.

Effects on oral and dental structures
Although systemic corticosteroids can induce cleft lip and palate formation in mice, there is little evidence that this unwanted effect occurs in humans. The main impact of systemic corticosteroids on the mouth is to cause an increased susceptibility to opportunistic infections. These include candidiasis and those due to herpes viruses. The anti-inflammatory and immunosuppressant properties of corticosteroids may afford the patient some degree of protection against periodontal breakdown. Paradoxically long-term systemic use can

precipitate osteoporosis. The latter is now regarded as a risk factor for periodontal disease.

Effects on patient management

The main unwanted effect of corticosteroid treatment is the suppression of the adrenal cortex and the possibility of an adrenal crisis when such patients are subjected to 'stressful events'. Whilst such suppression does occur physiologically, its clinical significance does appear to be overstated. As far as dentistry is concerned, there is increasing evidence that supplementary corticosteroids are not required. This would apply to all restorative procedures, periodontal surgery and the uncomplicated dental extractions. For more complicated dentoalveolar surgery, each case must be judged on its merits. An apprehensive patient may well require cover. It is important to monitor the patient's blood pressure before, during and for 30 minutes after the procedure. If diastolic pressure drops by more than 25%, then hydrocortisone 100 mg IV should be administered and the patient's blood pressure should continue to be monitored.

Patients should be screened regularly for oral infections such as fungal or viral infections. When these occur, they should be treated promptly with the appropriate chemotherapeutic agent. Likewise, any patient on corticosteroids that presents with an acute dental infection should be treated urgently as such infections can readily spread.

Drug interactions

Aspirin and NSAIDs should not be prescribed to patients on long-term corticosteroids. Both drugs are ulcerogenic and hence increase the risk of gastrointestinal bleeding and ulceration. The antifungal agent amphotericin increases the risk of corticosteroid-induced hypokalaemia, whilst ketoconazole inhibits corticosteroid hepatic metabolism.

Bethanechol chloride (Myotonine)

Description

A parasympathomimetic.

Indications

Urinary retention.

Effects on oral and dental structures

None reported.

Effects on patient management

Bethanechol frequently causes transient blurred vision, and patients may require more assistance than usual.

Drug interactions
None of any dental significance.

Biperiden (Akineton)

Description
An antimuscarinic drug.

Indications
Used in the management of Parkinsonism.

Effects on oral and dental structures
Xerostomia and glossitis can occur.

Effects on patient management
Xerostomia may increase caries incidence and thus a preventive regimen is important. If the xerostomia is severe artificial saliva may be indicated. Parkinsonism can lead to management problems as the patient may have uncontrollable movements. Short appointments are recommended.

Drug interactions
Absorption of ketoconazole is decreased. Side effects increase with concurrent medication with tricyclic and monoamine oxidase inhibitor antidepressants.

Biphasic isophane insulin (Human Mixtard, Pork Mixtard, Humulin, Insuman)

Description
A biphasic intermediate acting insulin.

Indications
Diabetes mellitus.

Effects on oral and dental structures
Biphasic isophane insulin can cause pain and swelling of the salivary glands.

Effects on patient management
The main concern with treating diabetic patients on biphasic isophane insulin is to avoid hypoglycaemia. Thus it is important to ensure that patients have taken their normal food and insulin prior to their dental appointment. Wherever possible treat diabetic patients in the first half of the morning and ensure that any treatment does not preclude them from eating. If an insulin-dependent diabetic requires a general anaesthetic, then patients should be referred to hospital.

Drug interactions
Aspirin and the NSAIDs can cause hypoglycaemia which could be a problem in a poorly-controlled insulin dependent diabetic. These analgesics should be used with caution in such patients. Systemic corticosteroids will antagonize the hypoglycaemia properties of insulin. If these drugs are required in an insulin-dependent diabetic, then consult the patient's physician before prescribing.

Bisacodyl

Description
A stimulant laxative.

Indications
Used in the management of constipation.

Effects on oral and dental structures
May produce an unpleasant taste.

Effects on patient management
Avoid the use of codeine and other opioid compounds as they exacerbate constipation.

Drug interactions
Prolonged use may produce a hypokalaemia and this may be exacerbated by potassium shifts due to corticosteroids and epinephrine in local anaesthetics.

Bisoprolol (Emcor, Monocor)

Description
A beta-adrenoceptor blocking drug.

Indications
Hypertension, angina.

Effects on oral and dental structures
Bisoprolol can cause xerostomia and lichenoid eruptions.

Effects on patient management
Xerostomia will make the dentate patient more susceptible to dental caries (especially root caries) and will cause problems with denture retention. If the xerostomia is severe, dentate patients should receive topical fluoride and be offered an artificial saliva. Postural hypotension may occur and patients may feel dizzy when the dental chair is restored to upright after they have been treated in the supine position.

Drug interactions
NSAIDs such as ibuprofen may antagonize the hypotensive action of bisoprolol: possible interaction between epinephrine and bisoprolol which may cause a slight transient increase in blood pressure. Do not exceed more than 3 cartridges of epinephrine containing local anaesthetic solution per adult patient.

Bleomycin

Description
A cytotoxic antibiotic.

Indications
Squamous cell carcinoma

Effects on oral and dental structures
Bleomycin causes bone marrow suppression with an accompanying thrombocytopenia and agranulocytosis. Bone marrow suppression can lead to troublesome oral ulceration, exacerbation of an existing periodontal condition and rapid spread of any residual (e.g. periapical) infections.

Effects on patient management
The effect of bleomycin on the bone marrow is transient and routine dental treatment is best avoided until the white blood cells and platelet counts start to recover. If emergency dental treatment such as an extraction is required then antibiotic cover may be required depending on the degree of myelosuppression. If the platelet count is low (<100,000) then the socket should be packed and sutured. Persistent bleeding may require a platelet transfusion.

Patients on chemotherapeutic agents such as bleomycin often neglect their oral hygiene and thus there could be an increase in both caries and periodontal disease. If time permits, patients about to go on chemotherapy should have a dental check up and any potential areas of infection should be treated. Similarly, to reduce the mucosal irritation (sensitivity) that often accompanies chemotherapy, it is advisable to remove any ill-fitting dentures and smooth over rough cusps or restorations.

Drug interactions
None of any dental significance.

Botulinum A Toxin (Botox, Dysport)

Description
A neurotoxic drug.

Indications
Used in the treatment of dystonias including hemifacial spasm and torticollis.

Effects on oral and dental structures
Xerostomia, pooling of saliva and dysphagia may occur when the toxin is used to treat torticollis.

Effects on patient management
Loss of muscle control will interfere with dental treatment. As the drug is only used short term xerostomia should not produce significant problems, however a preventive regimen may be considered.

Drug interactions
Effects of the toxin are increased by aminoglycoside antibacterials such as gentamicin.

Brinzolamide (Azopt)

Description
A topical carbonic anhydrase inhibitor.

Indications
Used in the treatment of glaucoma.

Effects on oral and dental structures
Taste disturbance and xerostomia may be produced.

Effects on patient management
Xerostomia may increase caries incidence and thus a preventive regimen is important. If the xerostomia is severe artificial saliva may be indicated.

Drug interactions
As this drug is used topically drug interactions in dentistry are unlikely. However, theoretically adverse effects may occur with drugs which interact with carbonic anhydrase inhibitors such as aspirin, procaine, carbamazepine, phenytoin, and corticosteroids (see acetazolamide).

Bromocriptine (Parlodel)

Description
A dopamine receptor stimulant.

Indications
Galactorrhoea, cyclical benign breast disease and for the treatment of prolactinomas.

Effects on oral and dental structures
Bromocriptine does cause xerostomia which increases the risk of dental caries, candidal infections and causes poor denture retention. If the xerostomia is severe, dentate patients should receive topical fluoride and be offered an artificial saliva. The drug also causes dyskenesias which can result in involuntary movements of lips, tongue, and jaws.

Effects on patient management
Bromocriptine-induced dyskenesias can cause problems with denture retention and make certain stages of denture construction (e.g. jaw registration) difficult. Postural hypotension is a particular problem in the early stages of dosing with bromocriptine. This can cause problems with operating on patients in the supine position and restoring the dental chair to the upright position.

Drug interactions
Erythromycin will raise the plasma concentration of bromocriptine, which increases the risk of adverse reactions.

Bromazepam (Lexotan)

Description
A benzodiazepine anxiolytic.

Indications
Used in the short term management of anxiety.

Effects on oral and dental structures
None reported but similar drugs produce xerostomia so this is a possibility.

Effects on patient management
Patients on alprazolam are anxious individuals and will require gentle sympathetic handling. The concurrent prescription of CNS inhibitors should be avoided.

Drug interactions
Enhancement of CNS inhibitors occurs, otherwise none relevant to dental patients.

Bromocriptine (Parlodel)

Description
A dopaminergic drug (an ergot derivative).

Indications
Used in the management of Parkinsonism.

Effects on oral and dental structures
Xerostomia can occur.

Effects on patient management
Xerostomia may increase caries incidence and thus a preventive regimen is important. If the xerostomia is severe artificial saliva may be indicated. This drug may cause postural hypotension, thus the patient should not be changed from the supine to the standing position too rapidly. Parkinsonism can lead to management problems as the patient may have uncontrollable movement. Short appointments are recommended.

Drug interactions
Concurrent use of erythromycin increases bromocriptine toxicity.

Brompheniramine maleate (Dimotane)

Description
An antihistamine.

Indications
Used in the treatment of allergies such as hay fever and urticaria.

Effects on oral and dental structures
Can produce xerostomia.

Effects on patient management
The patient may be drowsy which may interfere with co-operation. Xerostomia may increase caries incidence and thus a preventive regimen is important. If the xerostomia is severe artificial saliva may be indicated. This drug may cause thrombocytopenia, agranulocytosis, and anaemia. Thrombocytopenia may cause postoperative bleeding. If the platelet count is low (<100,000) then the socket should be packed and sutured. Persistent bleeding may require platelet transfusion. Agranulocytosis may affect healing adversely. Anaemia may result in poor healing. Any anaemia will need correction prior to elective general anaesthesia and sedation.

Drug interactions
Enhanced sedative effect with anxiolytic and hypnotic drugs. Tricyclic and monoamine oxidase inhibitor antidepressants increase antimuscarinic effects such as xerostomia. The photosensitive effect of tetracyclines is increased by brompheniramine.

Budesonide (Budenofalk, Entocort, Pulmicort)

Description
A corticosteroid drug.

Indications
Used in the management of Crohn's disease, ulcerative colitis and the prophylaxis of asthma.

Effects on oral and dental structures
Xerostomia and taste disturbance can occur; inhalational forms may cause candidiasis.

Effects on patient management
Adrenal crisis must be anticipated: this is due to adrenal suppression. Whilst such suppression does occur physiologically, its clinical significance does appear to be overstated. As far as dentistry is concerned, there is increasing evidence that supplementary corticosteroids are not required. This would apply to all restorative procedures, periodontal surgery and the uncomplicated dental extraction. For more complicated dentoalveolar surgery, each case must be judged on its merits. An apprehensive patient may well require cover. It is important to monitor the patient's blood pressure before, during and for 30 minutes after the procedure. If diastolic pressure drops by more than 25%, then hydrocortisone 100 mg IV should be administered and patient's blood pressure should continue to be monitored.

Patients may not be comfortable in the supine position if they have respiratory problems. If the patient suffers from asthma then aspirin-like compounds should not be prescribed as many asthmatic patients are allergic to these analgesics. Similarly, sulphite-containing compounds (such as preservatives in epinephrine-containing local anaesthetics) can produce allergy in asthmatic patients. Long-term use may lead to impaired wound healing. Xerostomia may increase caries incidence and thus a preventive regimen is important. If the xerostomia is severe artificial saliva may be indicated.

Drug interactions
None of importance in dentistry.

Bumetanide (Burinex)

Description
A loop diuretic.

Indications
Oedema, oliguria due to renal failure.

Effects on oral and dental structures
Loop diuretics can cause taste disturbances due to zinc chelation. They have also been cited as causing oral lichenoid eruptions.

Effects on patient management
Rarely causes bone marrow depression resulting in agranulocytosis (risk of oral ulceration and periodontal breakdown) and thrombocytopenia. If the platelet count is low (<100,000) then the socket should be packed and sutured. Persistent bleeding may require a platelet transfusion.

Drug interactions
Bumetanide, like many diuretics, causes a hypokalaemia which can be exacerbated by systemic amphotericin and epinephrine containing local anaesthetic solutions. No more than 3 cartridges should be administered per adult patient.

Bupivacaine (Marcain)

Description
An amide local anaesthetic.

Indications
Used to provide local anaesthesia, especially long-lasting anaesthesia after regional block injection.

Presentations
(i) 10 mL vials of 0.25%, 0.375%, 0.5% or 0.75% bupivacaine for injection (containing 25, 37.5, 50 and 75 mg bupivacaine respectively).

(ii) 10 mL vials of 0.25% and 0.5% bupivacaine with 1 : 200,000 epinephrine for injection (containing 25 and 50 mg bupivacaine respectively with 50 μg epinephrine).

Dose
Recommended maximum dose is 1.3 mg/kg with an absolute ceiling of 90 mg.

Contraindications
Allergy to amide local anaesthetics.

Precautions
Reduce the dose in hepatic disease. Epinephrine-containing solutions have additional precautions (see epinephrine).

Unwanted effects
Bupivacaine is more cardiotoxic than lidocaine.

Drug interactions

Success of bupivacaine when used as a regional (spinal) anaesthetic is reduced by concomitant administration of the anti-rheumatic drug indomethacin and in individuals who abuse alcohol (the mechanism is not understood). The depressant effect on the heart produced by bupivacaine is exacerbated by calcium-channel blockers but this is probably only important if accidental intravascular injection of the local anaesthetic occurs. As with lidocaine beta-blocking drugs, especially propranolol, increase the plasma concentration of bupivacaine. Serum levels of bupivacaine are also increased by diazepam. The toxicity of bupivacaine has been reported to be increased when used in combination with mepivacaine (probably due to displacement of bupivacaine from its binding sites).

Buprenorphine (Temgesic)

Description
An opioid analgesic.

Indications
Moderate to severe pain, perioperative analgesia.

Effects on oral and dental structures
Can cause xerostomia leading to an increased risk of root caries, candidal infections, and poor denture retention. If the xerostomia is severe, dentate patients should receive topical fluoride and be offered an artificial saliva.

Effects on patient management
Buprenorphine is a drug of dependence and can thus cause withdrawal symptoms if the medication is stopped abruptly. Such cessation of buprenorphine may account for unusual behavioural changes and poor compliance with dental treatment. The drug also depresses respiration and causes postural hypotension.

Drug interactions
Buprenorphine will enhance the sedative properties of midazolam and diazepam. Reduce the dose of the latter drug.

Buserelin (Suprecur)

Description
A gonadorelin analogue.

Indications
Endometriosis, prostate cancer.

Effects on oral and dental structures

Rare unwanted effects of buserelin include paraesthesia of the lips and oedema of the lips and tongue. The drug is also associated with dry mouth which increases the risk of dental caries, especially root caries, poor denture retention, and an increased susceptibility to candidal infection. If the xerostomia is severe, dentate patients should receive topical fluoride and be offered an artificial saliva.

Effects on patient management

Use of buserelin is associated with an increased risk of osteoporosis. The latter is now regarded as a significant risk factor for periodontal disease.

Drug interactions

None of any dental significance.

Buspirone hydrochloride (Buspar)

Description

An anxiolytic acting at serotonin receptors.

Indications

Used in the short term management of anxiety.

Effects on oral and dental structures

Xerostomia can occur.

Effects on patient management

Patient may be anxious and thus short appointments may be best. Xerostomia may increase caries incidence and thus a preventive regimen is important. If the xerostomia is severe artificial saliva may be indicated.

Drug interactions

May cause hypertension during concurrent use with monoamine oxidase inhibitors. Increased CNS depression occurs with alcohol and other CNS depressants.

Busulphan (Myleran)

Description

An alkylating agent.

Indications

Chronic myeloid leukaemia.

Effects on oral and dental structures

Busulphan causes bone marrow suppression with an accompanying thrombocytopenia and agranulocytosis. Bone marrow suppression can lead to troublesome oral ulceration, exacerbation of an existing periodontal condition, and rapid spread of any residual (e.g. periapical) infections.

Effects on patient management
The effect of busulphan on the bone marrow is transient and routine dental treatment is best avoided until the white blood cells and platelet counts start to recover. If emergency dental treatment such as an extraction is required then antibiotic cover may be necessary, depending on the degree of myelosuppression. If the platelet count is low (<100,000) then the socket should be packed and sutured. Persistent bleeding may require a platelet transfusion.

Patients on chemotherapeutic agents such as busulphan often neglect their oral hygiene and thus there could be an increase in both caries and periodontal disease. If time permits, patients about to go on chemotherapy should have a dental check up and any potential areas of infection should be treated. Similarly, to reduce the mucosal irritation (sensitivity) that often accompanies chemotherapy, it is advisable to remove any ill-fitting dentures and smooth over rough cusps or restorations.

Drug interactions
None of any dental significance.

Butobarbital (Butobarbitone) [Soneryl]

Description
A barbiturate hypnotic.

Indications
Only used in treatment of intractable insomnia in those already taking barbiturates.

Effects on oral and dental structures
Barbiturates may cause xerostomia and fixed drug eruptions.

Effects on patient management
Xerostomia may increase caries incidence and thus a preventive regimen is important. If the xerostomia is severe artificial saliva may be indicated. The patient may be drowsy and confused. As respiratory depression is produced by this drug, other drugs which produce such depression such as sedatives must be avoided in general practice.

Long term treatment with this drug may produce anaemia, agranulocytosis and thrombocytopenia. Thrombocytopenia may cause postoperative bleeding. If the platelet count is low (<100,000) then the socket should be packed and sutured. Persistent bleeding may require platelet transfusion. Anaemia and agranulocytosis may result in poor healing. Any anaemia will need correction prior to elective general anaesthesia and sedation.

Drug interactions
All barbiturates are enzyme-inducers and thus can increase the metabolism of concurrent medication. Drugs which are metabolized more rapidly in the presence of barbiturates include warfarin, carbamazepine, corticosteroids, and tricyclic antidepressants. The effects of other CNS depressants, including alcohol, are increased in the presence of barbiturates.

Cabergoline (Cabaser, Dostinex)

Description
A dopamine receptor stimulant.

Indications
Galactorrhoea, cyclical benign breast disease and for the treatment of prolactinomas.

Effects on oral and dental structures
Cabergoline does cause xerostomia which increases the risk of dental caries, candidal infections, and causes poor denture retention. If the xerostomia is severe, dentate patients should receive topical fluoride and be offered an artificial saliva. The drug also cause dyskenesias which can result in involuntary movements of lips, tongue, and jaws.

Effects on patient management
Cabergoline-induced dyskenesias can cause problems with denture retention and make certain stages of denture construction (e.g. jaw registration) difficult. Postural hypotension is a particular problem in the early stages of dosing with cabergoline. This can cause problems with operating on patients in the supine position and restoring the dental chair to upright.

Drug interactions
Erythromycin will raise the plasma concentration of cabergoline, which increases the risk of adverse reactions.

Calcitonin-porcine (Calcitare)

Description
A hormone secreted by parafollicular cells of the thyroid gland.

Indications
Paget's disease of bone, hypercalcaemia.

Effects on oral and dental structures
Can cause taste disturbances.

Effects on patient management
Nothing of significance.

Drug interactions
None of any dental significance.

Calcium salts

Description.
Examples include calcium gluconate, lactate, carbonate (Calcichew, Calcette), and phosphate (Ostram).

Indications
Hypocalcaemia, osteoporosis.

Effects on oral and dental structures
None reported.

Effects on patient management
Nothing of significance.

Drug interactions
Calcium salts chelate with tetracyclines and thus prevent absorption. Avoid concomitant use.

Candesartan (Amias)

Description
An angiotensin-II receptor antagonist.

Indications
Used as an alternative to ACE inhibitors where the latter cannot be tolerated.

Effects on oral and dental structures
Angioedema has been reported, but the incidence of this unwanted effect is much less than when compared to ACE inhibitors.

Effects on patient management
None of any significance.

Drug interactions
NSAIDs such as ibuprofen may reduce the antihypertensive action of candesartan.

Capreomycin (Capastat)

Description
An antituberculous drug.

Indications
Used in the treatment of tuberculosis.

Effects on oral and dental structures
None specific.

Effects on patient management
Only emergency dental treatment should be performed during active tuberculosis and care must be exercised to eliminate spread of tuberculosis between the patient and dental personnel, e.g. masks and glasses should be worn and where possible treatment should be performed under a rubber dam to reduce aerosol spread. This drug may cause thrombocytopenia and leucopenia. Thrombocytopenia may cause postoperative bleeding. If the platelet count is low (<100,000) then the socket should be packed and sutured. Persistent bleeding may require platelet transfusion. Leucopenia may affect healing adversely.

Drug interactions
There is an increased risk of ototoxicity with gentamicin and vancomycin.

Captopril (Acepril, Capoten)

Description
Captopril is an ACE inhibitor, that is, it inhibits renal angiotensin converting enzyme which is necessary to convert angiotensin I to the more potent angiotensin II. It is also available combined with a diuretic, hydrochlorothiazide (Capozide).

Indications
Mild to moderate hypertension, congestive heart failure and post myocardial infarction where there is left ventricular dysfunction.

Effects on oral and dental structures
Taste disturbances, angioedema, dry mouth, glossitis and lichenoid drug reactions may occur. Many of these unwanted effects are dose related and compounded if there is an impairment of renal function.

Effects on patient management
Captopril-induced angioedema is perhaps the most significant unwanted effect that impacts upon dental management, since dental procedures can induce the angioedema. Management of captopril-induced angioedema is problematic since the underlying mechanism is

poorly understood. Standard anti-anaphylactic treatment is of little value (epinephrine and hydrocortisone) since the angioedema is not mediated via mast cells or antibody/antigen interactions. Usually the angioedema subsides and patients on these drugs should be questioned as to whether they have experienced any problems with breathing or swallowing. This will alert the dental practitioner to the possible risk of this unwanted effect arising during dental treatment.

Captopril is also associated with suppression of bone marrow activity giving rise to possible neutropenia, agranulocytosis, thrombocytopenia, and aplastic anaemia. Patients on captopril who present with excessive bleeding of their gums, sore throats or oral ulceration should have a full haematological investigation. If the platelet count is low (<100,000) then the socket should be packed and sutured. Persistent bleeding may require a platelet transfusion. Captopril-induced xerostomia increases the risk of fungal infections (candidiasis) and caries, especially root caries. Antifungal treatment should be used when appropriate and topical fluoride (e.g. Duraphat) will reduce the risk of root surface caries.

Drug interactions
Non-steroidal anti-inflammatory drugs (NSAIDs) such as ibuprofen may reduce the antihypertensive effect of captopril.

Carbachol

Description
A parasympathomimetic.

Indications
Urinary retention.

Effects on oral and dental structures
None reported.

Effects on patient management
Carbachol frequently causes transient blurred vision and patients may require more assistance than usual.

Drug interactions
None of any dental significance.

Carbamazepine (Tegretol, Tegretol retard, Teril CR, Timonil retard)

Description
An anticonvulsant.

Indications

Used in the treatment of epilepsy and neuralgias.

Presentations

(i) Tablets containing 100, 200 or 400 mg.

(ii) Liquid containing 100 mg/5 mL.

(iii) 125 mg suppositories.

Dose

Adults: initially 100 mg one to two times daily up to 1 g daily.

Children: under one year maximum dose 200 mg daily; under five years maximum dose 400 mg daily; under ten years maximum dose 600 mg daily.

Contraindications

Bone marrow depression.

Cardiac conduction abnormalities.

Porphyria.

Concurrent (or recent) monoamine oxidase inhibitor antidepressant therapy.

Precautions

Liver, kidney and heart disease.

Glaucoma.

History of haematological changes during drug therapy.

Pregnancy and breastfeeding.

Unwanted effects

Oral side effects include xerostomia, glossitis and oral ulceration. Cervical lymphadenopathy may occur. If given to pregnant females this drug may cause cleft lip and palate in the foetus. Haematological disorders including anaemia, leucopenia, agranulocytosis, thrombocytopenia, and thromboembolism. Renal failure, proteinuria, hepatitis, and cardiac conduction abnormalities. Gastrointestinal upset including, nausea, vomiting, anorexia, constipation or diarrhoea. Neurological disturbances such as headache, confusion, aggression, ataxia drowsiness, dizziness, dyskenesias, paraesthesia, and depression. Metabolic imbalance such as hyponatraemia, osteomalacia, and oedema. Rash, photosensitivity, pulmonary hypersensitivity, and Stevens–Johnson syndrome. Impotence, alopecia, gynaecomastia and galactorrhoea. Arthralgia, fever epidermal necrolysis, and enlargement of lymph nodes.

Drug interactions

Effect of carbamazepine enhanced by acetazolamide, allopurinol, cimetidine, clarithromycin, danazol, dextropropoxyphene, diltiazem, erythromycin, fluvoxamine, gemfibrozil, isoniazid, nefazodone, omeprazole, quinine, ritonavir, and verapamil. The effect of carbamazepine is reduced by chloroquine, cinromide, cytotoxic drugs such as cisplatin, fluoxetine, fluvoxamine, isotretinoin, mefloquine, rifabutin, and viloxazine. The side effects of carbamazepine are enhanced by alcohol, other anticonvulsants, denzimol, dezinamide, lithium, and neuroleptic drugs such as chlorpromazine and possibly metronidazole, miconazole and terfenadine. Carbamazepine increases the toxic effects of lithium, enhances sodium loss with diuretics and increases vitamin D requirements.

Carbamazepine decreases the effects of amfebutamone, benzodiazepines, clozapine, cocaine (when used as a drug of abuse) corticosteroids, ciclosporin, digitoxin, doxycycline, felodipine, fentanyl, gestrinone, haloperidol, idinavir, isradipine, itraconazole, mebendazole, methadone, mianserin, nefazodone, nelfinavir, nicardipine, nicoumalone, nifedipine, non-depolarizing muscle relaxants, olanzapine, oral contraceptives, praziquantel, risperidone, paracetamol, saquinavir, sertindole, teniposide, theophylline, thyroxine, tibolone, toremifine, tramadol, tricyclic antidepressants, and warfarin.

Carbenoxolone sodium (Bioral gel, Bioplex, Pyrogastrone)

Description
An oleandane synthetic derivative of a licorice root component.

Indications
Used in the management of oesophageal inflammation and ulceration and as an oral preparation for the treatment of oral mucosal lesions such as aphthous ulceration.

Effects on oral and dental structures
An underlying condition of reflux can lead to erosion of the teeth, especially the palatal surfaces.

Effects on patient management
Patients may be uncomfortable in the fully supine position as a result of their underlying gastrointestinal disorder.

Drug interactions
Carbenoxolone, when taken systemically, can produce a hypokalaemia and thus any reduction in plasma potassium produced by corticosteroids and epinephrine (in local anaesthetics) will be additive.

Carbimazole (Neo-Mercazole)

Description
An anti-thyroid drug.

Indications
Hyperthyroidism.

Effects on oral and dental structures
Carbimazole has been cited as a cause of taste disturbances. It has also been reported as a cause of agranulocytosis which may result in mouth ulcers, an exacerbation of periodontal disease and an increased propensity to gingival bleeding.

Effects on patient management
Carbimazole-induced thrombocytopenia will cause impaired haemostasis after a dental surgical procedure. If the platelet count is low (<100,000) then the socket should be packed and sutured. Persistent bleeding may require a platelet transfusion.

Drug interactions
None of any dental significance.

Carbocisteine

Description
A mucolytic drug.

Indications
Used in chronic bronchitis and asthma.

Effects on oral and dental structures
None specific.

Effects on patient management
Patients may not be comfortable in the supine position if they have respiratory problems. If the patient suffers from asthma then aspirin-like compounds should not be prescribed as many asthmatic patients are allergic to these analgesics. Similarly, sulphite-containing compounds (such as preservatives in epinephrine-containing local anaesthetics) can produce allergy in asthmatic patients. The use of a rubber dam in patients with obstructive airway disease may further embarrass the airway. If a rubber dam is essential then supplemental oxygen via a nasal cannula may be required.

Drug interactions
None of importance in dentistry.

Carboplatin (Paraplatin)

Description
A platinum compound.

Indications
Small cell lung cancer.

Effects on oral and dental structures
Carboplatin causes bone marrow suppression with an accompanying thrombocytopenia and agranulocytosis. Bone marrow suppression can lead to troublesome oral ulceration, exacerbation of an existing periodontal condition and rapid spread of any residual (e.g. periapical) infections.

Effects on patient management
The effect of carboplatin on the bone marrow is transient and routine dental treatment is best avoided until the white blood cells and platelet counts start to recover. If emergency dental treatment such as an extraction is required then antibiotic cover may be necessary depending on the degree of myelosuppression. If the platelet count is low (<100,000) then the socket should be packed and sutured. Persistent bleeding may require a platelet transfusion.

Patients on chemotherapeutic agents such as carboplatin often neglect their oral hygiene and thus there could be an increase in both caries and periodontal disease. If time permits, patients about to go on chemotherapy should have a dental check up and any potential areas of infection should be treated. Similarly, to reduce the mucosal irritation (sensitivity) that often accompanies chemotherapy, it is advisable to remove any ill-fitting dentures and smooth over rough cusps or restorations.

Drug interactions
None of any dental significance.

Carmustine (BCNU)

Description
An alkylating agent.

Indications
Myeloma, lymphoma and brain tumours.

Effects on oral and dental structures
Carmustine causes bone marrow suppression with an accompanying thrombocytopenia and agranulocytosis. Bone marrow suppression can lead to troublesome oral ulceration, exacerbation of an existing periodontal condition and rapid spread of any residual (e.g. periapical) infections.

Effects on patient management
The effect of carmustine on the bone marrow is transient and routine dental treatment is best avoided until the white blood cells and platelet counts start to recover. If emergency dental treatment such as an extraction is required then antibiotic cover may be necessary depending on the degree of myelosuppression. If the platelet count is

low (<100,000) then the socket should be packed and sutured. Persistent bleeding may require a platelet transfusion.

Patients on chemotherapeutic agents such as carmustine often neglect their oral hygiene and thus there could be an increase in both caries and periodontal disease. If time permits, patients about to go on chemotherapy should have a dental check up and any potential areas of infection should be treated. Similarly, to reduce the mucosal irritation (sensitivity) that often accompanies chemotherapy, it is advisable to remove any ill-fitting dentures and smooth over rough cusps or restorations.

Drug interactions
None of any dental significance.

Carvedilol (Eucardic)

Description
A beta-adrenoceptor blocking drug.

Indications
Hypertension, angina and chronic heart failure (occasionally).

Effects on oral and dental structures
Carvedilol can cause xerostomia, oral lichenoid eruptions and paraesthesia of lips and nasal stuffiness. The latter will cause mouth breathing and contribute to the patient's dry mouth. Very rarely causes thrombocytopenia and leucopenia.

Effects on patient management
Xerostomia will make the dental patient more susceptible to dental caries (especially root caries) and will cause problems with denture retention. If the xerostomia is severe, dentate patients should receive topical fluoride and be offered an artificial saliva. Postural hypotension may occur and patients may feel dizzy when the dental chair is restored to upright after they have been treated in the supine position. Leucopenia may cause oral ulceration and increased periodontal breakdown. Thrombocytopenia will cause impaired haemostasis. If the platelet count is low (<100,000) then the socket should be packed and sutured. Persistent bleeding may require a platelet transfusion.

Drug interactions
NSAIDs such as ibuprofen may antagonize the hypotensive action of carvedilol; possible interaction between epinephrine and carvedilol which might cause a slight transient increase in blood pressure. Do not exceed more than 3 cartridges of epinephrine containing local anaesthetic solutions per adult patient.

Cefaclor (Distaclor, Distaclor MR)

Description
A beta-lactam antibiotic.

Indications
Used to treat Gram-positive and Gram-negative bacterial infections.

Effects on oral and dental structures
Candidiasis and glossitis may occur after prolonged use. Stevens–Johnson syndrome can occur.

Effects on patient management
Antifungal treatment may be needed. This drug may cause thrombocytopenia, agranulocytosis and anaemia. Thrombocytopenia may cause postoperative bleeding. If the platelet count is low (<100,000) then the socket should be packed and sutured. Persistent bleeding may require platelet transfusion. Agranulocytosis and anaemia may result in poor healing. Any anaemia will need correction prior to elective general anaesthesia and sedation.

Drug interactions
The efficacy of cephalosporins is reduced in combined therapy with tetracyclines or erythromycin. As with penicillin, probenecid decreases the excretion of the cephalosporins.

Cefadroxil (Baxan)

Description
A beta-lactam antibiotic.

Indications
Used to treat Gram-positive and Gram-negative bacterial infections.

Effects on oral and dental structures
Candidiasis and glossitis may occur after prolonged use. Stevens–Johnson syndrome can occur.

Effects on patient management
Antifungal treatment may be needed. This drug may cause thrombocytopenia, agranulocytosis and anaemia. Thrombocytopenia may cause postoperative bleeding. If the platelet count is low (<100,000) then the socket should be packed and sutured. Persistent bleeding may require platelet transfusion. Agranulocytosis and anaemia may result in poor healing. Any anaemia will need correction prior to elective general anaesthesia and sedation.

Drug interactions

The efficacy of cephalosporins is reduced in combined therapy with tetracyclines or erythromycin. The ion-exchange inhibitor cholestyramine reduces the absorption of cefadroxil. As with penicillin, probenecid decreases the excretion of the cephalosporins.

Cefalexin (Ceporex, Keflex)

Description
A beta-lactam antibiotic.

Indications
Occasionally used as an alternative to penicillin to treat dental infections in patients allergic to the latter drug.

Presentations
(i) 250 mg and 500 mg capsules and tablets.

(ii) As an oral suspension (125 mg/5 mL and 250 mg/5 mL).

Dose
Adults: 250 mg four times daily.
Children: a daily dose of 25 mg/kg (in divided doses).

Contraindications
Hypersensitivity (there is cross-sensitivity with penicillin in around 10% of those allergic to the latter drug).
Porphyria.

Precautions
Renal disease.

Unwanted effects
Candidiasis and glossitis.
Hypersensitivity.
Haemorrhage (due to hypoprothrombinaemia) and haematological disturbances including reduction in red cells, white cells, and platelets.
Gastrointestinal upset.
Hypokalaemia.
Hepatotoxicity.
Nephrotoxicity.
Neurological disturbances including restlessness, confusion, dizziness, and sleep disturbance.

Drug interactions
As with penicillin probenecid decreases the excretion of the cephalosporins. The ion-exchange inhibitor cholestyramine reduces the absorption of cefalexin. The efficacy of cefalexin is reduced in combined therapy with tetracyclines or erythromycin.

Cephalosporins

Description
Beta-lactam antibiotics.

Indications
Few if any indications for use in dentistry. Cefuroxime is occasionally used for surgical prophylaxis in oral and maxillofacial surgery.

Presentations
Formulations which might be used in dental practice include cefalexin which is available as 250 mg and 500 mg capsules and tablets and as an oral suspension (125 mg/5 mL and 250 mg/5 mL).

Cefuroxime is available as 125 mg and 250 mg tablets, 125 mg suspension and sachet and as vials containing 250 mg, 750 mg and 1.5 g for reconstitution for injection.

Dose
The normal oral dose of cefalexin is 250 mg four times daily. For children a daily dose of 25 mg/kg (in divided doses) is usual.

Cefuroxime for surgical prophylaxis is administered intravenously at a dose of 1.5 g at general anaesthetic induction.

Contraindications
Hypersensitivity (there is cross-sensitivity with penicillin in around 10% of those allergic to the latter drug).
Porphyria.

Precautions
Renal disease.

Unwanted effects
Candidiasis and glossitis.
Hypersensitivity.
Haemorrhage (due to hypoprothrombinaemia) and haematological disturbances including reduction in red cells, white cells, and platelets.
Gastrointestinal upset.
Hypokalaemia.
Hepatotoxicity.
Nephrotoxicity.
Neurological disturbances including restlessness, confusion, dizziness and sleep disturbance.

Drug interactions
A disulfiram-like (antabuse) reaction occurs with some of the cephalosporins (such as cefamandole) and alcohol. Cefamandole and cefazolin increase the anticoagulant effect of warfarin and nicoumalone. The efficacy of cephalosporins is reduced in combined therapy with

tetracyclines or erythromycin. As with penicillin, probenecid decreases the excretion of the cephalosporins. The ion-exchange inhibitor cholestyramine reduces the absorption of cefalexin and cefadroxil.

Antacids and H_2-receptor antagonist ulcer-healing drugs such as cimetidine and ranitidine reduce the absorption of some cephalosporins such as cefpodoxime. Cefalothin increases the nephrotoxicity of gentamicin and the nephrotoxic effects of cefaloridine is exacerbated by frusemide. Similarly, the nephrotoxic action of cefalothin is worsened by colistin. The combined use of cefotaxime and phenobarbitone appears to produce an increased number of exanthematous skin reactions.

Cefamandole (Kefadol)

Description
A beta-lactam antibiotic.

Indications
Used to treat Gram-positive and Gram-negative bacterial infections. Sometimes used in surgical prophylaxis.

Effects on oral and dental structures
Candidiasis and glossitis may occur after prolonged use. Stevens–Johnson syndrome can occur.

Effects on patient management
Antifungal treatment may be needed. This drug may cause thrombocytopenia, agranulocytosis, and anaemia. Thrombocytopenia may cause postoperative bleeding. If the platelet count is low (<100,000) then the socket should be packed and sutured. Persistent bleeding may require platelet transfusion. Agranulocytosis and anaemia may result in poor healing. Any anaemia will need correction prior to elective general anaesthesia and sedation.

Drug interactions
As with penicillin probenecid decreases the excretion of the cephalosporins. Cefamandole produces a disulfiram reaction with alcohol and increases the anticoagulant effect of warfarin and nicoumalone. The efficacy of cephalosporins is reduced in combined therapy with tetracyclines or erythromycin.

Cefazolin (Kefzol)

Description
A beta-lactam antibiotic.

Indications
Used to treat Gram-positive and Gram-negative bacterial infections and surgical prophylaxis.

Effects on oral and dental structures
Candidiasis and glossitis may occur after prolonged use. Stevens–Johnson syndrome can occur.

Effects on patient management
Antifungal treatment may be needed. This drug may cause thrombocytopenia, agranulocytosis, and anaemia. Thrombocytopenia may cause postoperative bleeding. If the platelet count is low (<100,000) then the socket should be packed and sutured. Persistent bleeding may require platelet transfusion. Agranulocytosis and anaemia may result in poor healing. Any anaemia will need correction prior to elective general anaesthesia and sedation.

Drug interactions
Cefazolin increases the anticoagulant effect of warfarin and nicoumalone. The efficacy of cephalosporins is reduced in combined therapy with tetracyclines or erythromycin. As with penicillin, probenecid decreases the excretion of the cephalosporins.

Cefixime (Suprax)

Description
A beta-lactam antibiotic.

Indications
Used to treat Gram-positive and Gram-negative bacterial infections.

Effects on oral and dental structures
Candidiasis and glossitis may occur after prolonged use. Stevens–Johnson syndrome can occur.

Effects on patient management
Antifungal treatment may be needed. This drug may cause thrombocytopenia, agranulocytosis, and anaemia. Thrombocytopenia may cause postoperative bleeding. If the platelet count is low (<100,000) then the socket should be packed and sutured. Persistent bleeding may require platelet transfusion. Agranulocytosis and anaemia may result in poor healing. Any anaemia will need correction prior to elective general anaesthesia and sedation.

Drug interactions
The efficacy of cephalosporins is reduced in combined therapy with tetracyclines or erythromycin. As with penicillin, probenecid decreases the excretion of the cephalosporins.

Cefodizime (Timecef)

Description
A beta-lactam antibiotic.

Indications
Used to treat Gram-positive and Gram-negative bacterial infections.

Effects on oral and dental structures
Candidiasis and glossitis may occur after prolonged use. Stevens–Johnson syndrome can occur.

Effects on patient management
Antifungal treatment may be needed. This drug may cause thrombocytopenia, agranulocytosis, and anaemia. Thrombocytopenia may cause postoperative bleeding. If the platelet count is low (<100,000) then the socket should be packed and sutured. Persistent bleeding may require platelet transfusion. Agranulocytosis and anaemia may result in poor healing. Any anaemia will need correction prior to elective general anaesthesia and sedation.

Drug interactions
The efficacy of cephalosporins is reduced in combined therapy with tetracyclines or erythromycin. As with penicillin, probenecid decreases the excretion of the cephalosporins.

Cefotaxime (Claforan)

Description
A beta-lactam antibiotic.

Indications
Used to treat Gram-positive and Gram-negative bacterial infections. Also used in surgical prophylaxis and the treatment of Haemophilus epiglottitis and meningitis.

Effects on oral and dental structures
Candidiasis and glossitis may occur after prolonged use. Stevens–Johnson syndrome can occur.

Effects on patient management
Antifungal treatment may be needed. This drug may cause thrombocytopenia, agranulocytosis, and anaemia. Thrombocytopenia may cause postoperative bleeding. If the platelet count is low (<100,000) then the socket should be packed and sutured. Persistent bleeding may require platelet transfusion. Agranulocytosis and anaemia may result in poor healing. Any anaemia will need correction prior to elective general anaesthesia and sedation.

Drug interactions

The combined use of cefotaxime and phenobarbitone appears to produce an increased number of exanthematous skin reactions. The efficacy of cephalosporins is reduced in combined therapy with tetracyclines or erythromycin. As with penicillin, probenecid decreases the excretion of the cephalosporins.

Cefoxitin (Mefoxin)

Description

A beta-lactam antibiotic.

Indications

Used to treat Gram-positive and Gram-negative bacterial infections and as surgical prophylaxis.

Effects on oral and dental structures

Candidiasis and glossitis may occur after prolonged use. Stevens–Johnson syndrome can occur.

Effects on patient management

Antifungal treatment may be needed. This drug may cause thrombocytopenia, agranulocytosis, and anaemia. Thrombocytopenia may cause postoperative bleeding. If the platelet count is low (<100,000) then the socket should be packed and sutured. Persistent bleeding may require platelet transfusion. Agranulocytosis and anaemia may result in poor healing. Any anaemia will need correction prior to elective general anaesthesia and sedation.

Drug interactions

The efficacy of cephalosporins is reduced in combined therapy with tetracyclines or erythromycin. As with penicillin, probenecid decreases the excretion of the cephalosporins.

Cefpirome (Cefrom)

Description

A beta-lactam antibiotic.

Indications

Used to treat Gram-positive and Gram-negative bacterial infections.

Effects on oral and dental structures

Candidiasis and glossitis may occur after prolonged use. Stevens-Johnson syndrome can occur.

Effects on patient management

Antifungal treatment may be needed. This drug may cause thrombocytopenia, agranulocytosis, and anaemia. Thrombocytopenia may cause postoperative bleeding. If the platelet count is low (<100,000) then the socket should be packed and sutured. Persistent bleeding may require platelet transfusion. Agranulocytosis and anaemia may result in poor healing. Any anaemia will need correction prior to elective general anaesthesia and sedation.

Drug interactions
The efficacy of cephalosporins is reduced in combined therapy with tetracyclines or erythromycin. As with penicillin, probenecid decreases the excretion of the cephalosporins.

Cefpodoxime (Orelox)

Description
A beta-lactam antibiotic.

Indications
Mainly used to treat respiratory and urinary tract infections.

Effects on oral and dental structures
Candidiasis and glossitis may occur after prolonged use. Stevens–Johnson syndrome can occur.

Effects on patient management
Antifungal treatment may be needed. This drug may cause thrombocytopenia, agranulocytosis, and anaemia. Thrombocytopenia may cause postoperative bleeding. If the platelet count is low (<100,000) then the socket should be packed and sutured. Persistent bleeding may require platelet transfusion. Agranulocytosis and anaemia may result in poor healing. Any anaemia will need correction prior to elective general anaesthesia and sedation.

Drug interactions
Antacids and H$_2$-receptor antagonist ulcer-healing drugs such as cimetidine and ranitidine reduce the absorption of cefpodoxime. The efficacy of cephalosporins is reduced in combined therapy with tetracyclines or erythromycin. As with penicillin, probenecid decreases the excretion of the cephalosporins.

Cefprozil (Cefzil)

Description
A beta-lactam antibiotic.

Indications
Mainly used to treat upper respiratory tract, soft tissue infections and otitis media.

Effects on oral and dental structures
Candidiasis and glossitis may occur after prolonged use. Stevens–Johnson syndrome can occur.

Effects on patient management
Antifungal treatment may be needed. This drug may cause thrombocytopenia, agranulocytosis, and anaemia. Thrombocytopenia may cause postoperative bleeding. If the platelet count is low (<100,000) then the socket should be packed and sutured. Persistent bleeding may require platelet transfusion. Agranulocytosis and anaemia may result in poor healing. Any anaemia will need correction prior to elective general anaesthesia and sedation.

Drug interactions
The efficacy of cephalosporins is reduced in combined therapy with tetracyclines or erythromycin. As with penicillin, probenecid decreases the excretion of the cephalosporins.

Cefradine (Velosef)

Description
A beta-lactam antibiotic.

Indications
Occasionally used as an alternative to penicillin to treat dental infections in patients allergic to the latter drug.

Presentations
 (i) 250 mg and 500 mg capsules and tablets.
 (ii) As a syrup (250 mg/5 mL).
(iii) As vials containing 500 mg or 1 g powder for reconstitution for injection.

Dose
Adults: 250 mg orally or 500 mg by injection (IM or slow IV) four times daily.
Child: a daily dose of 25 mg/kg orally or 50 mg/kg by injection (in divided doses).

Contraindications
Hypersensitivity (there is cross-sensitivity with penicillin in around 10% of those allergic to the latter drug).
Porphyria.

Precautions
Renal disease.

Unwanted effects
Candidiasis and glossitis.

Hypersensitivity.

Haemorrhage (due to hypoprothrombinaemia) and haematological disturbances including reduction in red cells, white cells, and platelets.

Gastrointestinal upset.

Hypokalaemia.

Hepatotoxicity.

Nephrotoxicity.

Neurological disturbances including restlessness, confusion, dizziness and sleep disturbance.

Drug interactions

As with penicillin, probenecid decreases the excretion of the cephalosporins. The efficacy of cefradine is reduced in combined therapy with tetracyclines or erythromycin.

Ceftazidime (Fortum, Kefadim)

Description
A beta-lactam antibiotic.

Indications
Used to treat Gram-positive and Gram-negative bacterial infections.

Effects on oral and dental structures
Candidiasis and glossitis may occur after prolonged use. Stevens–Johnson syndrome can occur.

Effects on patient management
Antifungal treatment may be needed. This drug may cause thrombocytopenia, agranulocytosis, and anaemia. Thrombocytopenia may cause postoperative bleeding. If the platelet count is low (<100,000) then the socket should be packed and sutured. Persistent bleeding may require platelet transfusion. Agranulocytosis and anaemia may result in poor healing. Any anaemia will need correction prior to elective general anaesthesia and sedation.

Drug interactions
The efficacy of cephalosporins is reduced in combined therapy with tetracyclines or erythromycin. As with penicillin, probenecid decreases the excretion of the cephalosporins.

Ceftriaxone (Rocephin)

Description
A beta-lactam antibiotic.

Indications
Used to treat Gram-positive and Gram-negative bacterial infections and for surgical prophylaxis.

Effects on oral and dental structures
Candidiasis and glossitis may occur after prolonged use. Stevens–Johnson syndrome can occur.

Effects on patient management
Antifungal treatment may be needed. This drug may cause thrombocytopenia, agranulocytosis, and anaemia. Thrombocytopenia may cause postoperative bleeding. If the platelet count is low (<100,000) then the socket should be packed and sutured. Persistent bleeding may require platelet transfusion. Agranulocytosis and anaemia may result in poor healing. Any anaemia will need correction prior to elective general anaesthesia and sedation.

Drug interactions
The efficacy of cephalosporins is reduced in combined therapy with tetracyclines or erythromycin. As with penicillin, probenecid decreases the excretion of the cephalosporins.

Cefuroxime (Zinacef, Zinnat)

Description
A beta-lactam antibiotic.

Indications
Cefuroxime is occasionally used for surgical prophylaxis in oral and maxillofacial surgery.

Presentations
  (i) 125 mg and 250 mg tablets.
 (ii) A suspension containing 125 mg/5 mL.
(iii) Sachets containing 125 mg.
 (iv) Vials containing 250 mg, 750 mg and 1.5 g powder for reconstitution for injection.

Dose
Cefuroxime for surgical prophylaxis is administered intravenously at a dose of 1.5 g at general anaesthetic induction.

Contraindications
Hypersensitivity (there is cross-sensitivity with penicillin in around 10% of those allergic to the latter drug).
Porphyria.

Precautions
Renal disease.

Unwanted effects
Candidiasis and glossitis (if used long term).

Hypersensitivity.

Haemorrhage (due to hypoprothrombinaemia) and haematological disturbances including reduction in red cells, white cells, and platelets.

Gastrointestinal upset.

Hypokalaemia.

Hepatotoxicity.

Nephrotoxicity.

Neurological disturbances including restlessness, confusion, dizziness and sleep disturbance.

Drug interactions
The efficacy of cefuroxime is reduced in combined therapy with tetra-cyclines or erythromycin. As with penicillin, probenecid decreases the excretion of the cephalosporins.

Celecoxib (Celebrex)

Description
A selective COX-2 inhibitor.

Indications
Pain and inflammation in osteoarthritis or rheumatoid arthritis.

Effects on oral and dental structures
Stomatitis, sinusitis and taste disturbances can occur.

Effects on patient management
If patient develops celecoxib-induced stomatitis then the drug should be stopped and a full blood count carried out.

Drug interactions
Celecoxib should not be given with other NSAIDs or aspirin since using such combinations will increase the risk of unwanted effects. The anticoagulant effects of both warfarin and heparin are enhanced by celecoxib and could increase the risk of haemorrhage. Celecoxib can antagonize the hypotensive effects of the ACE inhibitors (e.g. captopril, lisinopril). There is the additional increased risk of renal impairment and hyperkalaemia with these drugs and celecoxib. Antidiabetic drugs such as the sulphonylureas are extensively protein bound and can be displaced by celecoxib leading to hypoglycaemia. Celecoxib can increase the risk of gastrointestinal haemorrhage if given to patients taking antiplatelet drugs such as clopidogrel. Celecoxib should be

avoided in patients taking beta adrenoceptor blockers as there will be an antagonism of their hypotensive effect. Celecoxib may exacerbate heart failure, reduce glomerular filtration rate and increase plasma concentration of digoxin. Both celecoxib and corticosteroids (systemic) cause peptic ulceration therefore avoid the combination. The excretion of methotrexate is reduced by celecoxib which can lead to increased toxicity. Celecoxib reduces the excretion of the muscle relaxant baclofen. The excretion of lithium is reduced by celecoxib, thus increasing the risk of lithium toxicity.

Cerivastatin (Lipobay)

Description
A cholesterol lowering drug.

Indications
To reduce coronary events by lowering LDL cholesterol.

Effects on oral and dental structures
None reported.

Effects on patient management
None of any significance.

Drug interactions
None of any dental significance.

Certoparin (Alphaparin)

Description
A low molecular weight heparin.

Indications
Initial treatment and prevention of deep vein thrombosis and pulmonary embolism. Used to prevent blood coagulation in patients on haemodialysis. Certoparin and other low molecular weight heparins have a longer duration of action than heparin.

Effects on oral and dental structures
No direct effect, although if patients are repeatedly heparinized, they are susceptible to osteoporosis. This latter condition may make such patients susceptible to periodontal breakdown.

Effects on patient management
Certoparin can only be given parentally which reduces to impact of the drug in dental practice. However dentists, especially those working in a hospital environment, will encounter patients who are heparinized on a regular basis (e.g. renal dialysis patients). Bleeding is the main problem with treating such patients. This can arise as a

direct effect on the blood coagulation system or from a drug-induced immune-mediated thrombocytopenia. From the coagulation perspective, it is best to treat heparinized patients between treatments since the half-life of the drug is approximately 4 hours. If urgent treatment is required, then the anticoagulation effect of certoparin can be reversed with protamine sulphate 10 mg IV. If the platelet count is low (<100,000) then the socket should be packed and sutured. Persistent bleeding may require a platelet transfusion.

Drug interactions
Aspirin and parenteral NSAIDs (e.g. diclofenac and ketorolac) should be avoided in patients who are taking certoparin or heparinized on a regular basis. Such analgesics cause impairment of platelet aggregation which would compound a certoparin-induced thrombocytopenia and likewise cause serious problems with obtaining haemostasis.

Cetirizine hydrochloride (Zirtek)

Description
An antihistamine.

Indications
Used in the treatment of allergies such as hay fever.

Effects on oral and dental structures
May produce xerostomia, but this is less common compared to older antihistamines. Swelling of the tongue and orofacial dyskenesia may also occur although these are rare.

Effects on patient management
The patient may be drowsy which may interfere with co-operation. Xerostomia may increase caries incidence and thus a preventive regimen is important. If the xerostomia is severe artificial saliva may be indicated. Occasionally anaemia and thrombocytopenia occur which can affect postoperative healing and bleeding.

Drug interactions
Enhanced sedative effects occur with anxiolytic and hypnotic drugs. Tricyclic and monoamine oxidase inhibitor antidepressants increase antimuscarinic effects such as xerostomia.

Cetylpyridinium chloride (Merocet)

Description
An antiplaque agent.

Indications
Used as an aid to oral hygiene.

Presentations
(i) As a 0.05% solution.

(ii) Also in combination with benzocaine in an antiseptic lozenge.

Dose
10 ml twice daily as a rinse.

Contraindications
Allergy.

Precautions
None significant.

Unwanted effects
None significant.

Drug interactions
None of importance in dentistry.

Chloral hydrate (Chloral elixir, Chloral mixture, Welldorm)

Description
A hypnotic drug.

Indications
Sometimes used to treat insomnia and as an oral premedication in children and the elderly, but these days use is limited as benzodiazepines have superseded chloral derivatives.

Presentations
(i) Mixture of 500 mg in 5 mL.

(ii) 4% paediatric elixir.

(iii) Tablets containing 414 mg chloral hydrate.

Dose
In children 30–50 mg/kg up to a maximum of 1 g 30 minutes prior to treatment or before bedtime.

Contraindications
Heart disease, gastrointestinal irritation, liver and kidney impairment and porphyria. Pregnancy and breastfeeding.

Precautions
Respiratory disease.

Unwanted effects
Allergic reactions.
Mucosal irritation.

Non-thrombocytopaenic purpura.
Cardiac toxicity.
Liver damage.

Drug interactions

Like other CNS depressants, chloral hydrate interacts with alcohol and the effect may be more than additive. Some patients may experience a disulfiram (Antabuse)-type reaction if alcohol is taken with chloral hydrate. Chloral hydrate enhances the effects of warfarin. Chloral hydrate may have an additive effect with fluoxetine. The intravenous administration of frusemide to patients taking chloral hydrate can produce an unpleasant transient reaction, including hot flushes and tachycardia. This does not appear to happen after oral administration of the diuretic or following administration of the hypnotic to patients already receiving frusemide.

Chlorambucil (Leukeran)

Description

An alkylating agent.

Indications

Chronic lymphocytic leukaemia, non-Hodgkin's lymphoma, Hodgkin's disease, and ovarian cancer.

Effects on oral and dental structures

Chlorambucil causes bone marrow suppression with an accompanying thrombocytopenia and agranulocytosis. Bone marrow suppression can lead to troublesome oral ulceration, exacerbation of an existing periodontal condition and rapid spread of any residual (e.g. periapical) infections.

Effects on patient management

The effect of chlorambucil on the bone marrow is transient and routine dental treatment is best avoided until the white blood cells and platelet counts start to recover. If emergency dental treatment such as an extraction is required then antibiotic cover may be required depending on the degree of myelosuppression. If the platelet count is low (<100,000) then the socket should be packed and sutured. Persistent bleeding may require a platelet transfusion.

Patients on chemotherapeutic agents such as chlorambucil often neglect their oral hygiene and thus there could be an increase in both caries and periodontal disease. If time permits, patients about to go on chemotherapy should have a dental check up and any potential areas of infection should be treated. Similarly, to reduce the mucosal irritation (sensitivity) that often accompanies chemotherapy, it is advisable to remove any ill-fitting dentures and smooth over rough cusps or restorations.

Drug interactions
None of any dental significance.

Chloramphenicol (Chloromycetin, Kemicetine, Sno Phenicol)

Description
A broad spectrum antibiotic.

Indications
Used systemically only for life-threatening infections. Topically it is used as an anti-infective in the ears and eyes.

Effects on oral and dental structures
When used systemically it may produce stomatitis, glossitis, candidiasis, and Stevens–Johnson syndrome.

Effects on patient management
The patient will be extremely ill if this drug is being used systemically and thus only emergency treatments should be performed by the dentist. Chloramphenicol produces anaemia which will interfere with healing.

Drug interactions
Chloramphenicol enhances the anticoagulant effect of warfarin and nicoumalone. It also increases the risk of toxicity of phenytoin.

Chlordiazepoxide (Librium)

Description
A benzodiazepine anxiolytic.

Indications
Used in the short term management of anxiety and in alcohol withdrawal.

Effects on oral and dental structures
Xerostomia can occur.

Effects on patient management
Avoid concurrent prescription of CNS depressant agents. Sympathetic handling is required due to anxiety state or alcohol withdrawal. As use is only short term the xerostomia is unlikely to produce caries, however preventive regimens may be required. If the patient is in alcohol rehabilitation a pre-surgical clotting screen is advisable.

Drug interactions

As with all benzodiazepines, enhancement of other CNS depressants occurs. Ketoconazole decreases the elimination of chlordiazepoxide. Confusion, forgetfulness and lack of co-ordination may occur during combined therapy with amitryptiline. Concurrent use with the monoamine oxidase inhibitor phenelzine may produce chorea and severe oedema. Concurrent therapy with barbiturates can lead to barbiturate toxicity. Chlordiazepoxide increases the serum levels of phenytoin.

Chlorhexidine gluconate (Chlorohex, Corsodyl)

Description
An antiseptic drug.

Indications
This drug is used as an aid to oral hygiene and intra-oral wound healing.

Presentations
 (i) As a mouthwash containing either 0.12% or 0.2% chlorhexidine.
 (ii) As a gel containing 1% chlorhexidine.
(iii) As a spray containing 0.2% chlorhexidine.

Dose
10 ml of solution or up to 12 activations of the spray twice daily.

Contraindications
Allergy.

Precautions
Warn patients of tooth staining.

Unwanted effects
Mucosal irritation, desquamation, ulceration, taste alteration, reversible staining of teeth and tongue, and sialosis may occur.

Drug interactions
Toothpastes will reduce the substantivity properties of chlorhexidine thus these products should not be used together.

Chloroquine (Avloclor, Nivaquine, Paludrine/Avoclor)

Description
An antimalarial drug.

Indications
Used in the prophylaxis against malaria and in the suppression of rheumatoid arthritis and systemic lupus erythematosus.

Effects on oral and dental structures
Stomatitis, lichenoid reactions, oral ulceration, Stevens–Johnson syndrome, and blue-grey mucosal discolouration, especially of the palate, may occur.

Effects on patient management
This drug can cause anaemia, agranulocytosis, leucopenia and thrombocytopenia when used long term, such as in the treatment of rheumatoid arthritis and lupus erythematosus. Anaemia may result in poor healing. Any anaemia will need correction prior to elective general anaesthesia and sedation. Agranulocytosis and leucopenia will affect healing adversely and if severe prophylactic antibiotics should be prescribed to cover surgical procedures. Thrombocytopenia may cause postoperative bleeding. If the platelet count is low (<100,000) then the socket should be packed and sutured. Persistent bleeding may require platelet transfusion.

Drug interactions
Chloroquine reduces the absorption of ampicillin and may cause dystonic reactions such as facial grimacing if used in combination with metronidazole. The effects of anticonvulsant drugs are antagonized.

Chlorothiazide (Saluric)

Description
A thiazide diuretic.

Indications
Hypertension and oedema.

Effects on oral and dental structures
Thiazide diuretics can cause lichenoid eruptions in the mouth, xerostomia, and taste disturbances due to hyperzincuria.

Effects on patient management
Postural hypertension and rarely blood disorders, including agranulocytosis, neutropenia, and thrombocytopenia may be produced. The latter may have an effect on haemostasis after various dental surgical procedures. If the platelet count is low (<100,000) then the socket should be packed and sutured. Persistent bleeding may require a platelet transfusion.

Drug interactions
Long-term use and high doses of chlorothiazide can cause hypokalaemia, which can be exacerbated by systemic amphotericin and

epinephrine containing local anaesthetic solutions. No more than 3 cartridges should be administered per adult patient.

Chlorpheniramine maleate/Chlorphenamine maleate (Piriton)

Description
An antihistamine.

Indications
Used in the treatment of allergies such as hay fever, urticaria and in anaphylactic shock.

Effects on oral and dental structures
Can produce xerostomia.

Effects on patient management
The patient may be drowsy which may interfere with co-operation. Xerostomia may increase caries incidence and thus a preventive regimen is important. If the xerostomia is severe artificial saliva may be indicated. This drug may cause thrombocytopenia, agranulocytosis, and anaemia. Thrombocytopenia may cause postoperative bleeding. If the platelet count is low (<100,000) then the socket should be packed and sutured. Persistent bleeding may require platelet transfusion. Agranulocytosis may affect healing adversely. Anaemia may result in poor healing. Any anaemia will need correction prior to elective general anaesthesia and sedation.

Drug interactions
Enhanced sedative effects occur with anxiolytic and hypnotic drugs. Tricyclic and monoamine oxidase inhibitor antidepressants increase antimuscarinic effects such as xerostomia. Chlorpheniramine increases phenytoin toxicity.

Chlorpromazine hydrochloride (Largactil)

Description
A phenothiazine antipsychotic medication.

Indications
Used in the treatment of psychoses such as schizophrenia, short term anxiety, and occasionally as an anti-emetic drug.

Effects on oral and dental structures
Xerostomia and uncontrollable oro-facial muscle activity (tardive dyskenesia) may be produced. The oral mucosa may be discoloured and have a bluish-grey appearance. Stevens–Johnson syndrome and lichenoid reactions may occur with this drug.

Effects on patient management

Xerostomia may increase caries incidence and thus a preventive regimen is important. If the xerostomia is severe artificial saliva may be indicated. Uncontrollable muscle movement of jaws and tongue as well as the underlying psychotic condition may interfere with management as satisfactory co-operation may not be achieved readily. There may be problems with denture retention and certain stages of denture construction (e.g. jaw registration) can be difficult.

Postural hypotension often occurs with this drug, therefore rapid changes in patient position should be avoided. This drug can produce leucocytosis, agranulocytosis and anaemia which may interfere with postoperative healing.

Drug interactions

There is increased sedation when used in combination with CNS depressant drugs such as alcohol, opioid analgesics and sedatives. Combined therapy with tricyclic antidepressants increases the chances of cardiac arrhythmias and exacerbates antimuscarinic effects such as xerostomia. The photosensitive effect of tetracyclines is increased during combined therapy. When used in combination with carbamazepine neurotoxic effects are increased. This combination also increases the occurrence of Stevens–Johnson syndrome. There is a theoretical risk of hypotension being exacerbated by the epinephrine in dental local anaesthetics.

Chlorpropamide

Description

A sulphonylurea oral anti-diabetic drug.

Indications

Diabetes mellitus.

Effects on oral and dental structures

Chlorpropamide has been cited as causing oral lichenoid eruptions, erythema multiforme and orofacial neuropathy. The latter can manifest as tingling or burning in the lips and tongue. The drug is a rare cause of blood disorders and includes thrombocytopenia, agranulocytosis and aplastic anaemia. The blood disorders could cause oral ulceration, an exacerbation of periodontal disease and spontaneous bleeding from the gingival tissues. If the platelet count is low (<100,000) then the socket should be packed and sutured. Persistent bleeding may require a platelet transfusion.

Effects on patient management

The development of hypoglycaemia is the main problem associated with chlorpropamide. This problem is more common in the elderly.

Before commencing dental treatment, it is important to check that patients have had their normal food intake. If there is any doubt, give the patient a glucose drink. As with any diabetic patient try and treat in the first half of the morning and ensure the patient can eat after dental treatment. If a patient on chlorpropamide requires a general anaesthetic then refer to hospital.

Drug interactions
Aspirin and other NSAIDs enhance the hypoglycaemic actions of chlorpropamide. Antifungal agents such as fluconazole and miconazole increase plasma concentrations of chlorpropamide. Systemic corticosteroids will antagonize the hypoglycaemic properties of chlorpropamide. If these drugs are required, then consult the patient's physician before prescribing.

Chlorthalidone (Hygroton)

Description
A thiazide diuretic.

Indications
Hypertension, oedema, and diabetes.

Effects on oral and dental structures
Thiazide diuretics can cause lichenoid eruptions in the mouth, xerostomia, and taste disturbances due to hyperzincuria.

Effect on patient management
Postural hypotension and rarely blood disorders, including agranulocytosis, neutropenia and thrombocytopenia. The latter may have an effect on haemostasis after various dental surgical procedures. If the platelet count is low (<100,000) then the socket should be packed and sutured. Persistent bleeding may require a platelet transfusion.

Drug interactions
High doses of chlorthalidone can cause hypokalaemia which can be exacerbated by systemic amphotericin and epinephrine containing local anaesthetic solutions. No more than 3 cartridges should be administered per adult patient.

Cholestyramine (Questran)

Description
An anion-exchange resin.

Indications
A lipid-regulating drug that is used in the management of hypercholesterolaemia.

Effects on oral and dental structures

No direct effects, but anion-exchange resins do interfere with the absorption of vitamins A, D, and K and folic acid. Vitamin D deficiency in adults increases the risk of osteoporosis, which may increase a patient's susceptibility to periodontal breakdown. Poor absorption of vitamin K leads to hypoprothrombinaemia and thus an increased risk of bleeding. Folic acid deficiency can cause a glossitis and stomatitis. Cholestyramine is also associated with olfactory disturbances. Because there is a strong association between smell and taste, patients on this drug may also complain of taste disturbances.

Effects on patient management

Drug-induced hypoprothrombinaemia may lead to excessive bleeding after certain dental procedures if patient history puts them at risk from impaired haemostasis, check their INR. Some patients may require vitamin K supplements or in an emergency fresh frozen plasma to arrest any haemorrhage.

Drug interactions

Cholestyramine can interfere with the absorption of drugs from the gastrointestinal tract. If drugs used in dentistry are administered orally, then patients should be advised to take them one hour before or 4–6 hours after they have taken cholestyramine.

Ciclosporin (Neoral)

Description

An immunosuppressant.

Indications

To prevent graft rejection in organ transplantation; used in certain dermatological conditions such as atopic dermatitis and psoriasis and also in the treatment of rheumatoid arthritis.

Effects on oral and dental structures

Ciclosporin causes gingival overgrowth with about 30% of patients experiencing this unwanted effect. The immunosuppressant properties of ciclosporin could impact upon expression of periodontal disease (reduce breakdown), cause delayed healing, and make the patient more susceptible to opportunistic oral infections such as candida or herpetic infections. Organ transplant patients on ciclosporin are more prone to malignancy and lesions which can affect the mouth, including Kaposi's sarcoma and lip cancer. Hairy leukoplakia can also develop in these patients and again this is attributed to the immunosuppressant properties of ciclosporin.

Effects on patient management

Ciclosporin-induced gingival overgrowth is invariably treated surgically to restore gingival contour. All patients on immunosuppressant therapy should receive a regular oral screening because of the increased propensity to 'oral' and lip malignancies. Any suspicious lesion must be biopsied. Likewise signs of opportunistic oral infections must be treated promptly to avoid systemic complications. The delayed healing and increased susceptibility to infection does not warrant the use of prophylactic antibiotic cover before specific dental procedures.

Drug interactions

NSAIDs and amphotericin increase the risk of ciclosporin-induced nephrotoxicity. The antifungal agents, ketoconazole, miconazole, and fluconazole inhibit ciclosporin metabolism and hence increase the risk of unwanted effects.

Cidofovir (Vistide)

Description

A DNA polymerase chain inhibitor antiviral drug.

Indications

Used to treat retinitis caused by cytomegalovirus virus in AIDS.

Effects on oral and dental structures

None known.

Effects on patient management

Sensitive handling of the underlying disease state is essential. Excellent preventive dentistry and regular examinations are important in patients suffering from HIV, as dental infections are best avoided. HIV will interfere with postoperative healing and antibiotic prophylaxis prior to oral surgery may be advisable. Cidofovir may produce anaemia, neutropenia and thrombocytopenia. Anaemia may result in poor healing. Any anaemia will need correction prior to elective general anaesthesia and sedation. Neutropenia will affect healing adversely and if severe prophylactic antibiotics should be prescribed to cover surgical procedures. Thrombocytopenia may cause postoperative bleeding. If the platelet count is low (<100,000) then the socket should be packed and sutured. Persistent bleeding may require platelet transfusion.

Drug interactions

None of importance in dentistry.

Cilazapril (Vascace)

Description
An ACE inhibitor.

Indications
Essential hypertension, congestive heart failure.

Effects on oral and dental structures
Taste disturbances, angioedema, xerostomia, glossitis, stomatitis, and lichenoid eruption can occur.

Effect on patient management
Cilazapril-induced angioedema is perhaps the most significant unwanted effect that impacts upon dental management, since dental procedures can induce this unwanted effect. Management of cilazapril-induced angioedema is problematic since the underlying mechanisms are poorly understood. Standard anaphylactic treatment (epinephrine and hydrocortisone) is of little value since the angioedema is not mediated via mast cells or antibody/antigen interactions. Usually the angioedema subsides, however patients taking this drug should be questioned as to whether they have experienced any problems with breathing or swallowing. This will alert the dental practitioner to the possible risks of this unwanted effect arising during dental treatment.

Cilazapril-induced xerostomia will increase the risk of caries (especially root caries), candidal infections, and poor denture retention. Cilazapril is rarely associated with suppression of bone marrow activity, giving rise to possible agranulocytosis, and thrombocytopenia. Patients on cilazapril who present with excessive bleeding of their gums, sore throats or oral ulceration should have a full haematological investigation.

Drug interactions
NSAIDs such as ibuprofen may reduce the antihypertensive effect of cilazapril.

Cimetidine (Dyspamet, Tagamet)

Description
A histamine H_2-receptor antagonist.

Indications
Used in the management of gastric and duodenal ulcers and gastro-intestinal reflux.

Effects on oral and dental structures
The underlying condition of reflux can lead to erosion of the teeth, especially the palatal surfaces. H_2-receptor antagonists may cause pain and swelling of the salivary glands.

Effects on patient management

Patients may be uncomfortable in the fully supine position as a result of their underlying gastrointestinal disorder. Non steroidal anti-inflammatory drugs should be avoided due to gastric irritation. Similarly, high dose systemic steroids should not be prescribed in patients with gastrointestinal ulceration.

Long-term use of cimetidine may produce anaemia, neutropenia and thrombocytopenia. Anaemia may result in poor healing. Any anaemia will need correction prior to elective general anaesthesia and sedation. Neutropenia will affect healing adversely and if severe prophylactic antibiotics should be prescribed to cover surgical procedures. Thrombocytopenia may cause postoperative bleeding. If the platelet count is low (<100,000) then the socket should be packed and sutured. Persistent bleeding may require platelet transfusion.

The long-acting local anaesthetic agent bupivacaine may have increased toxicity in patients receiving cimetidine (see below). There is a theoretical interaction with lidocaine but this is not a concern when this drug is used as a dental local anaesthetic.

Drug interactions

Cimetidine may interfere with the metabolism of the long-acting local anaesthetic bupivacaine, leading to increased toxicity of this agent. Cimetidine inhibits the metabolism of benzodiazepines, opioid analgesics, the antibacterials erythromycin (which may lead to deafness), and metronidazole, the anticonvulsants carbamazepine, phenytoin, and valproate and tricyclic antidepressants. Cimetidine increases the activity of oral anticoagulants and inhibits the absorption of the antifungals ketoconazole and itraconazole.

Cinnarizine (Stugeron)

Description
An antihistamine.

Indications
Used in the treatment of vertigo, tinnitus, Ménière's disease, motion sickness, and nausea.

Effects on oral and dental structures
This drug can produce xerostomia.

Effects on patient management
Xerostomia may increase caries incidence and thus a preventive regimen is important. If the xerostomia is severe artificial saliva may be indicated.

Drug interactions
Xerostomia is exacerbated by other antimuscarinic agents such as antidepressants.

Cinoxacin (Cinobac)

Description
A quinolone antibiotic.

Indications
Used to treat urinary tract infections.

Effects on oral and dental structures
This drug can cause taste disturbance and Stevens–Johnson syndrome.

Effects on patient management
This drug may cause thrombocytopenia, leucopenia, and anaemia. Thrombocytopenia may cause postoperative bleeding. If the platelet count is low (<100,000) then the socket should be packed and sutured. Persistent bleeding may require platelet transfusion. Leucopenia and anaemia may result in poor healing. Any anaemia will need correction prior to elective general anaesthesia and sedation.

Drug interactions
Combined therapy with non-steroidal anti-inflammatory drugs increases the risk of convulsions.

Ciprofloxacin (Ciproxin)

Description
A quinolone antibiotic.

Indications
Used to treat respiratory and urinary tract infections and gonorrhoea.

Effects on oral and dental structures
This drug can cause candidiasis, stomatitis, xerostomia, taste disturbance, and Stevens–Johnson syndrome. When administered during dental development it can cause a greenish intrinsic staining of the teeth.

Effects on patient management
This drug may cause thrombocytopenia, leucopenia, and anaemia. Thrombocytopenia may cause postoperative bleeding. If the platelet count is low (<100,000) then the socket should be packed and sutured. Persistent bleeding may require platelet transfusion. Leucopenia and

anaemia may result in poor healing. Any anaemia will need correction prior to elective general anaesthesia and sedation.

Drug interactions
Ciprofloxacin increases the anticoagulant effect of warfarin and nicoumalone. Ciprofloxacin has been shown to both decrease and increase plasma levels of phenytoin. Combined therapy with non-steroidal anti-inflammatory drugs increases the risk of convulsions.

Cisapride (Prepulsid)

Description
A gastrointestinal motility stimulant.

Indications
Used in the management of gastrointestinal reflux, dyspepsia, and stasis.

Effects on oral and dental structures
Xerostomia may rarely occur. The underlying condition of reflux can lead to erosion of the teeth especially the palatal surfaces.

Effects on patient management
Patients may be uncomfortable in the fully supine position as a result of their underlying gastrointestinal disorder. Cisapride can produce anaemia, thrombocytosis and leucopenia. Anaemia may result in poor healing. Any anaemia will need correction prior to elective general anaesthesia and sedation. Leucopenia will affect healing adversely and if severe prophylactic antibiotics should be prescribed to cover surgical procedures. Thrombocytopenia may cause postoperative bleeding. If the platelet count is low (<100,000) then the socket should be packed and sutured. Persistent bleeding may require platelet transfusion. Selection of antimicrobial therapy is influenced by drug interactions with cisapride (see below). Similarly, oral benzodiazepine dosages may need to be reduced.

Drug interactions
Opioid analgesics antagonize the motility effects of cisapride. Tricyclic antidepressants, erythromycin, clarithromycin the antifungals fluconazole, itraconazole and ketoconazole and many antiviral drugs (including indinavir, nelfinavir, and ritonavir) inhibit the metabolism of cisapride and this can lead to ventricular arrhythmias. Concurrent therapy should be avoided. Cisapride increases the effects of benzodiazepines, oral anticoagulants, and of alcohol.

Cisplatin

Description
A platinum compound.

Indications
Ovarian cancer and testicular teratomas.

Effects on oral and dental structures
Cisplatin causes bone marrow suppression with an accompanying thrombocytopenia and agranulocytosis. Bone marrow suppression can lead to troublesome oral ulceration, exacerbation of an existing periodontal condition and rapid spread of any residual (e.g. periapical) infections.

Effects on patient management
The effect of cisplatin on the bone marrow is transient and routine dental treatment is best avoided until the white blood cells and platelet counts start to recover. If emergency dental treatment such as an extraction is required then antibiotic cover may be necessary depending on the degree of myelosuppression. If the platelet count is low (<100,000) then the socket should be packed and sutured. Persistent bleeding may require a platelet transfusion.

Patients on chemotherapeutic agents such as cisplatin often neglect their oral hygiene and thus there could be an increase in both caries and periodontal disease. If time permits, patients about to go on chemotherapy should have a dental check up and any potential areas of infection should be treated. Similarly, to reduce the mucosal irritation (sensitivity) that often accompanies chemotherapy, it is advisable to remove any ill-fitting dentures and smooth over rough cusps or restorations.

Drug interactions
None of any dental significance.

Citalopram (Cipramil)

Description
A selective serotonin reuptake inhibitor.

Indications
Used in the management of depression and panic disorders.

Effects on oral and dental structures
Both xerostomia and hypersalivation may occur. Taste disturbance may be produced.

Effects on patient management

Xerostomia may increase caries incidence and thus a preventive regimen is important. If the xerostomia is severe artificial saliva may be indicated. This drug may cause postural hypotension, thus the patient should not be changed from the supine to the standing position too rapidly.

Drug interactions

Combined therapy with other antidepressants should be avoided. Treatment with selective serotonin reuptake inhibitors should not begin until two weeks following cessation of monoamine oxidase inhibitor therapy. Selective serotonin reuptake inhibitors increase the anticoagulant effect of warfarin and antagonize the anticonvulsant effects of anti-epileptic medication.

Cladribine (Leustat)

Description

An antimetabolic.

Indications

Chronic lymphocytic leukaemia and hairy cell leukaemia.

Effects on oral and dental structures

Cladribine causes bone marrow suppression with an accompanying thrombocytopenia and agranulocytosis. Bone marrow suppression can lead to troublesome oral ulceration, exacerbation of an existing periodontal condition and rapid spread of any residual (e.g. periapical) infections.

Effects on patient management

The effect of cladribine on the bone marrow is transient and routine dental treatment is best avoided until the white blood cells and platelet counts start to recover. If emergency dental treatment is required such as an extraction then antibiotic cover may be required depending on the degree of myelosuppression. If the platelet count is low (<100,000) then the socket should be packed and sutured. Persistent bleeding may require a platelet transfusion.

Patients on chemotherapeutic agents such as cladribine often neglect their oral hygiene and thus there could be an increase in both caries and periodontal disease. If time permits, patients about to go on chemotherapy should have a dental check up and any potential areas of infection should be treated. Similarly, to reduce the mucosal irritation (sensitivity) that often accompanies chemotherapy, it is advisable to remove any ill-fitting dentures and smooth over rough cusps or restorations.

Drug interactions
None of any dental significance.

Clarithromycin (Klaricid, Klaricid XL)

Description
A macrolide antibiotic.

Indications
Used to treat respiratory and soft tissue infections.

Effects on oral and dental structures
Taste disturbance, glossitis, stomatitis, candidiasis, and Stevens–Johnson syndrome may occur.

Effects on patient management
Local treatment for stomatitis and candidiasis may be required.

Drug interactions
Clarithromycin probably enhances the anticoagulant effect of warfarin and nicoumalone. Clarithromycin increases the plasma concentration of carbamazepine.

Clemastine (Tavegil)

Description
An antihistamine.

Indications
Used in the treatment of allergies such as hay fever and urticaria.

Effects on oral and dental structures
Can produce xerostomia.

Effects on patient management
The patient may be drowsy which may interfere with co-operation. Xerostomia may increase caries incidence and thus a preventive regimen is important. If the xerostomia is severe artificial saliva may be indicated. This drug may cause thrombocytopenia, agranulocytosis, and anaemia. Thrombocytopenia may cause postoperative bleeding. If the platelet count is low (<100,000) then the socket should be packed and sutured. Persistent bleeding may require platelet transfusion. Agranulocytosis may affect healing adversely. Anaemia may result in poor healing. Any anaemia will need correction prior to elective general anaesthesia and sedation.

Drug interactions

Enhanced sedative effect with anxiolytic and hypnotic drugs. Tricyclic and monoamine oxidase inhibitor antidepressants increase antimuscarinic effects such as xerostomia.

Clindamycin (Dalacin C)

Description

A lincosamide antibacterial drug.

Indications

This is the first-choice agent for prophylaxis of endocarditis in those allergic to penicillin. Occasionally used in the management of dental infections that have progressed to bone in those allergic to penicillin.

Presentations

(i) 75 mg and 150 mg capsules.

(ii) A suspension containing 75 mg/5 mL.

(iii) 2 mL and 4 mL vials containing 150 mg/mL for injection.

Dose

(1) For management of infection

150–300 mg orally four times daily (child 3–6 mg/kg four times daily).

By intravenous infusion or deep intramuscular injection 0.6–2.7 kg daily over 2–4 doses (single doses over 600 mg by intravenous infusion only) (child 15–40 mg/kg daily over 3–4 doses).

(2) In prophylaxis of endocarditis

600 mg orally one hour preoperatively for prophylaxis when treatment under local anaesthesia. Under general anaesthesia 300 mg intravenously over 10 minutes at induction of anaesthesia followed by 150 mg orally 6 hours later.

Child under 5 years: 25% adult dose.

Child 5–10 years 50% adult dose.

Contraindications

Hypersensitivity.

Pre-existing diarrhoea.

Precautions

Stop therapy immediately if diarrhoea develops.

Liver and kidney disease.

Breastfeeding.

Unwanted effects

Facial oedema.

Gastrointestinal effects including the production of pseudomembranous colitis.

Hypersensitivity syndrome.
Altered liver function including jaundice.
Neuromuscular blockade.
Haematological effects reducing white cells and platelets.
Thrombophlebitis after intravenous administration.

Drug interactions
Renal failure may occur if used in combination with aminoglycoside antibiotics such as gentamycin. Clindamycin enhances neuromuscular blockade produced by pancuronium, suxamethonium, and pipecuronium. Clindamycin reduces the response to Vitamin K therapy and in patients receiving Vitamin K administration another antibiotic should be used.

Clobazam (Frisium)

Description
A benzodiazepine.

Indications
Used in the short term management of anxiety and as an add-on drug in the treatment of epilepsy.

Effects on oral and dental structures
This drug may produce xerostomia.

Effects on patient management
Sensitive handling is required as the patient may be anxious. The occurrence of fits must be anticipated and emergency anti-epileptic drugs (diazepam or midazolam) must be available.

Drug interactions
As with all benzodiazepines, enhancement of other CNS depressants will occur during combined therapy. Carbamazepine and phenytoin decrease the levels of clobazam in serum.

Clofazimine (Lamprene)

Description
An antileprotic drug.

Indications
Used in the treatment of leprosy.

Effects on oral and dental structures
This drug may cause a red discolouration of saliva and stomatitis.

Effects on patient management

It is extremely unlikely that patients taking this medication will attend out-patient dental practice, however an awareness of the underlying disease is important.

Drug interactions

None of importance in dentistry.

Clomethiazole [chlormethiazole] (Hemineverin)

Description

A hypnotic.

Indications

Used as a sedative and during alcohol withdrawal. Also used in the treatment of status epilepticus.

Effects on oral and dental structures

None known.

Effects on patient management

This drug can cause nasal congestion and increased nasal secretions which may make dental treatment (such as that under a rubber dam) difficult due to a reduction in the nasal airway.

Drug interactions

Can cause fatal CNS depression when combined with alcohol.

Clomifene (Clomid)

Description

An anti-oestrogen.

Indications

Anovulatory infertility.

Effects on oral and dental structures

None reported.

Effects on patient management

None of significance.

Drug interactions

None of any dental significance.

Clomipramine hydrochloride (Anafranil)

Description
A tricyclic antidepressant.

Indications
Used in the management of depressive illness, phobias, and narcolepsy.

Effects on oral and dental structures
Xerostomia and taste disturbance may occur.

Effects on patient management
Xerostomia may increase caries incidence and thus a preventive regimen is important. If the xerostomia is severe artificial saliva may be indicated. Postural hypotension and fainting may occur with this drug, therefore rapid changes in patient position should be avoided. This drug may cause thrombocytopenia, agranulocytosis, and leucopenia. Thrombocytopenia may cause postoperative bleeding. If the platelet count is low (<100,000) then the socket should be packed and sutured. Persistent bleeding may require platelet transfusion. Agranulocytosis and leucopenia may affect healing adversely.

Drug interactions
Increased sedation occurs with alcohol and sedative drugs such as benzodiazepines. This drug may antagonize the action of anticonvulsants such as carbamazepine and phenytoin. This drug increases the pressor effects of epinephrine. Nevertheless, the use of epinephrine-containing local anaesthetics is not contraindicated; however, epinephrine dose limitation is recommended.

Normal anticoagulant control by warfarin may be upset, both increases and decreases in INR have been noted during combined therapy with tricyclic antidepressants. Combined therapy with other antidepressants should be avoided and if prescribing another class of antidepressant a period of one to two weeks should elapse between changeover. Antimuscarinic effects such as xerostomia are increased when used in combination with other anticholinergic drugs such as antipsychotics.

Clonazepam (Rivotril)

Description
A benzodiazepine.

Indications
Used as an add-on drug in the treatment of epilepsy.

Effects on oral and dental structures
Xerostomia may occur, conversely hypersalivation is also possible.

Effects on patient management

Xerostomia may increase caries incidence and thus a preventive regimen is important. If the xerostomia is severe artificial saliva may be indicated. Epileptic fits are possible, especially if the patient is stressed, therefore sympathetic handling and perhaps sedation should be considered for stressful procedures. Emergency anticonvulsant medication (diazepam or midazolam) must be available. Clonazepam may cause excess bleeding, therefore local haemostatic measures may need to be employed after oral surgery.

Drug interactions

As with all benzodiazepines, enhancement of other CNS depressants will occur during combined therapy. Carbamazepine and phenytoin decrease the levels of clonazepam in serum.

Clonidine (Catapres, Dixarit)

Description

A centrally acting antihypertensive drug.

Indications

Hypertension and migraine.

Effects on oral and dental structures

Pain and swelling of the salivary glands and xerostomia may be produced. The latter leads to an increased risk of root caries, candidal infections, and poor denture retention. If the xerostomia is severe, dentate patients should receive topical fluoride and be offered an artificial saliva.

Effects on patient management

Nothing of dental significance.

Drug interactions

NSAIDs such as ibuprofen may enhance the hypotensive actions of clonidine.

Clopidogrel (Plavix)

Description

An antiplatelet drug.

Indications

Prevention of atherosclerotic events (stroke, myocardial infarction, and peripheral arterial disease).

Effects on oral and dental structures

Neutropenia is a rare unwanted effect associated with clopidogrel – this can give rise to oral ulceration and an increased risk of periodontal breakdown.

Effects on patient management

Increased risk of haemorrhage following any dental procedure associated with a risk of bleeding. Local measures (e.g. pack and suture) should be adopted. If this fails to control bleeding, then a platelet transfusion may be required.

Drug interactions

Aspirin and other NSAIDs reduce platelet aggregation and will enhance the antiplatelet actions of clopidogrel and lead to serious problems with haemostasis.

Clorazepate dipotassium

Description

A benzodiazepine.

Indications

Used in the short-term management of anxiety and during alcohol withdrawal. Also used as an adjunctive therapy in the management of epilepsy.

Effects on oral and dental structures

Xerostomia may occur.

Effects on patient management

Xerostomia may increase caries incidence and thus a preventive regimen is important. If the xerostomia is severe artificial saliva may be indicated. If patient is in alcohol rehabilitation a pre-surgical clotting screen is advisable.

Drug interactions

As with all benzodiazepines enhancement of other CNS depressants occurs.

Clozapine (Clozaril)

Description

An atypical antipsychotic drug.

Indications

Used in the treatment of schizophrenia.

Effects on oral and dental structures

Xerostomia and glossitis may be produced although hypersalivation and parotid gland enlargement may also occur. Uncontrollable oro-facial muscle activity may occur but this is less than with older antipsychotics.

Effects on patient management

This drug can produce a severe agranulocytosis and thus postoperative healing may be impaired. If the agranulocytosis is marked then prophylactic antibiotics should be used prior to surgery. Xerostomia may increase caries incidence and thus a preventive regimen is important. If the xerostomia is severe artificial saliva may be indicated. Uncontrollable muscle movement of jaws and tongue as well as the underlying psychotic condition may interfere with management as satisfactory co-operation may not be achieved readily. Postural hypotension may occur with this drug, therefore rapid changes in patient position should be avoided.

Drug interactions

There is increased sedation when used in combination with CNS depressant drugs such as alcohol, opioid analgesics, and sedatives. Carbamazepine and possibly phenytoin accelerate the metabolism of clozapine. Erythromycin may increase the leucocytosis produced by clozapine and may raise the plasma level of the antipsychotic. Combined therapy with tricyclic antidepressants increases the chances of cardiac arrhythmias and exacerbates antimuscarinic effects such as xerostomia.

Co-amoxiclav (Augmentin, Augmentin-Duo)

Description

A mixture of the broad spectrum beta-lactam antibacterial amoxicillin and the beta-lactamase inhibitor clavulanic acid.

Indications

Used to treat serious bacterial infection such as severe dental abscess causing cellulitis.

Presentations

(i) Tablets of 375 mg and 625 mg.

(ii) 375 mg dispersible tablets.

(iii) Oral suspensions of 156 mg/5 mL, 312 mg/5 mL and 457 mg/5 mL.

(iv) 600 mg and 1200 mg vials for reconstitution for injection.

Dose

Adults: 375 mg three times daily by mouth; by IV infusion 1200 mg three times daily.
Child under 6 years: 156 mg three times daily.
Child 6–12 years: 312 mg three times daily.

Contraindications

Hypersensitivity.
Liver dysfunction.

Precautions
Renal disease.
Glandular fever.
Chronic lymphatic leukaemia.
HIV.

Unwanted effects
Glossitis and tongue discolouration.
Candidiasis.
Hypersensitivity.
Gastrointestinal upset.
Pseudomembranous colitis.
Hypokalaemia.

Drug interactions
Amoxicillin reduces the excretion of the cytotoxic drug methotrexate, leading to increased toxicity of the latter drug which may cause death. There may be a reduced efficacy of oral contraceptives and other methods of contraception are advised during antibiotic therapy. Amoxicillin activity is decreased by tetracyclines. Amoxicillin rarely increases the prothrombin time when given to patients receiving warfarin. Probenecid significantly increases the half-life of amoxicillin. Nifedipine increases amoxicillin absorption but this is of little clinical importance. Amiloride decreases the absorption of amoxicillin but this is probably of little significance. The production of rashes is increased during concomitant treatment with allopurinol.

Co-beneldopa (Madopar, Maldopar CR)

Description
A dopaminergic drug. It is a mixture of levodopa and benserazide.

Indications
Used in the treatment of Parkinsonism.

Effects on oral and dental structures
Xerostomia and taste disturbance may occur.

Effects on patient management
General anaesthesia and sedation are affected (see drug interactions below). Xerostomia may increase caries incidence and thus a preventive regimen is important. If the xerostomia is severe artificial saliva may be indicated. This drug may cause postural hypotension, thus the patient should not be changed from the supine to the standing position too rapidly. Parkinsonism can lead to management problems as the patient may have uncontrollable movements. Short appointments are recommended.

Drug interactions
Combined use with volatile anaesthetics such as halothane increase the risk of cardiac arrhythmias. The effect of co-beneldopa is antagonized by some benzodiazepines including diazepam and by vitamin B6 (pyridoxine). Monoamine oxidase inhibitors should not be used concurrently as life-threatening hypertension may occur.

Cocaine

Description
An ester local anaesthetic and a drug of abuse.

Indications
Rarely used as a topical anaesthetic.

Presentations
As a topical preparation in the concentration range 4% to 10%.

Dose
The maximum dose is 1.5 mg/kg with a ceiling of 100 mg.

Contraindications
Allergy to ester local anaesthetics and parabens.

Precautions
The potential for misuse of cocaine mean that it should only be used on very rare occasions.

Unwanted effects
When abused cocaine can produce gingival bleeding due to thrombocytopenia. Repeated local application to the gingivae can produce oral ulceration, soft tissue and alveolar bone necrosis and localized dental caries (the latter being due to carbohydrate contaminants). Cocaine can produce psychological dependence, cardiotoxicity, and liver damage.

Drug interactions
Combined abuse with alcohol and barbiturates increases the likelihood of liver damage. Cocaine produces sympathomimetic synergism with epinephrine (adrenaline), thus epinephrine-containing local anaesthetic solutions should be avoided or used with caution in those who regularly abuse cocaine.

Co-careldopa (Sinemet, Sinemet plus, Sinemet CR, Half Sinemet)

Description
A dopaminergic drug. It is a mixture of levodopa and carbidopa.

Indications
Used in the treatment of Parkinsonism.

Effects on oral and dental structures
Xerostomia and taste disturbance may occur. Long term use can lead to Meige's syndrome (blepherospasm-oromandibular dystonia).

Effects on patient management
General anaesthesia and sedation are affected (see drug interactions below). Xerostomia may increase caries incidence and thus a preventive regimen is important. If the xerostomia is severe artificial saliva may be indicated. This drug may cause postural hypotension, thus the patient should not be changed from the supine to the standing position too rapidly. Parkinsonism can lead to management problems as the patient may have uncontrollable movement. Short appointments are recommended.

Drug interactions
Combined use with volatile anaesthetics such as halothane increase the risk of cardiac arrhythmias. The effect of co-careldopa is antagonized by some benzodiazepines, including diazepam, and by vitamin B6 (pyridoxine). Monoamine oxidase inhibitors should not be used concurrently as life-threatening hypertension may occur.

Codeine phosphate

Description
As opioid analgesic, also widely used as a constituent of compound analgesics.

Indications
Mild to moderate pain, also used to suppress cough.

Effects on oral and dental structures
Can cause xerostomia leading to an increased risk of root caries, candidal infections and poor denture retention. If the xerostomia is severe, dentate patients should receive topical fluoride and be offered an artificial saliva.

Effects on patient management
Although codeine phosphate is an opioid, it is not subjected to the same manner of abuse as say morphine. It has been used by drug addicts, usually when nothing more potent is available. If subject to abuse, it can cause withdrawal symptoms if stopped abruptly. Such cessation of codeine may account for unusual behavioural changes and poor compliance with dental treatment. Large doses of codeine phosphate can depress respiration and cause postural hypotension.

Drug interactions
Codeine phosphate will enhance the sedative properties of midazolam and diazepam. Reduce the dose of the latter.

Co-fluampicil (Magnapen)

Description
A mixture of the broad spectrum beta-lactam antibacterial ampicillin
and the beta-lactamase resistant antibacterial flucloxacillin.

Indications
Used to treat mixed bacterial infections which include beta-
lactamase producing staphylococci.

Presentations
(i) 500 mg capsules.

(ii) Syrup with 250 mg/5 mL.

(iii) 500 mg vials for reconstitution for injection.

Dose
500 mg four times daily.
Child under 10 years: 50% adult dose.

Contraindications
Hypersensitivity.

Precautions
Renal disease.
Glandular fever.
Chronic lymphatic leukaemia.
HIV.

Unwanted effects
Glossitis and tongue discolouration.
Candidiasis.
Hypersensitivity.
Gastrointestinal upset.
Hypokalaemia.
Pseudomembranous colitis.

Drug interactions
Co-fluampicil reduces the excretion of the cytotoxic drug methotrexate, leading to increased toxicity of the latter drug which may
cause death. There may be a reduced efficacy of oral contraceptives and
other methods of contraception are advised during antibiotic therapy.
Co-fluampicil activity is decreased by tetracyclines. Antagonism also
occurs with chloramphenicol and the neurological side effects of the
latter drug (e.g. deafness) are increased during combined therapy.

Chloroquine reduces the absorption of ampicillin. Co-fluampicil rarely increases the prothrombin time when given to patients receiving warfarin.

Ampicillin can increase the muscle weakness of patients with myasthenia gravis who are receiving anti-cholinergic drugs. Ampicillin reduces the efficacy of sulphasalazine which is used in the treatment of Crohn's disease. Probenecid significantly increases the half-life of ampicillin. Nifedipine increases ampicillin absorption but this is of little clinical importance. Amiloride decreases the absorption of ampicillin but this is probably of little significance. The production of rashes is increased during concomitant treatment with allopurinol. Large single doses of ampicillin (1 g) decrease the serum levels of the anti-hypertensive drug atenolol by half.

Colchicine

Description
An anti-inflammatory agent.

Indications
Acute gout and short-term prophylaxis.

Effects on oral and dental structures
Colchicine can interfere with the absorption of vitamin B12. Such a deficiency can cause stomatitis and glossitis.

Effects on patient management
None of any significance.

Drug interactions
None of any dental significance.

Colestipol hydrochloride (Colestid)

Description
An anion-exchange resin.

Indications
Hyperlipidaemias, particularly type IIa, in patients who have not responded adequately to diet or other measures to lower their serum lipids.

Effects on oral and dental structures
No direct effect, but anion-exchange resins do interfere with the absorption of vitamins A, D, and K and folic acid. Vitamin D deficiency in adults increase the risk of osteoporosis, which may increase a patient's susceptibility to periodontal breakdown. Poor absorption of vitamin K leads to hypoprothrombinaemia and thus an increased

risk of bleeding. Folic acid deficiency can cause glossitis and stomatitis. Colestipol is also associated with olfactory disturbances: because there is a strong association between smell and taste, patients on this drug may also complain of taste disturbances.

Effects on patient management
Drug-induced hypoprothrombinaemia may lead to excessive bleeding after certain dental procedures. If patient history puts them at risk from impaired haemostasis, check their INR. Some patients may require vitamin K supplements or, in an emergency, fresh frozen plasma to arrest any haemorrhage.

Drug interactions
Colestipol can interfere with the absorption of drugs from the gastrointestinal tract. If drugs used in dentistry are administered orally, then patients should be advised to take them one hour before or 4–6 hours after they have taken colestipol.

Colistin (Colomycin)

Description
A polymixin antibiotic.

Indications
Rarely indicated but may be used in preparation of the bowel for surgery or as an inhaler as an adjunct in treatment of Pseudomonas aeruginosa.

Effects on oral and dental structures
This drug produces peri-oral paraesthesia.

Effects on patient management
Patients receiving this drug are either awaiting surgery or are very ill and thus only emergency dental treatment is indicated.

Drug interactions
Nephrotoxicity is increased when used in combination with vancomycin and this should be avoided.

Contraceptive pill – combined oral contraceptives

Description
A combination of the female sex hormones oestrogen and progestogen.

Indications
Contraception and menstrual symptoms.

Effects on oral and dental structures
Oestrogen, and to a lesser extent progestogen, can exacerbate an existing gingivitis due to a combined hormone effect on the gingival vasculature. Oral pigmentation can also be enhanced by oestrogen. The hormone increases the production of beta-melanocyte stimulating hormone. This unwanted effect may be particularly marked in those patients with a high distribution of melanocytes in their gingival tissues. The use of oral contraceptives has been associated with a significant increase in the frequency of dry socket formation (alveolar osteitis) after third molar surgery. The probability of dry socket increases with the oestrogen dose in the oral contraceptive.

Effects on patient management
An exacerbation of an existing gingival inflammation may occur in some patients when they start the contraceptive pill. In such patients, it is important that plaque control measures are instituted to reduce, wherever possible, the inflammatory component. The increased frequency of dry sockets found in patients taking the pill can be minimized by carrying out the extractions during day 23–28 of the tablet cycle.

Drug interactions
Broad spectrum antibiotics such as tetracycline and ampicillin can cause pill failure due to their effect on the gut flora. These broad spectrum antibiotics can reduce the gut flora which is essential to breakdown the conjugated oestrogen/progestogen for subsequent reabsorption and the suppression of ovulation. If such antimicrobials are prescribed to patients taking oral contraceptives then they should be advised of the risk of pill failure – additional contraceptive precautions should be taken whilst taking the antibiotics and for 7 days after completion of the course. If the course of antibiotics exceeds 2 weeks, the bacterial flora develops antibiotic resistance and additional precautions become unnecessary.

Co-phenotrope (Lomotil)

Description
An antimotility drug combination of atropine sulphate and the opioid diphenoxylate hydrochloride.

Indications
Used in the acute treatment of diarrhoea.

Effects on oral and dental structures
The atropine component, although in low dose, may produce xerostomia in susceptible individuals.

Effects on patient management
This drug is used in the acute phase of diarrhoea, thus prolonged effects are unlikely. See drug interactions below.

Drug interactions
Due to the opioid component, other central nervous system depressants such as sedatives will have an exaggerated effect.

Cortisone acetate (Cortisyl)

Description
A corticosteroid.

Indications
Suppression of inflammation and allergic disorders. Used in the management of inflammatory bowel diseases, asthma, immunosuppression, and in various rheumatic diseases.

Effects on oral and dental structures
Although systemic corticosteroids can induce cleft lip and palate formation in mice, there is little evidence that this unwanted effect occurs in humans. The main impact of systemic corticosteroids on the mouth is to cause an increased susceptibility to opportunistic infections. These include candidiasis and those due to herpes viruses. The anti-inflammatory and immunosuppressant properties of corticosteroids may afford the patient some degree of protection against periodontal breakdown. Paradoxically long-term systemic use can precipitate osteoporosis. The latter is now regarded as a risk factor for periodontal disease.

Effects on patient management
The main unwanted effect of corticosteroid treatment is the suppression of the adrenal cortex and the possibility of an adrenal crisis when such patients are subjected to 'stressful events'. Whilst such suppression does occur physiologically, its clinical significance does appear to be overstated. As far as dentistry is concerned, there is increasing evidence that supplementary corticosteroids are not required. This would apply to all restorative procedures, periodontal surgery and uncomplicated dental extractions. For more complicated dentoalveolar surgery, each case must be judged on its merit. An apprehensive patient may well require cover. It is important to monitor the patient's blood pressure before, during and for 30 minutes after the procedure. If diastolic pressure drops by more than 25%, then hydrocortisone 100 mg IV should be administered and the patient's blood pressure should continue to be monitored.

Patients should be screened regularly for oral infections such as fungal or viral infections. When these occur, they should be treated promptly with the appropriate chemotherapeutic agent. Likewise, any patient on corticosteroids that presents with an acute dental infection should be treated urgently as such infections can readily spread.

Drug interactions

Aspirin and NSAIDs should not be prescribed to patients on long-term corticosteroids. Both drugs are ulcerogenic and hence increase the risk of gastrointestinal bleeding and ulceration. The antifungal agent amphotericin increases the risk of corticosteroid-induced hypokalaemia, whilst ketoconazole inhibits corticosteroid hepatic metabolism.

Co-trimoxazole (Septrin)

Description
A combination of the antibiotics sulfamethoxazole and trimethoprim.

Indications
Used in the treatment of respiratory and urinary tract infections, toxoplasmosis, and nocardiasis.

Effects on oral and dental structures
Stomatitis, glossitis and Stevens–Johnson syndrome, candidiasis, and salivary gland adenitis can occur.

Effects on patient management
This drug may cause thrombocytopenia, agranulocytosis, and anaemia. Thrombocytopenia may cause postoperative bleeding. If the platelet count is low (<100,000) then the socket should be packed and sutured. Persistent bleeding may require platelet transfusion. Agranulocytosis and anaemia may result in poor healing. Any anaemia will need correction prior to elective general anaesthesia and sedation.

Drug interactions
There is an increased chance of methaemoglobinaemia when used in combination with prilocaine, including topical use of the anaesthetic. The effects of the anticoagulants warfarin and nicoumalone are enhanced during combined therapy. The plasma concentration of phenytoin is increased by co-trimoxazole. Co-trimoxazole may counteract the beneficial effects of tricyclic antidepressants.

Cyclizine (Valoid)

Description
An antihistamine.

Indications

Used in the treatment of vertigo, labyrinthine disorders, motion sickness, and nausea.

Effects on oral and dental structures

This drug can produce xerostomia.

Effects on patient management

Xerostomia may increase caries incidence and thus a preventive regimen is important. If the xerostomia is severe artificial saliva may be indicated.

Drug interactions

Xerostomia is exacerbated by other antimuscarinic agents such as antidepressants.

Cyclophosphamide (Endoxana)

Description

An alkylating agent.

Indications

Chronic lymphocytic leukaemia, lymphomas, and solid tumour.

Effects on oral and dental structures

Cyclophosphamide causes bone marrow suppression with an accompanying thrombocytopenia and agranulocytosis. Bone marrow suppression can lead to troublesome oral ulceration, exacerbation of an existing periodontal condition and rapid spread of any residual (e.g. periapical) infections.

Effect on patient management

The effect of cyclophosphamide on the bone marrow is transient and routine dental treatment is best avoided until the white blood cells and platelet counts start to recover. If emergency dental treatment such as an extraction is required then antibiotic cover may be necessary depending on the degree of myelosuppression. If the platelet count is low (<100,000) then the socket should be packed and sutured. Persistent bleeding may require a platelet transfusion.

Patients on chemotherapeutic agents such as cyclophosphamide often neglect their oral hygiene and thus there could be an increase in both caries and periodontal disease. If time permits, patients about to go on chemotherapy should have a dental check up and any potential areas of infection should be treated. Similarly, to reduce the mucosal irritation (sensitivity) that often accompanies chemotherapy, it is advisable to remove any ill-fitting dentures and smooth over rough cusps or restorations.

Drug interactions
None of any dental significance.

Cycloserine

Description
An antituberculous drug.

Indications
Used in the treatment of tuberculosis.

Effects on oral and dental structures
None specific.

Effects on patient management
Only emergency dental treatment should be performed during active tuberculosis and care must be exercised to eliminate spread of tuberculosis between the patient and dental personnel, e.g. masks and glasses should be worn and where possible treatment should be performed under a rubber dam to reduce aerosol spread. This drug may produce anaemia which may result in poor healing. Any anaemia will need correction prior to elective general anaesthesia and sedation.

Drug interactions
There is an increased risk of phenytoin toxicity when used concurrently.

Cyproheptadine hydrochloride (Periactin)

Description
An antihistamine.

Indications
Used in the treatment of allergies such as hay fever and urticaria. Sometimes used in the management of migraine.

Effects on oral and dental structures
This drug can produce xerostomia.

Effects on patient management
The patient may be drowsy which may interfere with co-operation. Xerostomia may increase caries incidence and thus a preventive regimen is important. If the xerostomia is severe artificial saliva may be indicated. This drug may cause thrombocytopenia, leucopenia and anaemia. Thrombocytopenia may cause postoperative bleeding. If the platelet count is low (<100,000) then the socket should be packed and sutured. Persistent bleeding may require platelet transfusion. Leucopenia may affect healing adversely. Anaemia may result

in poor healing. Any anaemia will need correction prior to elective general anaesthesia and sedation.

Drug interactions
Enhanced sedative effects occur with anxiolytic and hypnotic drugs. Tricyclic and monoamine oxidase inhibitor antidepressants increase antimuscarinic effects such as xerostomia.

Cyproterone acetate (Androcur)

Description
An anti-androgen.

Indications
Used in the treatment of severe hypersexuality and male sexual deviation. Also used in the management of prostate cancer and in the treatment of acne and hirsutism in females.

Effects on oral and dental structures
Can induce osteoporosis which is now regarded as a risk factor for periodontal disease.

Effects on patient management
None of any significance.

Drug interactions
None of any dental significance.

Cytarabine (Cytosar)

Description
An antimetabolic.

Indications
Acute leukaemias.

Effects on oral and dental structures
Cytarabine causes bone marrow suppression with an accompanying thrombocytopenia and agranulocytosis. Bone marrow suppression can lead to troublesome oral ulceration, exacerbation of an existing periodontal condition and rapid spread of any residual (e.g. periapical) infections.

Effect on patient management
The effect of cytarabine on the bone marrow is transient and routine dental treatment is best avoided until the white blood cells and platelet counts start to recover. If emergency dental treatment such as an extraction is required then antibiotic cover may be necessary depending on the degree of myelosuppression. If the platelet count is low (<100,000)

then the socket should be packed and sutured. Persistent bleeding may require a platelet transfusion.

Patients on chemotherapeutic agents such as cytarabine often neglect their oral hygiene and thus there could be an increase in both caries and periodontal disease. If time permits, patients about to go on chemotherapy should have a dental check up and any potential areas of infection should be treated. Similarly, to reduce the mucosal irritation (sensitivity) that often accompanies chemotherapy, it is advisable to remove any ill-fitting dentures and smooth over rough cusps or restorations.

Drug interactions
None of any dental significance.

Dactinomycin

Description
A cytotoxic antibiotic.

Indications
Paediatric cancers.

Effects on oral and dental structures
Dactinomycin causes bone marrow suppression with an accompanying thrombocytopenia and agranulocytosis. Bone marrow suppression can lead to troublesome oral ulceration, exacerbation of an existing periodontal condition, and rapid spread of any residual (e.g. periapical) infections.

Effects on patient management
The effect of dactinomycin on the bone marrow is transient and routine dental treatment is best avoided until the white blood cells and platelet counts start to recover. If emergency dental treatment such as an extraction is required then antibiotic cover may be necessary depending on the degree of myelosuppression. If the platelet count is low (<100,000) then the socket should be packed and sutured. Persistent bleeding may require a platelet transfusion.

Patients on chemotherapeutic agents such as dactinomycin often neglect their oral hygiene and thus there could be an increase in both caries and periodontal disease. If time permits, patients about to go on chemotherapy should have a dental check up and any potential areas of infection should be treated. Similarly, to reduce the mucosal irritation (sensitivity) that often accompanies chemotherapy, it is advisable to smooth over rough cusps or restorations.

Drug interactions
None of any dental significance.

Dalteparin (Fragmin)

Description
A low molecular weight heparin.

Indications
Initial treatment and prevention of deep vein thrombosis and pulmonary embolism. Used to prevent blood coagulation in patients on haemodialysis. Dalteparin and other low molecular weight heparins have a longer duration of action than heparin.

Effects on oral and dental structures
No direct effect, although patients who are repeatedly heparinized are susceptible to osteoporosis. This latter condition may make such patients susceptible to periodontal breakdown.

Effects on patient management
Dalteparin can only be given parentally which reduces the impact of the drug in dental practice. However dentists, especially those working in a hospital environment, will encounter patients who are heparinized on a regular basis (e.g. renal dialysis patients). Bleeding is the main problem with treating such patients. This can arise as a direct effect on the blood coagulation system or from a drug-induced immune-mediated thrombocytopenia. From the coagulation perspective, it is best to treat heparinized patients between treatments since the half-life of the drug is approximately 4 hours. If urgent treatment is required, then the anticoagulation effect of dalteparin can be reversed with protamine sulphate 10 mg IV. If bleeding is due to thrombocytopenia then a platelet transfusion may be required.

Drug interactions
Aspirin and parenteral NSAIDs (e.g. diclofenac and ketorolac) should be avoided in patients who are taking dalteparin or are heparinized on a regular basis. Such analgesics cause impairment of platelet aggregation which would compound a dalteparin-induced thrombocytopenia and likewise cause serious problems with obtaining haemostasis.

Danaparoid (Orgaran)

Description
A heparinoid anticoagulant.

Indications
Prophylaxis of deep vein thrombosis in patients undergoing surgery. Used as an alternative to heparin where there is a history of thrombocytopenia.

Effects on oral and dental structures
No direct effect, although patients who are repeatedly heparinized are susceptible to osteoporosis. This latter condition may make such patients susceptible to periodontal breakdown.

Effects on patient management
Danaparoid can only be given parentally which reduces the impact of the drug in dental practice. However dentists, especially those working in a hospital environment, will encounter patients who are heparinized on a regular basis (e.g. renal dialysis patients). Bleeding is the main problem with treating such patients. This can arise as a direct effect on the blood coagulation system or from a drug-induced immune-mediate thrombocytopenia. From the coagulation perspective, it is best to treat heparinized patients between treatments since the half-life of the drug is approximately 4 hours. If urgent treatment is required, then the anticoagulation effect of dalteparin can be reversed with protamine sulphate 10 mg IV. If bleeding is due to thrombocytopenia then a platelet transfusion may be required.

Drug interactions
Aspirin and parenteral NSAIDs (e.g. diclofenac and ketorolac) should be avoided in patients who are taking dalteparin or are heparinized on a regular basis. Such analgesics cause impairment of platelet aggregation which would compound a dalteparin-induced thrombocytopenia and likewise cause serious problems with obtaining haemostasis.

Danazol

Description
An inhibitor of pituitary gonadotrophin.

Indications
Endometriosis, menorrhagia, severe cyclical mastalgia, benign breast cysts and gynaecomastia.

Effects on oral and dental structures
A rare unwanted effect of danazol is leucopenia and thrombocytopenia. Both can affect the expression of periodontal disease and also exacerbate gingival bleeding.

Effects on patient management
Danazol-induced thrombocytopenia can cause problems with prolonged bleeding following a dental surgical procedure. Always check patients susceptibility to prolonged bleeding or bruising. If prolonged bleeding does occur and fails to respond to local measures, then haemostasis can only be achieved with a platelet transfusion.

Drug interactions
None of any dental significance.

Dantron (Co-danthromer, Co-danthrusate)

Description
A stimulant laxative.

Indications
Used in the management of constipation in the terminally ill.

Effects on oral and dental structures
None specific.

Effects on patient management
As this drug is used only in the terminally ill it is unlikely to be encountered in dental practice. However, avoid the use of codeine and other opioid compounds as they exacerbate constipation.

Drug interactions
Prolonged use may produce a hypokalaemia and this may be exacerbated by potassium shifts due to corticosteroids and epinephrine in local anaesthetics.

Dapsone

Description
An antileprotic drug.

Indications
Used in the management of leprosy and dermatitis herpetiformis.

Effects on oral and dental structures
This drug may cause Stevens–Johnson syndrome and fixed drug eruptions.

Effects on patient management
This drug may cause leucopenia, agranulocytosis, and anaemia. Agranulocytosis and anaemia may result in poor healing. Any anaemia will need correction prior to elective general anaesthesia and sedation.

Drug interactions
None of importance in dentistry.

Daunorubicin (Cerubidin)

Description
A cytotoxic antibiotic.

Indications
Acute leukaemias and AIDS-related Kaposi's sarcoma.

Effects on oral and dental structures
Daunorubicin causes bone marrow suppression with an accompanying thrombocytopenia and agranulocytosis. Bone marrow suppression can lead to troublesome oral ulceration, exacerbation of an existing periodontal condition and rapid spread of any residual (e.g. periapical) infections.

Effect on patient management
The effect of daunorubicin on the bone marrow is transient and routine dental treatment is best avoided until the white blood cells and platelet counts start to recover. If emergency dental treatment is required such as an extraction then antibiotic cover may be required depending on the degree of myelosuppression. If the platelet count is low (<100,000) then the socket should be packed and sutured. Persistent bleeding may require a platelet transfusion.

Patients on chemotherapeutic agents such as daunorubicin often neglect their oral hygiene and thus there could be an increase in both caries and periodontal disease. If time permits, patients about to go on chemotherapy should have a dental check up and any potential areas of infection should be treated. Similarly, to reduce the mucosal irritation (sensitivity) that often accompanies chemotherapy, it is advisable to remove any ill-fitting dentures and smooth over rough cusps or restorations.

Drug interactions
None of any dental significance.

Deflazacort (Calcort)

Description
A corticosteroid.

Indications
Suppression of inflammation and allergic disorders. Used in the management of inflammatory bowel diseases, asthma, immunosuppression, and in various rheumatic diseases.

Effects on oral and dental structures
Although systemic corticosteroids can induce cleft lip and palate formation in mice, there is little evidence that this unwanted effect

occurs in humans. The main impact of systemic corticosteroids on the mouth is to cause an increased susceptibility to opportunistic infections. These include candidiasis and those due to herpes viruses. The anti-inflammatory and immunosuppressant properties of corticosteroids may afford the patient some degree of protection against periodontal breakdown. Paradoxically long-term systemic use can precipitate osteoporosis. The latter is now regarded as a risk factor for periodontal disease.

Effects on patient management

The main unwanted effect of corticosteroid treatment is the suppression of the adrenal cortex and the possibility of an adrenal crisis when such patients are subjected to 'stressful events'. Whilst such suppression does occur physiologically, its clinical significance does appear to be overstated. As far as dentistry is concerned, there is increasing evidence that supplementary corticosteroids are not required. This would apply to all restorative procedures, periodontal surgery and uncomplicated dental extractions. For more complicated dentoalveolar surgery, each case must be judged on its merit. An apprehensive patient may well require cover. It is important to monitor the patient's blood pressure before, during and for 30 minutes after the procedure. If diastolic pressure drops by more than 25%, then hydrocortisone 100 mg IV should be administered and the patient's blood pressure should continue to be monitored.

Patients should be screened regularly for oral infections such as fungal or viral infections. When these occur, they should be treated promptly with the appropriate chemotherapeutic agent. Likewise, any patient on corticosteroids that presents with an acute dental infection should be treated urgently as such infections can readily spread.

Drug interactions

Aspirin and NSAIDs should not be prescribed to patients on long-term corticosteroids. Both drugs are ulcerogenic and hence increase the risk of gastrointestinal bleeding and ulceration. The antifungal agent amphotericin increases the risk of corticosteroid-induced hypokalaemia, whilst ketoconazole inhibits corticosteroid hepatic metabolism.

Demeclocycline hydrochloride (Ledermycin)

Description

A tetracycline antibiotic.

Indications

Used to treat bacterial infection.

Effects on oral and dental structures
Can produce oral candidiasis, lichenoid reactions, fixed drug eruptions tooth staining, and discolouration of the tongue.

Effects on patient management
Antifungal therapy may be needed.

Drug interactions
Tetracyclines inhibit the absorption of iron and zinc. Chelation occurs with calcium salts thus combined intake should be avoided. Tetracyclines reduce the efficacy of penicillins and cephalosporins but may enhance the anticoagulant effect of warfarin and the other coumarin anticoagulants.

Desmopressin (DDAVP, Desmotabs)

Description
A synthetic posterior pituitary hormone.

Indications
Diabetes insipidus, primary nocturnal enuresis.

Effects on oral and dental structures
Can cause xerostomia leading to an increased risk of root caries, candidal infections and poor denture retention. If the xerostomia is severe, dentate patients should receive topical fluoride and be offered an artificial saliva.

Effects on patient management
Nothing of significance.

Drug interactions
None of any dental significance.

Dexamethasone (Decadron)

Description
A corticosteroid.

Indications
Suppression of inflammation and allergic disorders. Used in the management of inflammatory bowel diseases, asthma, immunosuppression, and in various rheumatic diseases.

Effects on oral and dental structures
Although systemic corticosteroids can induce cleft lip and palate formation in mice, there is little evidence that this unwanted effect occurs in humans. The main impact of systemic corticosteroids on the mouth is to cause an increased susceptibility to opportunistic

infections. These include candidiasis and those due to herpes viruses. The anti-inflammatory and immunosuppressant properties of corticosteroids may afford the patient some degree of protection against periodontal breakdown. Paradoxically long-term systemic use can precipitate osteoporosis. The latter is now regarded as a risk factor for periodontal disease.

Effects on patient management

The main unwanted effect of corticosteroid treatment is the suppression of the adrenal cortex and the possibility of an adrenal crisis when such patients are subjected to 'stressful events'. Whilst such suppression does occur physiologically, its clinical significance does appear to be overstated. As far as dentistry is concerned, there is increasing evidence that supplementary corticosteroids are not required. This would apply to all restorative procedures, periodontal surgery and uncomplicated dental extractions. For more complicated dentoalveolar surgery, each case must be judged on its merit. An apprehensive patient may well require cover. It is important to monitor the patient's blood pressure before, during and for 30 minutes after the procedure. If diastolic pressure drops by more than 25%, then hydrocortisone 100 mg IV should be administered and the patient's blood pressure should continue to be monitored.

Patients should be screened regularly for oral infections such as fungal or viral infections. When these occur, they should be treated promptly with the appropriate chemotherapeutic agent. Likewise, any patient on corticosteroids that presents with an acute dental infection should be treated urgently as such infections can readily spread.

Drug interactions

Aspirin and NSAIDs should not be prescribed to patients on long-term corticosteroids. Both drugs are ulcerogenic and hence increase the risk of gastrointestinal bleeding and ulceration. The antifungal agent amphotericin increases the risk of corticosteroid-induced hypokalaemia, whilst ketoconazole inhibits corticosteroid hepatic metabolism.

Dexamfetamine sulphate (Dexedrine)

Description

A central nervous stimulant.

Indications

Used in the management of hyperactivity in children and in narcolepsy.

Effects on oral and dental structures

This drug may produce xerostomia and a metallic taste.

Effects on patient management

Dose reduction of epinephrine in dental local anaesthetics is advisable (see drug interaction below). The underlying condition of hyperactivity may make compliance for prolonged procedures under local anaesthesia difficult. Xerostomia may increase caries incidence and thus a preventive regimen is important. If the xerostomia is severe artificial saliva may be indicated.

Drug interactions

Combined therapy with monoamine oxidase inhibitors can produce a hypertensive crisis. The unwanted effects of epinephrine in dental local anaesthetics will be enhanced during combined therapy. Dexamfetamine increases the analgesic effect and decreases the respiratory depressant action of the opioids. The sedative effects of antihistamines are antagonized by dexamfetamine.

Dextromoramide (Palfium)

Description

An opioid analgesic.

Indications

Severe pain.

Effects on oral and dental structures

Can cause xerostomia leading to an increased risk of root caries, candidal infections, and poor denture retention. If the xerostomia is severe, dentate patients should receive topical fluoride and be offered an artificial saliva.

Effects on patient management

Dextromoramide is a drug of dependence and can thus cause withdrawal symptoms if the medication is stopped abruptly. Such cessation of dextromoramide may account for unusual behavioural changes and poor compliance with dental treatment. The drug also depresses respiration and causes postural hypotension.

Drug interactions

Dextromoramide will enhance the sedative properties of midazolam and diazepam. Reduce the dose of both sedative agents.

Dextropropoxyphene hydrochloride

Description

An opioid analgesic, also used as a constituent of compound analgesics.

Indications

Mild to moderate pain.

Effects on oral and dental structures

Can cause xerostomia leading to an increased risk of root caries, candidal infections and poor denture retention. If the xerostomia is severe, dentate patients should receive topical fluoride and be offered an artificial saliva.

Effects on patient management

Contraindicated (either used singularly or as a compound analgesic) in patients with suicidal tendencies or those prone to addiction.

Drug interactions

Will enhance the sedative properties of midazolam and diazepam. Reduce the dose of both sedative agents.

Diamorphine (Heroin) hydrochloride

Description

An opioid analgesic.

Indications

Severe pain; pulmonary oedema.

Effects on oral and dental structures

Heroin may cause a thrombocytopaenia resulting in post-operative bleeding. A pre-operative platelet count is advisable. IV abuse may lead to cardiac valve damage and may make the patient susceptible to endocarditis. Cross-infection with hepatitis and HIV must be considered. Can cause xerostomia leading to an increased risk of root caries, candidal infections, and poor denture retention. If the xerostomia is severe, dentate patients should receive topical fluoride and be offered an artificial saliva. Pigmented lesions of the tongue are reported in heroin addicts who inhale. Histologically, the lesions are packed with melanocytes.

Effects on patient management

Diamorphine hydrochloride is a drug of dependence and can thus cause withdrawal symptoms if the medication is stopped abruptly. Such cessation of diamorphine hydrochloride may account for unusual behavioural changes and poor compliance with dental treatment. The drug also depresses respiration and causes postural hypotension.

Drug interactions

Diamorphine hydrochloride will enhance the sedative properties of midazolam and diazepam. Reduce the dose of both sedative agents.

Diazepam (Dialar, Diazemuls, Rimapam, Stesolid, Tensium, Valclair, Valium)

Description

A benzodiazepine sedative and anxiolytic drug with anticonvulsant properties.

Indications

Used in dental sedation and preoperative anxiolysis (although it has now been superseded by midazolam when intravenous techniques are employed: for oral sedation temazepam is the drug of choice). Also indicated in the emergency treatment of epilepsy in the dental surgery.

Presentations

(i) 2 mg, 5 mg, and 10 mg tablets.

(ii) Oral solutions of 2 mg/5 mL and 5 mg/5 mL.

(iii) Solution for injection 5 mg/mL.

(iv) 10 mg suppositories.

(v) Solutions for rectal administration 2 mg/mL and 4 mg/mL

Dose

(i) To treat anxiolysis
2 mg–10 mg three times daily.

(ii) As premedication prior to dental treatment
5–10 mg 1–2 hours prior to the appointment.

(iii) For intravenous dental sedation
incremental doses of 2.5 mg/minute until a satisfactory end-point (Verrill's sign which is drooping of the upper eyelid to cover half of the pupil). Midazolam has now superseded diazepam as the intravenous benzodiazepine for dental sedation.

(iv) In the emergency treatment of epilepsy (status epilepticus) in the dental surgery
5 mg over 1 minute increments intravenously repeated if necessary up to a dose of 20 mg.

Contraindications

Severe respiratory disease.
Severe liver disease.
Porphyria (although should be used in emergency management of status epilepticus).

Precautions

History of drug abuse.
Severe liver disease.
Severe muscle weakness (myasthenia gravis).
Pregnancy and breastfeeding.

Unwanted effects

Xerostomia.
Respiratory depression.
Hypotension.
Visual disturbances.

Headache.

Occasionally skin rashes (anaphylaxis is unusual).

Thrombophlebitis after intravenous use.

May produce condition similar to foetal alcohol syndrome including cleft lip and palate.

Drug dependence.

Sexual fantasy.

Drug interactions

There is synergy with all CNS depressant drugs (including alcohol and opioid analgesics) leading to an enhanced effect and thus combined use is best avoided. The antidepressant drugs fluoxetine and fluvoxamine enhance the effects of diazepam. Severe hypotension and respiratory depression may occur when diazepam is administered simultaneously with the antipsychotic drug clozapine and combined therapy is not recommended.

Cimetidine and omeprazole inhibit the metabolism of diazepam, thus increasing its sedative effect. In addition the gut motility stimulant cisapride and the anti-emetic drug metoclopramide enhance the action of oral diazepam. Similarly, oral contraceptives, the anti-alcohol drug disulfiram, the muscle relaxant baclofen, and the cannabinoid nabilone all increase the effect of diazepam. Beta-adrenergic drugs reduce metabolism of diazepam but there appears to be little clinical risk from combined therapy. Similarly, although paracetamol reduces the excretion of diazepam this is of no clinical importance.

The antibacterials isoniazid and ciprofloxacin inhibit the metabolism of diazepam whereas rifampicin increases metabolism of the benzodiazepine. Smoking increases the metabolism of diazepam. Diazepam affects the metabolism of phenytoin in an inconsistent manner, in some individuals the anticonvulsant plasma level is increased in others it is reduced. Carbamazepine possibly reduces the effects of diazepam, whereas sodium valproate enhances the effect of the benzodiazepine.

Diazepam can increase the effects of neuromuscular blockers tubocurarine, vecuronium, and atracurium. It reduces the effects of levodopa. Diazepam may increase the plasma concentration of the local anaesthetic bupivacaine. Flumazenil antagonizes the action of diazepam. Aminophylline also has some antagonistic properties. Caffeine can counteract some of the hypnotic effects of diazepam.

Diazoxide (Eudemine)

Description

An oral antidiabetic drug.

Indications
Chronic intractable hypoglycaemia.

Effects on oral and dental structures
Diazoxide has been cited as causing taste disturbances and dyskenesias. The latter can result in involuntary movement of the facial muscles (e.g. grimacing), lip smacking and tongue protrusion. Dyskinesias resolve on cessation of the drug.

Effects on patient management
Diazoxide can cause a thrombocytopenia. This can lead to impaired haemostasis after any dental surgical procedure. If the platelet count is low (<100,000) then the socket should be packed and sutured. Persistent bleeding may require a platelet transfusion.

Drug interactions
None of any dental significance.

Diclofenac sodium (Voltarol)

Description
A peripherally acting, non-steroidal anti-inflammatory analgesic.

Indications
Pain and inflammation associated with musculoskeletal disorders, e.g. rheumatoid arthritis, osteoarthritis and ankylosing spondylitis. Postoperative pain.

Effects on oral and dental structures
Patients on long-term NSAIDs such as diclofenac sodium may be afforded some degree of protection against periodontal breakdown. This arises from the drug's inhibitory action on prostaglandin synthesis. The latter is an important inflammatory mediator in the pathogenesis of periodontal breakdown.

Effects on patient management
Rare unwanted effects of diclofenac sodium include angioedema and thrombocytopenia. The latter may cause an increased bleeding tendency following any dental surgical procedure. If the platelet count is low (<100,000) then the socket should be packed and sutured. Persistent bleeding may require a platelet transfusion.

Drug interactions
Ibuprofen, aspirin and diflunisal should be avoided in patients taking diclofenac sodium due to an increase in unwanted effects, especially gastrointestinal ulceration, renal and liver damage. Systemic corticosteroids increase the risk of peptic ulceration and gastrointestinal bleeding.

Dicyclomine hydrochloride/Dicycloverine hydrochloride (Kolanticon, Merbentyl)

Description
An antimuscarinic drug.

Indications
Used for symptomatic relief in gastrointestinal disorders such as dyspepsia, diverticular disease, and irritable bowel syndrome.

Effects on oral and dental structures
Xerostomia may occur.

Effects on patient management
If use is prolonged xerostomia may increase caries incidence and thus a preventive regimen is important. If the xerostomia is severe artificial saliva may be indicated.

Drug interactions
Absorption of ketoconazole is decreased. Side effects increased with concurrent medication with tricyclic and monoamine oxidase inhibitor antidepressants.

Dicycloverine hydrochloride/Dicyclomine hydrochloride (Kolanticon, Merbentyl)

Description
An antimuscarinic drug.

Indications
Used for symptomatic relief in gastrointestinal disorders such as dyspepsia, diverticular disease, and irritable bowel syndrome.

Effects on oral and dental structures
Xerostomia may occur.

Effects on patient management
If use is prolonged xerostomia may increase caries incidence and thus a preventive regimen is important. If the xerostomia is severe artificial saliva may be indicated.

Drug interactions
Absorption of ketoconazole is decreased. Side effects increased with concurrent medication with tricyclic and monoamine oxidase inhibitor antidepressants.

Didanosine (Videx)

Description
A nucleoside reverse transcriptase inhibitor.

Indications
Used in the management of HIV infection.

Effects on oral and dental structures
Xerostomia, taste disturbance, and candidiasis can occur.

Effects on patient management
Sensitive handling of the underlying disease state is essential. Excellent preventive dentistry and regular examinations are important in patients suffering from HIV, as dental infections are best avoided. HIV will interfere with postoperative healing, and antibiotic prophylaxis prior to oral surgery may be advisable. This drug can produce a thrombocytopenia which may cause postoperative bleeding. If the platelet count is low (<100,000) then the socket should be packed and sutured. Persistent bleeding may require platelet transfusion. Xerostomia may increase caries incidence and thus a preventive regimen is important. If the xerostomia is severe artificial saliva may be indicated. Peripheral neuropathy is possible during relative analgesia in patients receiving didanosine (see below).

Drug interactions
Didanosine reduces the serum concentration of itraconazole. Ketoconazole and tetracyclines reduce the absorption of didanosine but this can be avoided by separating dosing by 2 hours. Concurrent treatment with metronidazole, sulfonamides or tetracyclines increases the risks of pancreatitis. Both metronidazole and nitrous oxide increase the risk of peripheral neuropathy.

Diethylstilbestrol (Stilboesterol)

Description
An oestrogen.

Indications
Prostate cancer (rarely), breast cancer in postmenopausal women.

Effects on oral and dental structures
Oestrogens may enhance the plaque-induced inflammatory responses in the gingival tissues.

Effects on patient management
Nothing of any significance.

Drug interactions
None of any dental significance.

Diflunisal (Dolobid)

Description
A peripherally acting, non-steroidal anti-inflammatory analgesic that is derived from salicylic acid.

Indications
Pain with a significant inflammatory component (e.g. postoperative pain after dental surgical procedures). Also used in the treatment of musculoskeletal disorder and dysmenorrhoea.

Presentations
A 250 mg tablet.

Dose
0.5–1 g every 12 hours. Not recommended for children.

Contraindications
Diflunisal is contraindicated in patients with a history of allergy to aspirin or any other NSAID. The drug should not be prescribed to asthmatics (can precipitate bronchoconstriction) or patients with a history of angioedema and urticaria. Diflunisal should not be prescribed to patients with active peptic ulceration (diflunisal is ulcerogenic) or to patients with haemorrhagic disorders because it will affect platelet aggregation. Diflunisal should be used with caution in patients who exhibit renal, cardiac or hepatic impairment since the repeated used of the drug can result in a deterioration in renal function.

Precautions
Elderly, breastfeeding mothers, and pregnancy.

Unwanted effects
Diflunisal is ulcerogenic although of all the NSAIDs, it has the lowest risk of gastrointestinal irritation. This unwanted effect can be further reduced by taking the drug with food or milk. Other rare unwanted effects include blood disorders, fluid retention, renal damage, eye changes and the precipitation of Stevens–Johnson syndrome. Patients who suffer from systemic lupus erythematosus may be susceptible to a NSAID induced aseptic meningitis. Excessive high doses of diflunisal can cause a metabolic acidosis if untreated, this can lead to a coma. Although diflunisal is an effective analgesic for the treatment of postoperative dental pain, its use after third molar surgery is associated with a high incidence of dry socket (alveolar osteitis) formation. This is thought to be due to an increased fibrinolytic action of the drug. Diflunisal has also been cited as a possible cause of drug-induced oral lichenoid reaction.

Drug interactions

Diflunisal should not be given with other NSAIDs or aspirin since using such combinations will increase the risk of unwanted effects. The anticoagulant effects of both warfarin and heparin are enhanced by diflunisal. The drug can antagonize the hypotensive effects of the ACE inhibitors (e.g. captopril, lisinopril). There is the additional increased risk of renal impairment and hyperkalaemia with these drugs and diflunisal. Antidiabetic drugs such as the sulphonylureas are extensively protein bound and can be displaced by diflunisal, leading to hypoglycaemia. Diflunisal can increase the risk of gastrointestinal haemorrhage if given to patients taking antiplatelet drugs such as clopidogrel. Diflunisal should be avoided in patients taking beta-adrenoceptor blockers as there will be an antagonism of their hypotensive effect. Diflunisal may exacerbate heart failure, reduce glomerular filtration rate and increase plasma concentration of digoxin. Both diflunisal and corticosteroids (systemic) cause peptic ulceration therefore avoid the combination. The excretion of methotrexate is reduced by diflunisal which can lead to increased toxicity. Diflunisal reduces the excretion of the muscle relaxant baclofen. The excretion of lithium is reduced by diflunisal, thus increasing the risk of lithium toxicity.

Digoxin (Lanoxin)

Description

A cardiac glycoside that was originally obtained from the leaves of the foxglove (Digitalis).

Indications

In the treatment of cardiac failure in association with atrial fibrillation.

Effects on oral and dental structures

Has been known to cause pain similar to trigeminal neuralgia in the lower third of the face.

Effects on patient management

Digoxin is a drug with a low therapeutic index and a slight increase in plasma concentrations can cause digoxin toxicity. Hypokalaemia predisposes to digoxin toxicity and epinephrine containing local anaesthetic solutions can cause hypokalaemia. No more than 3 cartridges should be used at any one time on adult patients taking digoxin.

Drug interactions

NSAIDs, such as ibuprofen, may exacerbate heart failure, reduce GFR and increase plasma concentrations of digoxin. Erythromycin enhances the action of digoxin. Systemic amphotericin can cause a hypokalaemia which enhances digoxin toxicity. Non-steroidal anti-inflammatory drugs (e.g. ibuprofen) may exacerbate heart failure and increase plasma concentrations of digoxin leading to toxicity. Systemic amphotericin will exacerbate a digoxin-induced hypokalaemia.

Dihydrocodeine tartrate (DF118)

Description
An opioid analgesic.

Indications
Moderate to severe pain.

Presentations
(i) 30 mg tablet.

(ii) Oral solution, 10 mg/ml.

(iii) IM injection, 50 mg/ml.

Dose – Oral
Adults: 30 mg every 4–6 hours.
Children: over 4 years, 0.5–1 mg/kg every 4–6 hours.

Dose – Deep subcutaneous or intramuscular injection
Adults: 50 mg every 4–6 hours.
Children: over 4 years, 0.5–1 mg/kg every 4–6 hours.

Contraindications
All opioids are addictive and hence dihydrocodeine may be requested specifically by a drug addict, irrespective of their level of pain. The drug depresses respiration and so should be avoided in patients with any form of respiratory impairment (e.g. chronic obstructive pulmonary disease). Dihydrocodeine should be used with caution in those who suffer from hypotension, hypothyroidism and prostatic hypertrophy. The drug should be avoided during pregnancy and whilst breastfeeding. Similarly avoid in patients with both renal and hepatic impairment. Dihydrocodeine should not be used in patients who have a suspected head injury or raised intracranial pressure. The respiratory depressant properties of dihydrocodeine will raise the intracranial pressure further and the action of the drug on the pupillary reflex to light will mask signs of the level of consciousness.

Precautions
Elderly and debilitated patients.

Unwanted effects
Dihydrocodeine is associated with a high prevalence of unwanted effects which include nausea, vomiting, constipation, drowsiness, dysphoria, impaired micturition, dry mouth, uteric or biliary spasm, sweating, facial flushing, bradycardia and tachycardia. Whilst dihydrocodeine is classified as an analgesic, its efficacy in the treatment of

postoperative dental pain is uncertain. Indeed, studies have shown that the drug can make the pain worse. Thus in view of the large range of unwanted effects and its uncertain efficacy, there must remain significant questions over the value of this drug in dental practice.

Drug interactions
Nothing of any significance.

Dihydroergotamine mesilate (Migranal)

Description
An ergot alkaloid drug.

Indications
Used in the treatment of acute migraine.

Effects on oral and dental structures
None specific to this drug, which is administered intranasally.

Effects on patient management
Any precipitator of migrainous attacks, such as the dental light shining in the eyes or sudden noises, should be avoided.

Drug interactions
Erythromycin increases the toxicity of ergot alkaloids.

Diloxanide furoate (Furamide) [Entamizole is diloxanide in combination with metronidazole]

Description
An antiprotozoal drug.

Indications
Used as an amoebicide.

Effects on oral and dental structures
None reported.

Effects on patient management
None specific.

Drug interactions
None of importance in dentistry.

Diltiazem (Tildiem, Adizem, Angitil, Calicard, Dilzem, Slozem, Viazem, Zemtard)

Description
A calcium-channel blocker.

Indications
Supraventricular arrhythmias, angina prophylaxis and hypertension.

Effects on oral and dental structures
Diltiazem can cause gingival overgrowth, especially in the anterior part of the mouth. It also causes taste disturbances arising from inhibiting calcium-channel activity necessary for the normal function of taste and smell receptors.

Effects on patient management
None of any significance.

Drug interactions
Diltiazem can inhibit the metabolism of midazolam, thus causing an increase in plasma concentration and an increased sedative action. A lower titrated dose of midazolam may be necessary for dental sedation.

Dimenhydrinate (Dramamine)

Description
An antihistamine.

Indications
Used in the treatment of vertigo, labyrinthine disorders, motion sickness, and nausea.

Effects on oral and dental structures
This drug can produce xerostomia.

Effects on patient management
Xerostomia may increase caries incidence and thus a preventive regimen is important. If the xerostomia is severe artificial saliva may be indicated.

Drug interactions
Xerostomia is exacerbated by other antimuscarinic agents such as antidepressants.

Diphenhydramine hydrochloride

Description
An antihistamine.

Indications
Used as a hypnotic and as a constituent of cough and decongestant medications. Also used to treat allergic rhinitis and as a topical anaesthetic in some countries.

Effects on oral and dental structures
Can produce xerostomia.

Effects on patient management
The patient may be drowsy which may interfere with co-operation. Xerostomia may increase caries incidence and thus a preventive regimen is important. If the xerostomia is severe artificial saliva may be indicated. This drug may cause thrombocytopenia, agranulocytosis and anaemia. Thrombocytopenia may cause postoperative bleeding. If the platelet count is low (<100,000) then the socket should be packed and sutured. Persistent bleeding may require platelet transfusion. Agranulocytosis may affect healing adversely. Anaemia may result in poor healing. Any anaemia will need correction prior to elective general anaesthesia and sedation.

Drug interactions
Enhanced sedative effect with anxiolytic and hypnotic drugs. Tricyclic and monoamine oxidase inhibitor antidepressants increase antimuscarinic effects such as xerostomia.

Diphenylpyraline hydrochloride

Description
An antihistamine.

Indications
Used as a hypnotic and as a constituent of cough and decongestant medications.

Effects on oral and dental structures
Can produce xerostomia.

Effects on patient management
The patient may be drowsy which may interfere with co-operation. Xerostomia may increase caries incidence and thus a preventive regimen is important. If the xerostomia is severe artificial saliva may be indicated. This drug may cause thrombocytopenia, agranulocytosis, and anaemia. Thrombocytopenia may cause postoperative bleeding.

If the platelet count is low (<100,000) then the socket should be packed and sutured. Persistent bleeding may require platelet transfusion. Agranulocytosis may affect healing adversely. Anaemia may result in poor healing. Any anaemia will need correction prior to elective general anaesthesia and sedation.

Drug interactions
Enhanced sedative effect with anxiolytic and hypnotic drugs. Tricyclic and monoamine oxidase inhibitor.

Dipipanone (Diconal)

Description
An opioid analgesic.

Indications
Moderate to severe pain.

Effects on oral and dental structures
Can cause xerostomia leading to an increased risk of root caries, candidal infections and poor denture retention. If the xerostomia is severe, dentate patients should receive topical fluoride and be offered an artificial saliva.

Effects on patient management
Dipipanone is a drug of dependence and can thus case withdrawal symptoms if the medication is stopped abruptly. Such cessation of dipipanone may account for unusual behavioural changes and poor compliance with dental treatment. The drug also depresses respiration and cause postural hypotension.

Drug interactions
Dipipanone will enhance the sedative properties of midazolam and diazepam. Reduce the dose of both sedation agents.

Dipyridamole (Persantin)

Description
An antiplatelet drug.

Indications
Prevention of atherosclerotic events (stroke, myocardial infarction, and peripheral arterial disease).

Effects on oral and dental structures
None of any significance.

Effects on patient management
Increased risk of haemorrhage following any dental procedure associated with a risk of bleeding. Local measures (e.g. pack and suture) should be adopted. If this fails to control bleeding, then a platelet transfusion may be required.

Drug interactions
Aspirin and other NSAIDs reduce platelet aggregation and will enhance the antiplatelet actions of dipyridamole and lead to serious problems with haemostasis.

Disopyramide (Rythmodan)

Description
A class Ia antidysrhythmic drug.

Indications
Post myocardial infarction ventricular arrhythmia.

Effects on oral and dental structures
May cause xerostomia due to an antimuscarinic action – leading to increased risk of root caries, candidal infections, and poor denture retention. If the xerostomia is severe, dentate patients should receive topical fluoride and be offered an artificial saliva.

Effects on patient management
Disopyramide can cause hypoglycaemia. The drug has also been cited as causing agranulocytosis (high risk of oral ulceration and periodontal breakdown) and thrombocytopenia (impaired haemostasis). If the platelet count is low (<100,000) then the socket should be packed and sutured. Persistent bleeding may require a platelet transfusion.

Drug interactions
Erythromycin can increase plasma concentrations of disopyramide.

Distigmine bromide (Ubretid)

Description
A parasympathomimetic.

Indications
Urinary retention.

Effects on oral and dental structures
None reported.

Effects on patient management
Distigmine bromide frequently causes transient blurred vision and patients may require more assistance than usual.

Drug interactions
Nothing of any dental significance.

Disulfiram (Antabuse)

Description
An anti-alcohol drug.

Indications
Used in the management of alcohol dependence.

Effects on oral and dental structures
Halitosis and metallic taste may be produced.

Effects on patient management
History of alcohol dependence may cause bleeding disorders and affect drug metabolism.

Drug interactions
Obviously alcohol should be avoided. Combined therapy with metronidazole produces psychosis and confusion. Disulfiram enhances the effects of benzodiazepines, warfarin, phenytoin, and tricyclic antidepressants.

Docetaxel (Taxotere)

Description
An antineoplastic drug.

Indications
Advanced or metastatic breast cancer.

Effects on oral and dental structures
Docetaxel causes bone marrow suppression with an accompanying thrombocytopenia and agranulocytosis. Bone marrow suppression can lead to troublesome oral ulceration, exacerbation of an existing periodontal condition and rapid spread of any residual (e.g. periapical) infections.

Effects on patient management
The effect of docetaxel on the bone marrow is transient and routine dental treatment is best avoided until the white blood cells and platelet counts start to recover. If emergency dental treatment such as an extraction is required then antibiotic cover may be necessary depending on the degree of myelosuppression. If the platelet count is

low (<100,000) then the socket should be packed and sutured. Persistent bleeding may require a platelet transfusion.

Patients on chemotherapeutic agents such as docetaxel often neglect their oral hygiene and thus there could be an increase in both caries and periodontal disease. If time permits, patients about to go on chemotherapy should have a dental check up and any potential areas of infection should be treated. Similarly, to reduce the mucosal irritation (sensitivity) that often accompanies chemotherapy, it is advisable to remove any ill-fitting dentures and smooth over rough cusps or restorations.

Drug interactions
None of any dental significance.

Docusate sodium (Dioctyl, Docusol, Fletcher's Enemette, Norgalax Micro-enema)

Description
A stimulant laxative.

Indications
Used in the management of constipation.

Effects on oral and dental structures
May produce an unpleasant taste.

Effects on patient management
Avoid the use of codeine and other opioid compounds as they exacerbate constipation.

Drug interactions
Docusate may decrease the efficacy of aspirin. Prolonged use may produce a hypokalaemia and this may be exacerbated by potassium shifts due to corticosteroids and epinephrine in local anaesthetics.

Domperidone (Motilium) [Also found in combination with paracetamol in Domperamol]

Description
An anti-emetic drug.

Indications
Used in the management of nausea, vomiting, and short term treatment of dyspepsia. Also used in combination with paracetamol in anti-migraine drugs.

Effects on oral and dental structures
This drug can produce xerostomia.

Effects on patient management
As the drug is only used short term xerostomia should not produce significant problems, however a preventive regimen may be considered. The underlying condition may increase the incidence of dental erosion, especially of the palatal surfaces of teeth. Patients may be uncomfortable in the fully supine position as a result of their underlying gastrointestinal disorder.

Drug interactions
This drug accelerates the absorption of paracetamol, enhancing its effect. Opioids antagonize the gastrointestinal effects of domperidone.

Donepezil hydrochloride (Aricept)

Description
An anticholinesterase drug.

Indications
Used in the management of Alzheimer's disease.

Effects on oral and dental structures
Xerostomia, lingual swelling, gingivitis, bad taste and occasionally toothache can be produced.

Effects on patient management
Xerostomia may increase caries incidence and thus a preventive regimen is important. If the xerostomia is severe artificial saliva may be indicated. Thrombocytopenia may cause postoperative bleeding. If the platelet count is low (<100,000) then the socket should be packed and sutured. Persistent bleeding may require platelet transfusion. Non-steroidal anti-inflammatory drugs are best avoided in postoperative pain control (see drug interaction below).

Drug interactions
Gastrointestinal effects of non-steroidal anti-inflammatory drugs exacerbated. Ketoconazole inhibits metabolism of donepezil.

Dornase alpha (Pulmozyne)

Description
A mucolytic drug.

Indications
Used in cystic fibrosis.

Effects on oral and dental structures
Can produce pharyngitis and sinusitis.

Effects on patient management
Patients may not be comfortable in the supine position due to their respiratory problems.

Drug interactions
None of importance in dentistry.

Dorzolamide (Cosopt, Trusopt)

Description
A topical carbonic anhydrase inhibitor.

Indications
Used in the treatment of glaucoma.

Effects on oral and dental structures
A bitter taste may be produced.

Effects on patient management
Patient may require reassurance that taste disturbance is due to drug therapy. Other carbonic anhydrase inhibitors can produce xerostomia; this should be considered as a possibility and caries prevention regimens encouraged.

Drug interactions
As this drug is used topically drug interactions in dentistry are unlikely. However theoretically adverse effects may occur with drugs which interact with carbonic anhydrase inhibitors, such as aspirin, procaine, carbamazepine, phenytoin, and corticosteroids (see acetazolamide).

Dosulepin hydrochloride/Dothiepin hydrochloride (Prothiaden)

Description
A tricyclic antidepressant.

Indications
Used in the management of depressive illness.

Effects on oral and dental structures
Xerostomia may occur.

Effects on patient management
Xerostomia may increase caries incidence and thus a preventive regimen is important. If the xerostomia is severe artificial saliva may

be indicated. Postural hypotension may occur with this drug, therefore rapid changes in patient position should be avoided. This drug may cause thrombocytopenia, agranulocytosis and leucopenia. Thrombocytopenia may cause postoperative bleeding. If the platelet count is low (<100,000) then the socket should be packed and sutured. Persistent bleeding may require platelet transfusion. Agranulocytosis and leucopenia may affect healing adversely.

Drug interactions
Increased sedation occurs with alcohol and sedative drugs such as benzodiazepines. This drug may antagonize the action of anticonvulsants such as carbamazepine and phenytoin. This drug increases the pressor effects of epinephrine. Nevertheless, the use of epinephrine-containing local anaesthetics is not contraindicated. However, epinephrine dose limitation is recommended.

Normal anticoagulant control by warfarin may be upset, both increases and decreases in INR have been noted during combined therapy with tricyclic antidepressants. Combined therapy with other antidepressants should be avoided and if prescribing another class of antidepressant a period of one to two weeks should elapse between changeover. Antimuscarinic effects such as xerostomia are increased when used in combination with other anticholinergic drugs such as antipsychotics.

Dothiepin hydrochloride/Dosulepin hydrochloride (Prothiaden)

Description
A tricyclic antidepressant.

Indications
Used in the management of depressive illness.

Effects on oral and dental structures
Xerostomia may occur.

Effects on patient management
Xerostomia may increase caries incidence and thus a preventive regimen is important. If the xerostomia is severe artificial saliva may be indicated. Postural hypotension may occur with this drug, therefore rapid changes in patient position should be avoided. This drug may cause thrombocytopenia, agranulocytosis, and leucopenia. Thrombocytopenia may cause postoperative bleeding. If the platelet count is low (<100,000) then the socket should be packed and sutured. Persistent bleeding may require platelet transfusion. Agranulocytosis and leucopenia may affect healing adversely.

Drug interactions

Increased sedation occurs with alcohol and sedative drugs such as benzodiazepines. This drug may antagonize the action of anticonvulsants such as carbamazepine and phenytoin. This drug increases the pressor effects of epinephrine. Nevertheless, the use of epinephrine-containing local anaesthetics is not contraindicated; however, epinephrine dose limitation is recommended.

Normal anticoagulant control by warfarin may be upset, both increases and decreases in INR have been noted during combined therapy with tricyclic antidepressants. Combined therapy with other antidepressants should be avoided and if prescribing another class of antidepressant a period of one to two weeks should elapse between changeover. Antimuscarinic effects such as xerostomia are increased when used in combination with other anticholinergic drugs such as antipsychotics.

Doxazosin (Cardura)

Description
An alpha-adrenoceptor blocking drug.

Indications
Hypertension and benign prostatic hyperplasia.

Effects on oral and dental structures
None reported.

Effects on patient management
This drug may produce postural hypotension and rarely thrombocytopenia which could cause impaired haemostasis after a dental surgical procedure. If the platelet count is low (<100,000) then the socket should be packed and sutured. Persistent bleeding may require a platelet transfusion.

Drug interactions
NSAIDs such as ibuprofen and systemic corticosteroids may antagonize the hypotensive effect of doxazosin.

Doxycycline (Vibramycin, Vibramycin-D)

Description
A tetracycline antibiotic.

Indications
Occasionally used in the treatment of sinusitis.

Presentations
(i) 50 mg tablets.

(ii) 50 mg capsules.

(iii) 100 mg dispersible tablet.

Dose
200 mg on the first day then 100 mg daily.

Contraindications
Pregnancy.
Breastfeeding.
Children under 12 years.
Kidney disease.
Systemic lupus erythematosus.

Precautions
Liver disease.

Unwanted effects
Staining of teeth and bones.
Opportunistic fungal infections ('tetracycline sore mouth').
Lichenoid reactions.
Fixed drug eruptions.
Stevens–Johnson syndrome.
Hypersensitivity.
Photosensitivity.
Facial pigmentation.
Headache and visual disturbances.
Anaemia.
Hepatotoxicity.
Pancreatitis.
Gastrointestinal upset including pseudomembranous colitis.

Drug interactions
As tetracycline chelates calcium and other cations a number of drugs (and foodstuffs such as dairy products) which contain cations reduce the absorption of tetracycline. Among the drugs which reduce the absorption of tetracycline are the ACE-inhibitor quinapril, antacids, calcium, and zinc salts, ulcer-healing drugs such as sucralfate and the ion-exchange resin colestipol. Similarly tetracyclines inhibit the absorption of iron and zinc.

Tetracyclines reduce the efficacy of penicillins and cephalosporins. Tetracyclines raise blood urea levels and this effect is exacerbated with combined therapy with diuretics. Tetracyclines may enhance the anticoagulant effect of warfarin and the other coumarin anticoagulants. Tetracyclines may interfere without the action of oral contraceptives and alternative methods of contraception should be advised during therapy. Tetracyclines have a hypoglycaemic effect and their administration to patients receiving insulin or oral hypoglycaemics should be avoided.

Tetracyclines may increase the serum levels of digoxin, theophylline and the anti-malarial medication mefloquine. Tetracycline may also increase the risk of methotrexate toxicity. The serum levels of doxycycline are reduced by alcohol, phenytoin, carbamazepine, barbiturates, and rifampicin. These interactions can interfere with the efficacy of the antibiotic. Combined therapy with ergotamine can produce ergotism (the most dramatic effect of ergotism is vasospasm which can cause gangrene).

Patients who use a contact lens cleaner containing thiomersal have reported ocular irritation during tetracycline therapy. Cranial hypertension leading to headache and dizziness may result with the combined use of tetracycline and retinoids.

Doxepin (Sinequan)

Description
A tricyclic antidepressant.

Indications
Used in the management of depressive illness.

Effects on oral and dental structures
Xerostomia, taste disturbance, and stomatitis may occur.

Effects on patient management
Xerostomia may increase caries incidence and thus a preventive regimen is important. If the xerostomia is severe artificial saliva may be indicated. Postural hypotension may occur with this drug, therefore rapid changes in patient position should be avoided. This drug may cause thrombocytopenia, agranulocytosis, and leucopenia. Thrombocytopenia may cause postoperative bleeding. If the platelet count is low (<100,000) then the socket should be packed and sutured. Persistent bleeding may require platelet transfusion. Agranulocytosis and leucopenia may affect healing adversely.

Drug interactions
Increased sedation occurs with alcohol and sedative drugs such as benzodiazepines. This drug may antagonize the action of anticonvulsants such as carbamazepine and phenytoin. This drug increases the pressor effects of epinephrine. Nevertheless, the use of epinephrine-containing local anaesthetics is not contraindicated; however, epinephrine dose limitation is recommended.

Normal anticoagulant control by warfarin may be upset, both increases and decreases in INR have been noted during combined therapy with tricyclic antidepressants. Combined therapy with other antidepressants should be avoided and if prescribing another class of antidepressant a period of one to two weeks should elapse between changeover. Antimuscarinic effects such as xerostomia are increased when used in combination with other anticholinergic drugs such as antipsychotics.

Doxylamine

Description
An antihistamine.

Indications
Found in compound analgesic, cough and decongestant medications.

Effects on oral and dental structures
Can produce xerostomia.

Effects on patient management
The patient may be drowsy which may interfere with co-operation. Xerostomia may increase caries incidence and thus a preventive regimen is important. If the xerostomia is severe artificial saliva may be indicated. This drug may cause thrombocytopenia, agranulocytosis and anaemia. Thrombocytopenia may cause postoperative bleeding. If the platelet count is low (<100,000) then the socket should be packed and sutured. Persistent bleeding may require platelet transfusion. Agranulocytosis may affect healing adversely. Anaemia may result in poor healing. Any anaemia will need correction prior to elective general anaesthesia and sedation.

Drug interactions
Enhanced sedative effect with anxiolytic and hypnotic drugs. Tricyclic and monoamine oxidase inhibitor antidepressants increase antimuscarinic effects such as xerostomia.

Droperidol (Droleptan)

Description
A butyrophenone antipsychotic drug.

Indications
Used in the treatment of mania, as a major tranquillizer and as an anti-emetic medication during anti-cancer chemotherapy.

Effects on oral and dental structures
Dry and painful mouth, involuntary movements of oro-facial musculature and facial oedema may be produced. Droperidol-induced swelling and cyanosis of the tongue has been reported.

Effects on patient management
Xerostomia may increase caries incidence and thus a preventive regimen is important. If the xerostomia is severe artificial saliva may

be indicated. The underlying psychosis may also cause problems in management. Involuntary muscle movements, e.g. of the tongue, will interfere with operative dentistry. Postural hypotension may occur with this drug, therefore rapid changes in patient position should be avoided.

Drug interactions

Enhanced sedative effects occur with any central nervous system depressant, including opioid analgesics and alcohol. There is a theoretical risk of hypotension with epinephrine in dental local anaesthetics. Combined therapy with tricyclic antidepressants increases the chances of cardiac arrhythmias and exacerbates antimuscarinic effects such as xerostomia. The photosensitive effect of tetracyclines may be increased during combined therapy.

Efavirenz (Sustiva)

Description
A non-nucleoside reverse transcriptase inhibitor antiviral drug.

Indications
Used in the management of HIV infection.

Effects on oral and dental structures
May produce xerostomia, taste disturbance, and Stevens–Johnson syndrome.

Effects on patient management
Sensitive handling of the underlying disease state is essential. Excellent preventive dentistry and regular examinations are important in patients suffering from HIV infection as dental infections are best avoided. HIV will interfere with postoperative healing and antibiotic prophylaxis prior to oral surgery may be advisable.

Drug interactions
Efavirenz prolongs the action of midazolam and concurrent use is best avoided. The action of warfarin may be increased.

Eformoterol fumarate/Formoterol fumarate (Foradil, Oxis)

Description
A beta$_2$-adrenoceptor stimulant.

Indications
Used in the management of asthma and reversible obstructive airway disease.

Effects on oral and dental structures

Xerostomia, taste alteration and mucosal irritation may occur.

Effects on patient management

Patients may not be comfortable in the supine position if they have respiratory problems. Aspirin-like compounds should not be prescribed as many asthmatic patients are allergic to these analgesics. Similarly, sulphite-containing compounds (such as preservatives in epinephrine-containing local anaesthetics) can produce allergy in asthmatic patients. Xerostomia may increase caries incidence and thus a preventive regimen is important. If the xerostomia is severe artificial saliva may be indicated. The use of a rubber dam in patients with obstructive airway disease may further embarrass the airway. If a rubber dam is essential then supplemental oxygen via a nasal cannula may be required.

Drug interactions

The hypokalaemia which may result from large doses of eformoterol may be exacerbated by a reduction in potassium produced by high doses of steroids and by epinephrine in dental local anaesthetics.

Enalapril (Innovace)

Description

Enalapril is an ACE inhibitor, that is it inhibits renal angiotensin converting enzyme which is necessary to convert angiotensin I to the more potent angiotensin II.

Indications

Mild to moderate hypertension, congestive heart failure and post myocardial infarction where there is left ventricular dysfunction.

Effects on oral and dental structures

Enalapril can cause taste disturbances, angioedema, dry mouth, glossitis, and lichenoid drug reactions. Many of these unwanted effects are dose related and compounded if there is an impairment of renal function. Enalapril-induced xerostomia increases the risk of fungal infections (candidiasis) and caries, especially root caries. Antifungal treatment should be used when appropriate and topical fluoride (e.g. Duraphat) will reduce the risk of root surface caries.

Effects on patient management

Enalapril-induced angioedema is perhaps the most significant unwanted effect that impacts upon dental management, because dental procedures can induce the angioedema. Management of enalapril-induced angioedema is problematic because the underlying mechanisms are poorly understood. Standard anti-anaphylactic treatment is of little value (epinephrine and hydrocortisone) because the angioedema is not mediated via mast cells or antibody/antigen interactions. Usually the angioedema subsides and patients on these drugs should be questioned as to whether they have experienced any problems with breathing or swallowing. This will alert the dental practitioner to the possible risk of this unwanted effect arising during dental treatment.

Enalapril is also associated with suppression of bone marrow activity giving rise to possible neutropenia, agranulocytosis, thrombocytopenia, and aplastic anaemia. Patients on enalapril who present with excessive bleeding of their gums, sore throats or oral ulceration should have a full haematological investigation.

Drug interactions
Non-steroidal anti-inflammatory drugs (NSAIDs) such as ibuprofen may reduce the antihypertensive effect of enalapril.

Enoxaparin (Clexane)

Description
A low molecular weight heparin.

Indications
Initial treatment and prevention of deep vein thrombosis and pulmonary embolism. Used to prevent blood coagulation in patients with haemodialysis. Enoxaparin and other low molecular weight heparins have a longer duration of action than heparin.

Effects on oral and dental structures
No direct effect, although patients who are repeatedly heparinized are susceptible to osteoporosis. This latter condition may make such patients susceptible to periodontal breakdown.

Effects on patient management
Enoxaparin can only be given parenterally which reduces the impact of the drug in dental practice. However dentists, especially those working in a hospital environment, will encounter patients who are heparinized on a regular basis (e.g. renal dialysis patients). Bleeding is the main problem with treating such patients. This can arise as a direct effect on the blood coagulation system or from a drug-induced immune–mediated thrombocytopenia. From the coagulation perspective, it is the best to treat heparinized patients between treatments since the half-life of the drug is approximately 4 hours. If urgent treatment is required, then the anticoagulation effect of enoxaparin can be reversed with protamine sulphate 10 mg IV. If bleeding is due to thrombocytopenia then a platelet transfusion may be required.

Drug interactions
Aspirin and parenteral NSAIDs (e.g. diclofenac and ketorolac) should be avoided in patients who are taking enoxaparin or are heparinized on a regular basis. Such analgesics cause impairment of platelet aggregation, which would compound a heparin-induced thrombocytopenia and likewise cause serious problems with obtaining haemostasis.

Entacapone (Comtess)

Description
A selective reversible inhibitor of catechol-O-methyl transferase.

Indications
Used as an adjunctive treatment in Parkinsonism.

Effects on oral and dental structures
Xerostomia may be produced.

Effects on patient management
Xerostomia may increase caries incidence and thus a preventive regimen is important. If the xerostomia is severe artificial saliva may be indicated. Entacapone can produce anaemia. Anaemia may result in poor healing. Any anaemia will need correction prior to elective general anaesthesia and sedation. Parkinsonism can lead to management problems as the patient may have uncontrollable movement. Short appointments are recommended. The effect of epinephrine is enhanced, therefore dose-reduction of epinephrine-containing local anaesthetics is advised.

Drug interactions
See epinephrine above. Concomitant use with tricyclic and monoamine oxidase inhibitors is not advised.

Epinephrine (adrenaline)

Description
A catecholamine sympathomimetic agent.

Indications
Used in dental local anaesthetic solutions to increase their efficacy and duration and to aid in haemostasis.

Presentations
Epinephrine is contained in local anaesthetic solutions in concentrations of 1 : 80,000 (12.5 µg/mL), 1 : 100,000 (10 µg/mL) and 1 : 200,000 (5 µg/mL).

Dose

The maximum recommended dose over one visit in dental local anaesthetic solutions is 200 μg.

Contraindications

Severe cardiac disease such as uncontrolled arrhythmias and unstable angina are contraindications to the use of epinephrine. The unusual catecholamine-secreting tumour of the adrenal gland known as phaeochromocytoma and thyroid storm (an acute hyperthyroid episode) are other contraindications to epinephrine in dental local anaesthesia.

Precautions

Dose reduction is wise when cardiac disease exists (see also drug interactions below).

Unwanted effects

Excessive dosage or inadvertent intravascular injection will produce symptoms of fear and anxiety such as tachycardia and tremors. Systolic blood pressure can rise and diastolic blood pressure may fall. Epinephrine, even at doses used in dentistry, can produce a hypokalaemia (reduction in plasma potassium) and this can lead to cardiac arrhythmias.

Drug interactions

Many drug interactions with epinephrine are theoretical, however some have been shown to produce effects that are clinically important. Tricyclic antidepressant drugs increase the pressor effects of epinephrine twofold; as the pressor effects are negligible at the doses used in dental local anaesthetics then simple dose reduction is all that is required.

Adrenergic beta-blocking drugs such as propranolol can lead to unopposed increases in systolic blood pressure and dose reduction of epinephrine-containing local anaesthetics is advised. Non-potassium sparing diuretics exacerbate the hypokalaemia produced by epinephrine and this is apparent at the doses used in dental local anaesthesia; thus for patients receiving such diuretic therapy epinephrine dose reduction is advised. The volatile anaesthetics such as halothane increase cardiac sensitivity to the effects of epinephrine and a 50% dose reduction in the amount of catecholamine used is advised. Any agent with sympathomimetic properties has the potential to increase the toxicity of epinephrine and among these agents are drugs of abuse such as cocaine, cannabis, and amphetamines.

Ephedrine hydrochloride

Description
An adrenoceptor stimulant.

Indications
Used in the treatment of reversible airway obstruction and the management of nasal congestion.

Effects on oral and dental structures
May produce xerostomia.

Effects on patient management
Patients may not be comfortable in the supine position if they have respiratory problems. If the patient is suffering from asthma then aspirin-like compounds should not be prescribed as many asthmatic patients are allergic to these analgesics. Similarly, sulphite-containing compounds (such as preservatives in epinephrine-containing local anaesthetics) can produce allergy in asthmatic patients. Xerostomia may increase caries incidence and thus a preventive regimen is important. If the xerostomia is severe artificial saliva may be indicated. The use of a rubber dam in patients with obstructive airway disease may further embarrass the airway. If a rubber dam is essential then supplemental oxygen via a nasal cannula may be required.

Drug interactions
The adrenergic effects of epinephrine in dental local anaesthetics will be enhanced by ephedrine, so dose reduction should be considered. A hypertensive crisis can occur with concurrent use of monoamine oxidase inhibitors. Ephedrine increases the metabolism of dexamethasone. There is an increased chance of dysrhythmia with halogenated general anaesthetic agents.

Epirubicin (Pharmorubicin)

Description
A cytotoxic antibiotic.

Indications
Breast and bladder cancer.

Effects on oral and dental structures
Epirubicin causes bone marrow suppression with an accompanying thrombocytopenia and agranulocytosis. Bone marrow suppression can lead to troublesome oral ulceration, exacerbation of an existing periodontal condition and rapid spread of any residual (e.g. periapical) infections.

Effects on patient management

The effect of epirubicin on the bone marrow is transient and routine dental treatment is best avoided until the white blood cells and platelet counts start to recover. If emergency dental treatment such as an extraction is required then antibiotic cover may be necessary depending on the degree of myelosuppression. If the platelet count is low (<100,000) then the socket should be packed and sutured. Persistent bleeding may require a platelet transfusion.

Patients on chemotherapeutic agents such as epirubicin often neglect their oral hygiene and thus there could be an increase in both caries and periodontal disease. If time permits, patients about to go on chemotherapy should have a dental check up and any potential areas of infection should be treated. Similarly, to reduce the mucosal irritation (sensitivity) that often accompanies chemotherapy, it is advisable to remove any ill-fitting dentures and smooth over rough cusps or restorations.

Drug interactions

None of any dental significance.

Eprosartan (Teveten)

Description

An angiotensin II receptor antagonist.

Indications

Used as an alternative to ACE inhibitors where the latter cannot be tolerated.

Effects on oral and dental structures

Angioedema has been reported, but the incidence of this unwanted effect is much less than when compared to ACE inhibitors.

Effect on patient management

None of any significance.

Drug interactions

NSAIDs such as ibuprofen may reduce the antihypertensive action of eprosartan.

Ergotamine tartrate (Cafegot, Lingraine, Migril)

Description

An ergot alkaloid drug.

Indications

Used in the treatment of acute migraine.

Effects on oral and dental structures
Oral ulceration due to local irritation may occur.

Effects on patient management
Any precipitator of migrainous attacks such as the dental light shining in the eyes or sudden noises should be avoided.

Drug interactions
Erythromycin increases the toxicity of ergot alkaloids.

Erythromycin (Erymax, Erythrocin, Erythroped, Ilosone, Tiloryth)

Description
A macrolide antibiotic.

Indications
Used to treat bacterial infections such as acute dental abscesses, especially in those allergic to penicillin.

Presentations
(i) 250 mg and 500 mg tablets.

(ii) 250 mg capsules.

(iii) Oral suspensions of 125 mg/5 mL, 250 mg/5 mL and 500 mg/5 mL.

(iv) 1 g powder for reconstitution for intravenous infusion.

Dose
250–500 mg four times a day.
Child under 8 years 50% adult dose.

Contraindications
Estolate formulations are contra-indicated in liver disease.

Precautions
Liver and renal disease.
Porphyria.
Prolongation of the Q–T interval on ECGs.

Unwanted effects
Hypersensitivity reactions.
Rarely may cause gingival overgrowth.
Gastrointestinal upsets.
Pseudomembranous colitis.
Jaundice.
Cardiac arrhythmias and chest pain.
Hearing loss.
Exacerbation of muscle weakness in myasthenia gravis.

Drug interactions

Erythromycin has a number of important drug interactions. It enhances the anticoagulant effects of warfarin and nicoumalone. Serious arrhythmias can occur if erythromycin is prescribed to patients receiving the anti-histamines terfenadine and astemizole, the anti-abuse drug levacetylmethadol and the gut motility stimulant cisapride. Concurrent therapy with these drugs should be avoided. The serum level of another anti-histamine, loratidine is also raised by erythromycin. The effect of digoxin is enhanced by erythromycin. Erythromycin increases the plasma levels of the anticonvulsant carbamazepine, the analgesic alfentanil, the anti-arrhythmics disopyramide and quinidine, the antipsychotic clozapine, the benzodiazepines midazolam, triazolam and alprazolam, the beta-blocker nadolol, the calcium-channel blocker felodipine, cyclosporin, methylprednisolone, theophylline, the dopaminergics bromocriptine and cabergoline, the immunosuppressant tacrolimus, and the anti-gout medication colchicine. In addition the toxic effects of the cytotoxic medication vinblastine are increased and combined therapy is not recommended. Erythromycin may interact with antidiabetic medications. Combined therapy with chlorpropamide may produce liver damage and concurrent use with glibenclamide may precipitate hypoglycaemia.

Erythromycin has been shown to increase the absorption of the hypnotic zopiclone so that its effect is more rapid. In addition erythromycin may increase the absorption of the monoamine oxidase inhibitor phenelzine which might cause hypotension. Combined therapy with the plasma lipoprotein lowering drug lovastatin has precipitated diffuse muscle weakness.

Acute ergotism can be precipitated by combined use of erythromycin and ergotamine (the most dramatic effect of ergotism is vasospasm which can cause gangrene). Erythromycin may interfere with oral contraceptives and other methods of contraception are advised during therapy. The ulcer-healing drug cimetidine increases the plasma concentration of erythromycin increasing the toxicity of the antibacterial.

Estramustine phosphate (Estracyt)

Description
An alkylating agent.

Indications
Prostate cancer.

Effects on oral and dental structures
Estramustine phosphate causes bone marrow suppression with an accompanying thrombocytopenia and agranulocytosis. Bone marrow

suppression can lead to troublesome oral ulceration, exacerbation of an existing periodontal condition and rapid spread of any residual (e.g. periapical) infections.

Effects on patient management

The effect of estramustine phosphate on the bone marrow is transient and routine dental treatment is best avoided until the white blood cells and platelet counts start to recover. If emergency dental treatment such as an extraction is required then antibiotic cover may be necessary depending on the degree of myelosuppression. If the platelet count is low (<100,000) then the socket should be packed and sutured. Persistent bleeding may require a platelet transfusion.

Patients on chemotherapeutic agents such as estramustine phosphate often neglect their oral hygiene and thus there could be an increase in both caries and periodontal disease. If time permits, patients about to go on chemotherapy should have a dental check up and any potential areas of infection should be treated. Similarly, to reduce the mucosal irritation (sensitivity) that often accompanies chemotherapy, it is advisable to remove any ill-fitting dentures and smooth over rough cusps or restorations.

Drug interactions

None of any dental significance.

Ethambutol hydrochloride

Description

An antituberculous drug.

Indications

Used in the treatment of tuberculosis.

Effects on oral and dental structures

Taste disturbance and Stevens–Johnson syndrome may occur with this drug.

Effects on patient management

Only emergency dental treatment should be performed during active tuberculosis and care must be exercised to eliminate spread of tuberculosis between the patient and dental personnel, e.g. masks and glasses should be worn and where possible treatment should be performed under a rubber dam to reduce aerosol spread. This drug may cause thrombocytopenia which can cause postoperative bleeding. If the platelet count is low (<100,000) then the socket should be packed and sutured. Persistent bleeding may require platelet transfusion.

Drug interactions

None of importance in dentistry.

Ethinylestradiol

Description
An oestrogen.

Indications
Prostate cancer (rarely), breast cancer in postmenopausal women.

Effects on oral and dental structures
Oestrogens may enhance the plaque-induced inflammatory responses in the gingival tissues.

Effects on patient management
Nothing of any significance.

Drug interactions
None of any dental significance.

Ethosuximide (Emeside, Zarontin)

Description
An anticonvulsant drug.

Indications
Used in the management of epilepsy.

Effects on oral and dental structures
Gingival bleeding, rarely gingival overgrowth, Stevens–Johnson syndrome and systemic lupus erythematosus may be produced.

Effects on patient management
Epileptic fits are possible especially if the patient is stressed, therefore sympathetic handling and perhaps sedation should be considered for stressful procedures. Emergency anticonvulsant medication (diazepam or midazolam) must be available. Postoperative haemorrhage is possible due to thrombocytopenia and although not usually severe, local measures such as packing sockets and suturing should be considered.

Drug interactions
The effects and toxicity of ethosuximide are increased by other anticonvulsants and isoniazid. The action of ethosuximide is inhibited by antidepressants and antipsychotic drugs.

Etodolac (Lodine)

Description
A peripherally acting, non-steroidal anti-inflammatory analgesic.

Indications
Pain and inflammation associated with musculoskeletal disorders, e.g. rheumatoid arthritis, osteoarthritis, and ankylosing spondylitis.

Effects on oral and dental structures
Patients on long-term NSAIDs such as etodolac may be afforded some degree of protection against periodontal breakdown. This arises from the drug's inhibitory action on prostaglandin synthesis. The latter is an important inflammatory mediator in the pathogenesis of periodontal breakdown.

Effects on patient management
Rare unwanted effects of etodolac include angioedema and thrombocytopenia. The latter may cause an increased bleeding tendency following any dental surgical procedure. If the platelet count is low (<100,000) then the socket should be packed and sutured. Persistent bleeding may require a platelet transfusion

Drug interactions
Ibuprofen, aspirin and diflunisal should be avoided in patients taking etodolac due to an increase in unwanted effects, especially gastrointestinal ulceration, renal, and liver damage. Systemic corticosteroids increase the risk of peptic ulceration and gastrointestinal bleeding.

Etoposide (Vepesid)

Description
A vinca alkaloid.

Indications
Small cell carcinoma of the bronchus, lymphomas, and testicular cancers.

Effects on oral and dental structures
Etoposide causes bone marrow suppression with an accompanying thrombocytopenia and agranulocytosis. Bone marrow suppression can lead to troublesome oral ulceration, exacerbation of an existing periodontal condition and rapid spread of any residual (e.g. periapical) infections.

Effects on patient management
The effect of etoposide on the bone marrow is transient and routine dental treatment is best avoided until the white blood cells and platelet

counts start to recover. If emergency dental treatment such as an extraction is required then antibiotic cover may be necessary depending on the degree of myelosuppression. If the platelet count is low (<100,000) then the socket should be packed and sutured. Persistent bleeding may require a platelet transfusion.

Patients on chemotherapeutic agents such as etoposide often neglect their oral hygiene and thus there could be an increase in both caries and periodontal disease. If time permits, patients about to go on chemotherapy should have a dental check up and any potential areas of infection should be treated. Similarly, to reduce the mucosal irritation (sensitivity) that often accompanies chemotherapy, it is advisable to remove any ill-fitting dentures and smooth over rough cusps or restorations.

Drug interactions
None of any dental significance.

Exemestan (Arosmasin)

Description
A non-steroidal aromatase inhibitor.

Indications
Advanced postmenopausal breast cancer.

Effects on oral and dental structures
Nothing reported.

Effects on patient management
Nothing of any significance.

Drug interactions
None of any dental significance.

Famciclovir (Famvir)

Description
An antiviral drug.

Indications
Used in the treatment of herpes zoster and genital herpetic infections.

Presentations
125 mg, 250 mg and 500 mg tablets.

Dose
Adults: 750 mg daily either as a single dose or in 3 doses.
Child: not recommended for use in children.

Contraindications
Hypersensitivity, children.

Precautions
Renal and liver disease, pregnancy and breastfeeding. Maintenance of adequate fluid intake is required with high doses.

Unwanted effects
Fever, gastrointestinal upset, dizziness, confusion, and hallucinations, headache and sinusitis, rash.

Drug interactions
Famciclovir may increase the toxicity of pethidine. Probenicid increases the plasma concentration of famciclovir.

Famotidine (Pepcid)

Description
An antihistamine H_2-antagonist.

Indications
Used in the management of gastric and duodenal ulcers.

Effects on oral and dental structures
Xerostomia and taste disturbance may be produced.

Effects on patient management
Patients may be uncomfortable in the fully supine position as a result of their underlying gastrointestinal disorder. Non-steroidal anti-inflammatory drugs should be avoided due to gastrointestinal irritation. Similarly, high dose systemic steroids should not be prescribed in patients with gastrointestinal ulceration. This drug may produce thrombocytopenia which may cause postoperative bleeding. Local measures to reduce haemorrhage (such as suturing and packing extraction sockets) should be considered. Similarly, it can cause a neutropenia which can affect healing adversely. When the neutropenia is marked prophylactic antibiotics should be prescribed to cover surgical procedures.

Drug interactions
Famotidine decreases the effectiveness of the antifungals ketoconazole and itraconazole.

Felodipine (Plendil)

Description
A calcium-channel blocker.

Indications
Hypertension and angina prophylaxis.

Effects on oral and dental structures
Felodipine can cause gingival overgrowth, especially in the anterior part of the mouth. It also causes taste disturbances arising from an inhibition of calcium-channel activity that is necessary for the normal function of taste and smell receptors.

Effects on patient management
Nothing of any significance.

Drug interactions
Erythromycin inhibits the metabolism of felodipine and thus causes an increase in plasma concentration.

Fenbufen (Lederfen)

Description
A peripherally acting, non-steroidal anti-inflammatory analgesic.

Indications
Pain and inflammation associated with musculoskeletal disorders, e.g. rheumatoid arthritis, osteoarthritis, and ankylosing spondylitis.

Effects on oral and dental structures
Patients on long-term NSAIDs such as fenbufen may be afforded some degree of protection against periodontal breakdown. This arises from the drug's inhibitory action on prostaglandin synthesis. The latter is an important inflammatory mediator in the pathogenesis of periodontal breakdown. Fenbufen can cause (albeit rarely) erythema multiforme and Stevens–Johnson syndrome. Both conditions can effect the oral mucosa and lips causing bullous formation and ulceration.

Effects on patient management
Rare unwanted effects of fenbufen include angioedema and thrombocytopenia. The latter may cause an increased bleeding tendency following any dental surgical procedure. If the platelet count is low (<100,000) then the socket should be packed and sutured. Persistent bleeding may require a platelet transfusion.

Drug interactions
Ibuprofen, aspirin and diflunisal should be avoided in patients taking fenbufen due to an increase in unwanted effects, especially gastrointestinal ulceration, renal and liver damage. Systemic corticosteroids increase the risk of peptic ulceration and gastrointestinal bleeding.

Fenoprofen (Fenopron)

Description
A peripherally acting, non-steroidal anti-inflammatory analgesic.

Indications
Pain and inflammation associated with musculoskeletal disorders, e.g. rheumatoid arthritis, osteoarthritis, and ankylosing spondylitis.

Effects on oral and dental structures
Patients on long-term NSAIDs such as fenoprofen may be afforded some degree of protection against periodontal breakdown. This arises from the drug's inhibitory action on prostaglandin synthesis. The latter is an important inflammatory mediator in the pathogenesis of periodontal breakdown.

Effects on patient management
Rare unwanted effects of fenoprofen include angioedema and thrombocytopenia. The latter may cause an increased bleeding tendency following any dental surgical procedure. If the platelet count is low (<100,000) then the socket should be packed and sutured. Persistent bleeding may require a platelet transfusion.

Drug interactions
Ibuprofen, aspirin and diflunisal should be avoided in patients taking fenoprofen due to an increase in unwanted effects, especially gastrointestinal ulceration, renal and liver damage. Systemic corticosteroids increase the risk of peptic ulceration and gastrointestinal bleeding.

Fenoterol hydrobromide (Berotec)

Description
A beta$_2$-adrenoceptor stimulant.

Indications
Used in the management of reversible airway obstruction and asthma.

Effects on oral and dental structures
Xerostomia and taste alteration may occur.

Effects on patient management
Patients may not be comfortable in the supine position if they have respiratory problems. Aspirin-like compounds should not be prescribed as many asthmatic patients are allergic to these analgesics. Similarly, sulphite-containing compounds (such as preservatives in epinephrine-containing local anaesthetics) can produce allergy in

asthmatic patients. Xerostomia may increase caries incidence and thus a preventive regimen is important. If the xerostomia is severe artificial saliva may be indicated. The use of a rubber dam in patients with obstructive airway disease may further embarrass the airway. If a rubber dam is essential then supplemental oxygen via a nasal cannula may be required.

Drug interactions
The hypokalaemia which may result from large doses of salbutamol may be exacerbated by a reduction in potassium produced by high doses of steroids and by epinephrine in dental local anaesthetics.

Fentanyl (Durogesic)

Description
An opioid analgesic that is administered via a self-adhesive patch.

Indications
Chronic intractable pain due to cancer.

Effects on oral and dental structures
Can cause xerostomia leading to an increased risk of root caries, candidal infections and poor denture retention. If the xerostomia is severe, dentate patients should receive topical fluoride and be offered an artificial saliva.

Effects on patient management
Fentanyl is a drug of dependence and can thus case withdrawal symptoms if the medication is stopped abruptly. Such cessation of fentanyl may account for unusual behavioural changes and poor compliance with dental treatment. The drug also depresses respiration and causes postural hypotension.

Drug interactions
Fentanyl will enhance the sedative properties of midazolam and diazepam. Reduce the dose of both sedation agents. Avoid additional use of opioids if patient is on a fentanyl patch.

Ferrous fumarate (Fersaday, Fersamal)

Description
An iron salt.

Indications
Iron deficiency anaemia.

Effects on oral and dental structures
None reported.

Effects on patient management
Nothing of significance.

Drug interactions
Iron salts chelate tetracyclines which in turn prevent their absorption. The two drugs should not be given together.

Ferrous gluconate

Description
An iron salt.

Indications
Iron deficiency anaemia.

Effects on oral and dental structures
None reported.

Effects on patient management
Nothing of significance.

Drug interactions
Iron salts chelate tetracyclines which in turn prevent their absorption. The two drugs should not be given together.

Ferrous glycine sulphate (Plesmet)

Description
An iron salt.

Indications
Iron deficiency anaemia.

Effects on oral and dental structures
None reported.

Effect on patient management
Nothing of significance.

Drug interactions
Iron salts chelate tetracyclines which in turn prevent their absorption. The two drugs should not be given together.

Ferrous sulphate (Feospan, Ferrograd)

Description
An iron salt.

Indications
Iron deficiency anaemia.

Effects on oral and dental structures
None reported.

Effect on patient management
Nothing of significance.

Drug interactions
Iron salts chelate tetracyclines which in turn prevent their absorption. The two drugs should not be given together.

Fexofenadine hydrochloride (Telfast)

Description
An antihistamine.

Indications
Used in the treatment of allergies such as hay fever.

Effects on oral and dental structures
None specific.

Effects on patient management
None specific.

Drug interactions
Plasma levels of fexofenadine increased by erythromycin and ketoconazole.

Finasteride (Proscar)

Description
An anti-androgen.

Indications
Benign prostatic hyperplasia.

Effects on oral and dental structures
Finasteride can cause hypersensitivity reactions that often result in swelling of the lips.

Effects on patient management
Nothing of any significance.

Drug interactions
None of any dental significance.

Flavoxate hydrochloride (Urispass 200)

Description
An antimuscarinic drug.

Indications
Urinary frequency, urgency and incontinence, neurogenic bladder instability, and nocturnal enuresis.

Effects on oral and dental structures
Dry mouth is one of the main unwanted effects of flavoxate hydrochloride. This will increase the risk of dental caries (especially root caries), impede denture retention and the patient will be more prone to candidal infections. If the xerostomia is severe, dentate patients should receive topical fluoride and be offered an artificial saliva. A rare unwanted effect of flavoxate hydrochloride is angioedema which can affect the floor of the mouth, the tongue, and the lips.

Effects on patient management
Patients on flavoxate hydrochloride may become disorientated and suffer from blurred vision.

Drug interactions
None of any dental significance.

Flecainide acetate (Tambocor)

Description
Class Ic antidysrhythmic drug.

Indications
Life-threatening ventricular tachycardia.

Effects on oral and dental structures
None reported.

Effect on patient management
Nothing of any significance.

Drug interactions
None of any dental significance.

Flucloxacillin (Floxapen)

Description
A penicillinase-resistant beta-lactam antibacterial drug.

Indications
Used to treat penicillinase-producing staphylococcal infections such as facial cellulitis.

Presentations
 (i) As 250 mg and 500 mg tablets.
 (ii) As 250 mg and 500 mg capsules.
 (iii) An oral solution (125 mg/5 mL and 250 mg/5 mL) (Penicillin V).
 (iv) As vials containing 250 mg, 500 mg or 1 g of powder for reconstitution for intramuscular or intravenous administration.

Dose
Adult: 250 mg four times a day orally or IM; 250 mg–1 g four times daily by IV infusion.
Child: under 2 years 25% adult dose.
Child: 2–10 years 50% adult dose.

Contraindications
Hypersensitivity.

Precautions
Renal disease.
Porphyria.

Unwanted effects
Hypersensitivity reactions.
Gastrointestinal upset.
Hepatitis and cholestatic jaundice.

Drug interactions

Penicillins reduce the excretion of the cytotoxic drug methotrexate, leading to increased toxicity of the latter drug which may cause death. There may be a reduced efficacy of oral contraceptives and other methods of contraception are advised during antibiotic therapy. Penicillin activity is decreased by tetracyclines.

Fluconazole (Diflucan)

Description
A triazole antifungal agent.

Indications
Used to treat oral fungal infections.

Presentations
(i) An oral suspension for reconstitution with water (50 mg/5 mL).

(ii) A 50 mg capsule.

Dose
In adults 50–100 mg daily for 7–14 days (in children 3 mg/kg daily).

Contraindications
Previous hypersensitivity (plus see important drug interactions below). Best avoided during pregnancy and when breastfeeding.

Precautions
Use with caution in patients with renal and hepatic disease.

Unwanted effects
Hypersensitivity reactions.
Gastrointestinal problems.
Hypokalaemia.

Drug interactions
There are a number of important drug interactions with fluconazole. Unlike the situation with some other antifungals such as miconazole, normal doses of fluconazole do not interfere with the antihistamine terfenadine, however large doses of the antifungal may cause an interaction which could lead to cardiac dysryhthmias. Fluconazole enhances the anticoagulant effect of warfarin even after topical use. Fluconazole increases the anti-epileptic effects of phenytoin and increases the plasma concentrations of the sulphonylurea oral hypoglycaemics. It may also increase the plasma concentration of midazolam. Fluconazole also increases the plasma concentration of ciclosporin by inhibiting the metabolism of this immunosuppressant. Fluconazole also inhibits the metabolism of the anti-spasmodic drug cisapride and this can lead to ventricular arrhythmias. Fluconazole may

reduce the efficacy of oral contraceptives, although the evidence is not conclusive. The plasma concentration of the bronchodilator theophylline is increased by fluconazole. The plasma level of the tricyclic antidepressant drug nortriptyline may be increased by fluconazole although the clinical importance of this is unknown. Fluconazole increases the plasma levels of the antiviral agent zidovudine and this may lead to increased side effects of the latter drug.

Rifampicin increases the elimination of fluconazole and this might lead to a reduction in antifungal action. When fluconazole is used concurrently with amphotericin combined activity is less than when amphotericin is used alone.

Flucytosine (Ancotil)

Description
An antifungal agent.

Indications
Used as an adjunctive treatment in severe candidiasis.

Effects on oral and dental structures
Stomatitis and gingival bleeding can occur.

Effects on patient management
This drug can produce a thrombocytopenia. Thrombocytopenia may cause postoperative bleeding. If the platelet count is low (<100,000) then the socket should be packed and sutured. Persistent bleeding may require platelet transfusion. Leucopenia may also occur leading to impaired healing.

Drug interactions
Increased toxicity occurs with concurrent administration of amphotericin.

Fludarabine phosphate (Fludara)

Description
An antimetabolic drug.

Indications
B-cell lymphocytic leukaemia.

Effects on oral and dental structures
Fludarabine phosphate causes bone marrow suppression with an accompanying thrombocytopenia and agranulocytosis. Bone marrow suppression can lead to troublesome oral ulceration, exacerbation of an existing periodontal condition and rapid spread of any residual (e.g. periapical) infections.

Effects on patient management

The effect of fludarabine phosphate on the bone marrow is transient and routine dental treatment is best avoided until the white blood cells and platelet counts start to recover. If emergency dental treatment such as an extraction is required then antibiotic cover may be necessary depending on the degree of myelosuppression. If the platelet count is low (<100,000) then the socket should be packed and sutured. Persistent bleeding may require a platelet transfusion.

Patients on chemotherapeutic agents such as fludarabine phosphate often neglect their oral hygiene and thus there could be an increase in both caries and periodontal disease. If time permits, patients about to go on chemotherapy should have a dental check up and any potential areas of infection should be treated. Similarly, to reduce the mucosal irritation (sensitivity) that often accompanies chemotherapy, it is advisable to remove any ill-fitting dentures and smooth over rough cusps or restorations.

Drug interactions

None of any dental significance.

Fludrocortisone acetate (Florinef)

Description

A mineralocorticoid.

Indications

Replacement therapy in patients with Addison's disease or who have undergone adrenalectomy.

Effects on oral and dental structures

Although systemic corticosteroids can induce cleft lip and palate formation in mice, there is little evidence that this unwanted effect occurs in humans. The main impact of systemic corticosteroids on the mouth is to cause an increased susceptibility to opportunistic infections. These include candidiasis and those due to herpes viruses. The anti-inflammatory and immunosuppressant properties of corticosteroids may afford the patient some degree of protection against periodontal breakdown.

Effects on patient management

Patients who suffer from Addison's disease or who have undergone adrenalectomy will require supplementary corticosteroids to prevent an adrenal crisis when subjected to a 'stressful episode'. Certain dental procedures, especially those of a surgical nature, may be considered stressful and hence will require supplementary corticosteroid (hydrocortisone 100 mg in 30 minutes before the procedure). If supplementary corticosteroids are given, then it is essential to monitor the patient's blood pressure, before, during and for up to 30 minutes postoperatively. A fall in diastolic pressure of more than 25% will require further corticosteroids.

Patients should be regularly screened for oral infections such as fungal or viral infections. When these occur, they should be treated promptly with the appropriate chemotherapeutic agent. Likewise, any patient on corticosteroids that presents with an acute dental infection should be treated urgently as such infection can readily spread.

Drug interactions
Aspirin and NSAIDs should not be prescribed to patients on long-term corticosteroids. Both drugs are ulcerogenic and hence increase the risk of gastrointestinal bleeding and ulceration. The antifungal agent amphotericin increases the risk of corticosteroid-induced hypokalaemia, whilst ketoconazole inhibits corticosteroid hepatic metabolism.

Flumazenil (Anexate)

Description
A benzodiazepine antagonist.

Indications
Used to reverse benzodiazepine sedation (during an emergency – should not be used routinely).

Presentations
As an intravenous solution; 5 mL containing 100 µg/mL.

Dose
200 µg over 15 seconds then 100 µg at 1 minute intervals. Maximum dose 1 mg.

Contraindications
Epilepsy.

Precautions
When used with a long-acting benzodiazepine re-sedation will occur. Liver disease.

Unwanted effects
Anxiety.
Flushing.
Nausea and vomiting.
Convulsions.

Drug interactions
Flumazenil counteracts the sedative and amnesic effects of benzodiazepines. It also antagonizes the action of the imadazopyridine zolpidem.

Flunitrazepam (Rohypnol)

Description
A benzodiazepine hypnotic.

Indications
Used as a short term treatment of insomnia.

Effects on oral and dental structures
Xerostomia can occur.

Effects on patient management
The main interaction in the management of patients receiving any benzodiazepine therapy is the use of benzodiazepine sedation. During short term use an additive effect will be noted, after long term benzodiazepine therapy tolerance occurs and large doses of benzodiazepines may be needed to achieve sedation. Also the confusion and amnesia that benzodiazepines produce may necessitate the presence of an escort. As this drug is only used for a short time the xerostomia is unlikely to be a major problem, nevertheless a preventive regimen may be required.

Drug interactions
As with all benzodiazepines, enhanced effects occur with combined therapy with other CNS depressants such as alcohol, other hypnotic or sedative agents, and opioid analgesics.

Fluorouracil (Efudix)

Description
An antimetabolic drug.

Indications
Breast cancer, gastrointestinal tract cancers; applied topically for certain pre-malignant skin conditions.

Effects on oral and dental structures
Fluorouracil causes bone marrow suppression with an accompanying thrombocytopenia and agranulocytosis. Bone marrow suppression can lead to troublesome oral ulceration, exacerbation of an existing periodontal condition and rapid spread of any residual (e.g. periapical) infections.

Effects on patient management
The effect of fluorouracil on the bone marrow is transient and routine dental treatment is best avoided until the white blood cells and platelet counts start to recover. If emergency dental treatment such as an extraction is required then antibiotic cover may be necessary

depending on the degree of myelosuppression. If the platelet count is low (<100,000) then the socket should be packed and sutured. Persistent bleeding may require a platelet transfusion.

Patients on chemotherapeutic agents such as fluorouracil often neglect their oral hygiene and thus there could be an increase in both caries and periodontal disease. If time permits, patients about to go on chemotherapy should have a dental check up and any potential areas of infection should be treated. Similarly, to reduce the mucosal irritation (sensitivity) that often accompanies chemotherapy, it is advisable to remove any ill-fitting dentures and smooth over rough cusps or restorations.

Drug interactions
Metronidazole inhibits the hepatic metabolism of fluorouracil, which increases the drug's toxicity.

Fluoxetine (Prozac)

Description
A selective serotonin reuptake inhibitor.

Indications
Used in the management of depression, bulimia, and obsessive compulsive disorder.

Effects on oral and dental structures
Xerostomia and taste alteration may occur.

Effects on patient management
Xerostomia may increase caries incidence and thus a preventive regimen is important. If the xerostomia is severe artificial saliva may be indicated. Fluoxetine can produce anaemia and thrombocytopenia. Anaemia may result in poor healing. Any anaemia will need correction prior to elective general anaesthesia and sedation. Thrombocytopenia may cause postoperative bleeding. If the platelet count is low (<100,000) then the socket should be packed and sutured. Persistent bleeding may require platelet transfusion. Gingival bleeding may also occur as a result of thrombocytopenia.

Drug interactions
Combined therapy with other antidepressants should be avoided. Treatment with selective serotonin reuptake inhibitors should not begin until two weeks following cessation of monoamine oxidase inhibitor therapy. Fluoxetine increases the plasma concentration of diazepam. Selective serotonin reuptake inhibitors increase the anticoagulant effect of warfarin. Selective serotonin reuptake inhibitors antagonize the anticonvulsant effects of anti-epileptic medication.

Fluoxetine increases the plasma concentration of carbamazepine and phenytoin.

Flupentixol (Depixol, Fluanxol)

Description
A thioxanthene antipsychotic medication.

Indications
Used in the treatment of psychoses such as schizophrenia, as an antidepressant and as an anxiolytic.

Effects on oral and dental structures
Xerostomia and uncontrollable oro-facial muscle activity (tardive dyskenesia) may be produced.

Effects on patient management
Xerostomia may increase caries incidence and thus a preventive regimen is important. If the xerostomia is severe artificial saliva may be indicated. Uncontrollable muscle movement of jaws and tongue as well as the underlying psychotic condition may interfere with management as satisfactory co-operation may not be achieved readily. There may be problems with denture retention and certain stages of denture construction (e.g. jaw registration) can be difficult. Postural hypotension often occurs with this drug, therefore rapid changes in patient position should be avoided.

Drug interactions
There is increased sedation when used in combination with CNS depressant drugs such as alcohol, opioid analgesics, and sedatives. Combined therapy with tricyclic antidepressants increases the chances of cardiac arrhythmias and exacerbates antimuscarinic effects such as xerostomia. There is a theoretical risk of hypotension being exacerbated by the epinephrine in dental local anaesthetics.

Flupentixol decanoate (Depixol, Depixol Conc, Depixol Low Volume)

Description
A thioxanthene antipsychotic medication.

Indications
Used as a depot injection in the treatment of psychoses such as schizophrenia.

Effects on oral and dental structures
Xerostomia and uncontrollable oro-facial muscle activity (tardive dyskenesia) may be produced.

Effects on patient management
Xerostomia may increase caries incidence and thus a preventive regimen is important. If the xerostomia is severe artificial saliva may be indicated. Uncontrollable muscle movement of jaws and tongue as well as the underlying psychotic condition may interfere with management as satisfactory co-operation may not be achieved readily. There may be problems with denture retention and certain stages of denture construction (e.g. jaw registration) can be difficult. Postural hypotension often occurs with this drug, therefore rapid changes in patient position should be avoided.

Drug interactions
There is increased sedation when used in combination with CNS depressant drugs such as alcohol, opioid analgesics, and sedatives. Combined therapy with tricyclic antidepressants increases the chances of cardiac arrhythmias and exacerbates antimuscarinic effects such as xerostomia. There is a theoretical risk of hypotension being exacerbated by the epinephrine in dental local anaesthetics.

Fluphenazine hydrochloride (Moditen, Modecate)

Description
A phenothiazine antipsychotic medication.

Indications
Used in the treatment of psychoses such as schizophrenia and mania.

Effects on oral and dental structures
Xerostomia and uncontrollable oro-facial muscle activity (tardive dyskenesia) may be produced. The oral mucosa may be discoloured and have a bluish-grey appearance. Stevens–Johnson syndrome and lichenoid reactions may occur with this drug.

Effects on patient management
Xerostomia may increase caries incidence and thus a preventive regimen is important. If the xerostomia is severe artificial saliva may be indicated. Uncontrollable muscle movement of jaws and tongue as well as the underlying psychotic condition may interfere with management as satisfactory co-operation may not be achieved readily. There may be problems with denture retention and certain stages of denture construction (e.g. jaw registration) can be difficult. Postural hypotension may occur with this drug, therefore rapid changes in patient position should be avoided.

Drug interactions
There is increased sedation when used in combination with CNS depressant drugs such as alcohol, opioid analgesics, and sedatives.

Combined therapy with tricyclic antidepressants increases the chances of cardiac arrhythmias and exacerbates antimuscarinic effects such as xerostomia. When combined with carbamazepine there is an increased chance of Stevens–Johnson syndrome. There is a theoretical risk of hypotension being exacerbated by the epinephrine in dental local anaesthetics.

Flurazepam (Dalmane)

Description
A benzodiazepine hypnotic.

Indications
Used as a short term treatment of insomnia.

Effects on oral and dental structures
Xerostomia may occur.

Effects on patient management
The main interaction in the management of patients receiving any benzodiazepine therapy is the use of benzodiazepine sedation. During short term use an additive effect will be noted, after long term benzodiazepine therapy tolerance occurs and large doses of benzodiazepines may be needed to achieve sedation. Also the confusion and amnesia that benzodiazepines produce may necessitate the presence of an escort. As this drug is only used for a short time the xerostomia is unlikely to be a major problem, nevertheless a preventive regimen may be required.

Drug interactions
As with all benzodiazepines, enhanced effects occur with combined therapy with other CNS depressants such as alcohol, other hypnotic or sedative agents, and opioid analgesics.

Flurbiprofen (Froben)

Description
A peripherally acting, non-steroidal anti-inflammatory analgesic.

Indications
Pain and inflammation associated with musculoskeletal disorders, e.g. rheumatoid arthritis, osteoarthritis, and ankylosing spondylitis. Dysmenorrhoea and postoperative analgesia.

Effects on oral and dental structures
Patients on long-term NSAIDs such as flurbiprofen may be afforded some degree of protection against periodontal breakdown. This arises from the drug's inhibitory action on prostaglandin synthesis. The latter is an important inflammatory mediator in the pathogenesis

of periodontal breakdown. The drug has also been implicated for inducing oral lichenoid eruptions and oral ulceration.

Effects on patient management
Rare unwanted effects of flurbiprofen include angioedema and thrombocytopenia. The latter may cause an increased bleeding tendency following any dental surgical procedure. If the platelet count is low (<100,000) then the socket should be packed and sutured. Persistent bleeding may require a platelet transfusion.

Drug interactions
Ibuprofen, aspirin, and diflunisal should be avoided in patients taking flurbiprofen due to an increase in unwanted effects, especially gastrointestinal ulceration, renal, and liver damage. Systemic corticosteroids increase the risk of peptic ulceration and gastrointestinal bleeding.

Fluticasone propionate (Accuhaler, Diskhaler, Evohaler, Nebules, Flixonase, Flixotide, Seretide, Ultralanum)

Description
A corticosteroid.

Indications
Used in the prophylaxis of asthma, in allergic rhinitis and inflammatory skin disorders such as eczema.

Effects on oral and dental structures
The inhalational forms may produce xerostomia and candidiasis.

Effects on patient management
The patient may be at risk of adrenal crisis under stress. This is due to adrenal suppression. Whilst such suppression does occur physiologically, its clinical significance does appear to be overstated. As far as dentistry is concerned, there is increasing evidence that supplementary corticosteroids are not required. This would apply to all restorative procedures, periodontal surgery, and the uncomplicated dental extraction. For more complicated dento-alveolar surgery, each case must be judged on its merits. An apprehensive patient may well require cover. It is important to monitor the patient's blood pressure before, during and for 30 minutes after the procedure. If diastolic pressure drops by more than 25%, then hydrocortisone 100 mg IV should be administered and the patient's blood pressure should continue to be monitored.

Patients may not be comfortable in the supine position if they have respiratory problems. If the patient suffers from asthma then aspirin-like compounds should not be prescribed as many asthmatic patients are allergic to these analgesics. Similarly, sulphite-containing compounds (such as preservatives in epinephrine-containing local anaesthetics) can produce allergy in asthmatic patients. Xerostomia may increase caries incidence and thus a preventive regimen is important. If the xerostomia is severe artificial saliva may be indicated.

Drug interactions
When used topically, including by inhalation, drug interactions of relevance to dentistry are not a concern.

Fluvastatin (Lescol)

Description
A cholesterol lowering drug.

Indications
To reduce coronary events by lowering LDL cholesterol.

Effects on oral and dental structures
None reported.

Effects on patient management
Nothing of any significance.

Drug interactions
None of any dental significance.

Fluvoxamine maleate (Faverin)

Description
A selective serotonin reuptake inhibitor.

Indications
Used in the management of depression and obsessive compulsive disorder.

Effects on oral and dental structures
Both xerostomia and hypersalivation can be produced. Taste alteration and dysphagia may occur.

Effects on patient management
Xerostomia may increase caries incidence and thus a preventive regimen is important. If the xerostomia is severe artificial saliva may be indicated. Fluvoxamine may cause postural hypotension, thus rapid changes in patient position should be avoided. Dose reduction during benzodiazepine sedation may be needed (see drug interactions below).

Drug interactions
Combined therapy with other antidepressants should be avoided. Treatment with selective serotonin reuptake inhibitors should not begin until two weeks following cessation of monoamine oxidase inhibitor therapy. Fluvoxamine increases the plasma concentration of benzodiazepines. Selective serotonin reuptake inhibitors increase the anticoagulant effect of warfarin. Selective serotonin reuptake inhibitors antagonize the anticonvulsant effects of anti-epileptic medication. Fluvoxamine increases the plasma concentration of carbamazepine and phenytoin.

Folic acid

Indications
Folate deficiency, megaloblastic anaemia, taken during pregnancy to prevent neural tube defects.

Effects on oral and dental structures
None reported.

Effects on patient management
Nothing of significance.

Drug interactions
None of any dental significance.

Formestane (Lentaron)

Description
A non-steroidal aromatase inhibitor.

Indications
Advanced postmenopausal breast cancer.

Effects on oral and dental structures
Nothing reported.

Effects on patient management
Nothing of any significance.

Drug interactions
None of any dental significance.

Formoterol fumarate/Eformoterol fumarate (Foradil, Oxis)

Description
A beta$_2$-adrenoceptor stimulant.

Indications
Used in the management of asthma and reversible obstructive airway disease.

Effects on oral and dental structures
Xerostomia, taste alteration, and mucosal irritation may occur.

Effects on patient management
Patients may not be comfortable in the supine position if they have respiratory problems. Aspirin-like compounds should not be prescribed as many asthmatic patients are allergic to these analgesics. Similarly, sulphite-containing compounds (such as preservatives in epinephrine-containing local anaesthetics) can produce allergy in asthmatic patients. Xerostomia may increase caries incidence and thus a preventive regimen is important. If the xerostomia is severe artificial saliva may be indicated. The use of a rubber dam in patients with obstructive airway disease may further embarrass the airway. If a rubber dam is essential then supplemental oxygen via a nasal cannula may be required.

Drug interactions
The hypokalaemia which may result from large doses of salbutamol may be exacerbated by a reduction in potassium produced by high doses of steroids and by epinephrine in dental local anaesthetics.

Foscarnet sodium (Foscavir)

Description
A DNA polymerase and reverse transcriptase antiviral drug.

Indications
Used in the management of retinitis caused by cytomegalovirus in AIDS and in the management of herpetic infections in the immuno-compromised.

Effects on oral and dental structures
Xerostomia, taste disturbance, oral ulceration, glossitis, stomatitis, and facial swelling may be produced.

Effects on patient management
Xerostomia may increase caries incidence, and as patients receiving this drug will probably be severely immunocompromised excellent

preventive dentistry is essential to thwart dental infection. If the xerostomia is severe artificial saliva may be indicated. This drug produces anaemia, leucopenia, and thrombocytopenia. Anaemia may result in poor healing. Any anaemia will need correction prior to elective general anaesthesia and sedation. Leucopenia will affect healing adversely and if severe prophylactic antibiotics should be prescribed to cover surgical procedures. Thrombocytopenia may cause postoperative bleeding. If the platelet count is low (<100,000) then the socket should be packed and sutured. Persistent bleeding may require platelet transfusion.

Drug interactions
None of importance in dentistry.

Fosfestrol tetrasodium (Honvan)

Description
An oestrogen.

Indications
Prostate cancer (rarely), breast cancer in postmenopausal women.

Effects on oral and dental structures
Oestrogens may enhance the plaque-induced inflammatory responses in the gingival tissues.

Effects on patient management
Nothing of any significance.

Drug interactions
None of any dental significance.

Fosinopril (Staril)

Description
Fosinopril is an ACE inhibitor, that is it inhibits the renal angiotensin converting enzyme which is necessary to convert angiotensin I to the more potent angiotensin II.

Indications
Mild to moderate hypertension, congestive heart failure and post myocardial infarction where there is left ventricular dysfunction.

Effects on oral and dental structures
Fosinopril can cause taste disturbances, angioedema, dry mouth, glossitis, and lichenoid drug reactions. Many of these unwanted effects are dose related and compounded if there is an impairment of renal function. Fosinopril-induced xerostomia increases the risk of

fungal infections (candidiasis) and caries, especially root caries. Antifungal treatment should be used when appropriate and topical fluoride (e.g. Duraphat) will reduce the risk of root surface caries.

Effects on patient management
Fosinopril-induced angioedema is perhaps the most significant unwanted effect that impacts upon dental management, since dental procedures can induce the angioedema. Management of fosinopril-induced angioedema is problematic since the underlying mechanisms are poorly understood. Standard anti-anaphylactic treatment is of little value (epinephrine and hydrocortisone) since the angioedema is not mediated via mast cells or antibody/antigen interactions. Usually the angioedema subsides and patients on these drugs should be questioned as to whether they have experienced any problems with breathing or swallowing. This will alert the dental practitioner to the possible risk of this unwanted effect arising during dental treatment.

Fosinopril is also associated with suppression of bone marrow activity giving rise to possible neutropenia, agranulocytosis, thrombocytopenia and aplastic anaemia. Patients on fosinopril who present with excessive bleeding of their gums, sore throats or oral ulceration should have a full haematological investigation.

Drug interactions
Non-steroidal anti-inflammatory drugs (NSAIDs) such as ibuprofen may reduce the antihypertensive effect of fosinopril.

Fosphenytoin sodium (Pro Epanutin)

Description
This is a pro-drug for phenytoin.

Indications
Only used when oral administration of phenytoin is not possible.

Effects on oral and dental structures
Used only as a temporary substitute for phenytoin. Most of the side effects of chronic phenytoin use, such as developmental dental defects, gingival overgrowth, and taste disturbance may be seen. Stevens–Johnson syndrome may be produced by fosphenytoin.

Effects on patient management
It is unlikely that a patient receiving this drug will be receiving dental treatment. However, the side effects of phenytoin would be expected. Epileptic fits are possible especially if the patient is stressed, therefore sympathetic handling and perhaps sedation should be considered for stressful procedures. Emergency anticonvulsant medication (diazepam or midazolam) must be available. Phenytoin can produce agranulocytosis, anaemia, and thrombocytopenia. Agranulocytosis and anaemia

may result in poor healing. Any anaemia will need correction prior to elective general anaesthesia and sedation. Thrombocytopenia may cause postoperative bleeding. If the platelet count is low (<100,000) then the socket should be packed and sutured. Persistent bleeding may require platelet transfusion.

Both lidocaine and phenytoin have a depressant effect on the heart and intravenous lidocaine and phenytoin have been known to cause heart block. The use of high doses of lidocaine should thus be avoided in dental practice in patients taking this anticonvulsant.

Drug interactions

Effects of phenytoin are increased by aspirin (and possibly other non-steroidals including ibuprofen), chloramphenicol, dextropropoxyphene, fluconazole, isoniazid, metronidazole, miconazole, and sulphonamide antimicrobials. Effects of phenytoin are reduced by chronic heavy alcohol consumption, aciclovir, and folic acid. Phenytoin has a mixed interaction with benzodiazepines. The effect of the anticonvulsant is increased by chlordiazepoxide, clonazepam, and diazepam. Conversely clonazepam and diazepam can also decrease the plasma concentration of phenytoin. Phenytoin reduces the effects of anticoagulants including warfarin, corticosteroids, doxycycline, fentanyl, itraconazole, ketoconazole, oral contraceptives, and possibly paracetamol. Phenytoin possibly increases the toxic effects of pethidine. See the effect of lidocaine mentioned above.

Frusemide (Lasix)

Description
A loop diuretic.

Indications
Pulmonary oedema, oliguria due to renal failure.

Effects on oral and dental structures
Loop diuretics can cause taste disturbances due to zinc chelation, and have also been implicated in causing oral lichenoid eruptions.

Effects on patient management
Rarely cause bone marrow depression resulting in agranulocystosis (high risk of oral ulceration and periodontal breakdown) and thrombocytopenia (impaired haemostasis). If the platelet count is low (<100,000) then the socket should be packed and sutured. Persistent bleeding may require a platelet transfusion.

Drug interactions
Frusemide, like many diuretics, causes hypokalaemia which can be exacerbated by amphotericin and epinephrine containing local anaesthetic agents. No more than 3 cartridges per adult patient.

Gabapentin (Neurontin)

Description
A GABA analogue anticonvulsant drug.

Indications
Used as an add-on drug in epilepsy.

Effects on oral and dental structures
Xerostomia, gingivitis, stomatitis, and Stevens–Johnson syndrome may be produced.

Effects on patient management
Xerostomia may increase caries incidence and thus a preventive regimen is important. If the xerostomia is severe artificial saliva may be indicated. Epileptic fits are possible, especially if the paitent is stressed, therefore sympathetic handling and perhaps sedation should be considered for stressful procedures. Emergency anticonvulsant medication (diazepam or midazolam) must be available.

Drug interactions
None of importance in dentistry.

Ganciclovir (Cymevene)

Description
A DNA polymerase inhibitor antiviral drug.

Indications
Used to treat life-threatening cytomegalovirus infections or as a prophylaxis during immunosuppressive therapy.

Effects on oral and dental structures
Oral ulceration, taste disturbance, and xerostomia can occur.

Effects on patient management
Xerostomia may increase caries incidence and patients taking this medication are severely immunocompromised, therefore effective preventive dentistry is important to avoid dental infections. If the xerostomia is severe artificial saliva may be indicated. This drug produces anaemia, leucopenia, and thrombocytopenia. Anaemia may result in poor healing. Any anaemia will need correction prior to elective general anaesthesia and sedation. Leucopenia will affect healing adversely and if severe, prophylactic antibiotics should be prescribed to cover surgical procedures. Thrombocytopenia may cause postoperative bleeding. If the platelet count is low (<100,000) then the socket should be packed and sutured. Persistent bleeding may require platelet transfusion.

Drug interactions

Combined therapy with carbamazepine will increase the risk of haematological problems.

Gemcitabine (Gemzar)

Description

An antimetabolic drug.

Indications

For palliative treatment in patients with locally advanced or metastatic non-small cell lung and pancreatic cancer.

Effects on oral and dental structures

Gemcitabine causes bone marrow suppression with an accompanying thrombocytopenia and agranulocytosis. Bone marrow suppression can lead to troublesome oral ulceration, exacerbation of an existing periodontal condition and rapid spread of any residual (e.g. periapical) infections.

Effect on patient management

The effect of gemcitabine on the bone marrow is transient and routine dental treatment is best avoided until the white blood cells and platelet counts start to recover. If emergency dental treatment such as an extraction is required then antibiotic cover may be necessary depending on the degree of myelosuppression. If the platelet count is low (<100,000) then the socket should be packed and sutured. Persistent bleeding may require a platelet transfusion.

Patients on chemotherapeutic agents such as gemcitabine often neglect their oral hygiene and thus there could be an increase in both caries and periodontal disease. If time permits, patients about to go on chemotherapy should have a dental check up and any potential areas of infection should be treated. Similarly, to reduce the mucosal irritation (sensitivity) that often accompanies chemotherapy, it is advisable to remove any ill-fitting dentures and smooth over rough cusps or restorations.

Drug interactions

None of any dental significance.

Gentamicin (Cidomycin, Genticin)

Description

An aminoglycoside antibiotic.

Indications

The only use in dentistry is in endocarditis prophylaxis.

Presentations

(i) Vials containing the drug at doses of 5 mg/mL, 10 mg/mL, and 40 mg/mL.

(ii) A 100 mL infusion at a dose of 800 mg/mL.

Dose

In the prophylaxis of endocarditis 120 mg is administered intravenously at the induction of general anaesthesia in combined therapy with amoxicillin, vancomycin or teicoplanin. In children under ten years the dose of gentamicin is 2 mg/kg.

Contraindications

Hypersensitivity.
Pregnancy.
Myasthenia gravis.
Hypermagnesia in infants.

Precautions

Renal disease.
History of deafness.

Unwanted effects

Disturbances of hearing and balance.
Nephrotoxicity.
Pseudomembranous colitis during prolonged use.
Inhibition of neuromuscular transmission.
Thrombocytopenia.

Drug interactions

The ototoxic effect of gentamicin is exacerbated by vancomycin, loop diuretics, and the cytotoxic drug cisplatin. Nephrotoxicity is increased when gentamicin is used in combination with amphotericin B, clindamycin, cefalothins, and ciclosporins. The risk of hypocalcaemia produced by bisphophonates, which are used in the management of Paget's disease of bone, is increased by gentamicin.

The neuromuscular blockade produced by non-depolarizing muscle relaxants and by botulinum toxin is enhanced by gentamicin. The effects of neostigmine and pyridostigmine are antagonized by gentamicin. Gentamicin interacts with extended spectrum penicillins such as carbenicillin and piperacillin in such a way that it is chemically inactivated. This is only a problem if the drugs are mixed together in an infusion or are administered to patients with impaired renal function. Hypomagnesia may occur during combined therapy with cytotoxic agents such as thioguanine, daunorubicin, and cytarabine. Gentamicin reduces the response to Vitamin K therapy and in patients receiving Vitamin K administration another antibiotic should be used.

Gestrinone (Dimetriose)

Description
An inhibitor of pituitary gonadotrophin.

Indications
Endometriosis.

Effects on oral and dental structure
None reported.

Effects on patient management
Nothing of any significance.

Drug interactions
None of any dental significance.

Glibenclamide (Daonil, Euglucon)

Description
A sulphonylurea oral anti-diabetic.

Indications
Diabetes mellitus.

Effects on oral and dental structures
Glibenclamide has been cited as causing oral lichenoid eruptions, erythema multiforme, and oro-facial neuropathy. The latter can manifest as tingling or burning in the lips and tongue. The drug is a rare cause of blood disorders including thrombocytopenia, agranulocytosis and aplastic anaemia. The blood disorders could cause oral ulceration, an exacerbation of periodontal disease and spontaneous bleeding from the gingival tissues. If the platelet count is low (<100,000) then the socket should be packed and sutured. Persistent bleeding may require a platelet transfusion.

Effects on patient management
The development of hypoglycaemia is the main problem associated with glibenclamide. This problem is more common in the elderly. Before commencing dental treatment, it is important to check that the patients have had their normal food intake. If there is any doubt, give the patient a glucose drink. As with any diabetic patient try and treat in the first half of the morning and ensure the patient can eat after dental treatment. If a patient on glibenclamide requires a general anaesthetic then refer to hospital.

Drug interactions
Aspirin and other NSAIDs enhance the hypoglycaemic actions of glibenclamide. Antifungal agents such as fluconazole and miconazole

increase plasma concentrations of glibenclamide. Systemic corticosteroids will antagonize the hypoglycaemic properties of glibenclamide. If these drugs are required, then consult the patient's physician before prescribing.

Gliclazide (Diamicron)

Description
A sulphonylurea oral anti-diabetic.

Indications
Diabetes mellitus.

Effects on oral and dental structures
Gliclazide has been cited as causing oral lichenoid eruptions, erythema multiforme, and orofacial neuropathy. The latter can manifest as tingling or burning in the lips and tongue. The drug is a rare cause of blood disorders including thrombocytopenia, agranulocytosis, and aplastic anaemia. The blood disorders could cause oral ulceration, an exacerbation of periodontal disease and spontaneous bleeding from the gingival tissues. If the platelet count is low (<100,000) then the socket should be packed and sutured. Persistent bleeding may require a platelet transfusion.

Effects on patient management
The development of hypoglycaemia is the main problem associated with gliclazide. This problem is more common in the elderly. Before commencing dental treatment, it is important to check that the patients have had their normal food intake. If there is any doubt, give the patient a glucose drink. As with any diabetic patient try and treat in the first half of the morning and ensure the patient can eat after dental treatment. If a patient on gliclazide requires a general anaesthetic then refer to hospital.

Drug interactions
Aspirin and other NSAIDs enhance the hypoglycaemic actions of gliclazide. Antifungal agents such as fluconazole and miconazole increase plasma concentrations of gliclazide. Systemic corticosteroids will antagonize the hypoglycaemic properties of gliclazide. If these drugs are required, then consult the patient's physician before prescribing.

Glimepiride (Amaryl)

Description
A sulphonylurea oral anti-diabetic.

Indications
Diabetes mellitus.

Effects on oral and dental structures

Glimepiride has been cited as causing oral lichenoid eruptions, erythema multiforme and orofacial neuropathy. The latter can manifest as tingling or burning in the lips and tongue. The drug is a rare cause of blood disorders including thrombocytopenia, agranulocytosis, and aplastic anaemia. The blood disorders could cause oral ulceration, an exacerbation of periodontal disease and spontaneous bleeding from the gingival tissues. If the platelet count is low (<100,000) then the socket should be packed and sutured. Persistent bleeding may require a platelet transfusion.

Effects on patient management

The development of hypoglycaemia is the main problem associated with glimepiride. This problem is more common in the elderly. Before commencing dental treatment, it is important to check that the patients have had their normal food intake. If there is any doubt, give the patient a glucose drink. As with any diabetic patient try and treat in the first half of the morning and ensure the patient can eat after dental treatment. If a patient on glimepiride requires a general anaesthetic then refer to hospital.

Drug interactions

Aspirin and other NSAIDs enhance the hypoglycaemic actions of glimepiride. Antifungal agents such as fluconazole and miconazole increase plasma concentrations of glimepiride. Systemic corticosteroids will antagonize the hypoglycaemic properties of glimepiride. If these drugs are required, then consult the patient's physician before prescribing.

Glipizide (Glibenese)

Description

A sulphonylurea oral anti-diabetic.

Indications

Diabetes mellitus.

Effects on oral and dental structures

Glipizide has been cited as causing oral lichenoid eruptions, erythema multiforme and orofacial neuropathy. The latter can manifest as tingling or burning in the lips and tongue. The drug is a rare cause of blood disorders including thrombocytopenia, agranulocytosis, and aplastic anaemia. The blood disorders could cause oral ulceration, an exacerbation of periodontal disease and spontaneous bleeding from the gingival tissues. If the platelet count is low (<100,000) then the socket should be packed and sutured. Persistent bleeding may require a platelet transfusion.

Effects on patient management

The development of hypoglycaemia is the main problem associated with glipizide. This problem is more common in the elderly. Before commencing dental treatment, it is important to check that the patients have had their normal food intake. If there is any doubt, give the patient a glucose drink. As with any diabetic patient try and treat in the first half of the morning and ensure the patient can eat after dental treatment. If a patient on glipizide requires a general anaesthetic then refer to hospital.

Drug interactions

Aspirin and other NSAIDs enhance the hypoglycaemic actions of glipizide. Antifungal agents such as fluconazole and miconazole increase plasma concentrations of glipizide. Systemic corticosteroids will antagonize the hypoglycaemic properties of glipizide. If these drugs are required, then consult the patient's physician before prescribing.

Gliquidone (Glurenorm)

Description

A sulphonylurea oral anti-diabetic.

Indications

Diabetes mellitus.

Effects on oral and dental structures

Gliquidone has been cited as causing oral lichenoid eruptions, erythema multiforme and orofacial neuropathy. The latter can manifest as tingling or burning in the lips and tongue. The drug is a rare cause of blood disorders including thrombocytopenia, agranulocytosis, and aplastic anaemia. The blood disorders could cause oral ulceration, an exacerbation of periodontal disease and spontaneous bleeding from the gingival tissues. If the platelet count is low (<100,000) then the socket should be packed and sutured. Persistent bleeding may require a platelet transfusion.

Effects on patient management

The development of hypoglycaemia is the main problem associated with gliquidone. This problem is more common in the elderly. Before commencing dental treatment, it is important to check that the patients have had their normal food intake. If there is any doubt, give the patient a glucose drink. As with any diabetic patient try and treat in the first half of the morning and ensure the patient can eat after dental treatment. If a patient on gliquidone requires a general anaesthetic then refer to hospital.

Drug interactions
Aspirin and other NSAIDs enhance the hypoglycaemic actions of gliquidone. Antifungal agents such as fluconazole and miconazole increase plasma concentrations of gliquidone. Systemic corticosteroids will antagonize the hypoglycaemic properties of gliquidone. If these drugs are required, then consult the patient's physician before prescribing.

Glyceril trinitrate

Description
A vasodilator that is available as a sublingual spray, tablets, or transdermal patch.

Indications
Prophylaxis and treatment of angina: left ventricular failure.

Effects on oral and dental structures
None reported.

Effects on patient management
Postural hypotension may occur: dry mouth may reduce the sublingual absorption of glyceryl trinitrate.

Drug interactions
None of any dental significance.

Goserelin

Description
A gonadorelin analogue.

Indications
Endometriosis, prostate cancer.

Effects on oral and dental structures
Rare unwanted effects of goserelin include paraesthesia of the lips and oedema of the lips and tongue. The drug is also associated with dry mouth which increases the risk of dental caries, especially root caries, poor denture retention and an increased susceptibility to candidal infection. If the xerostomia is severe, dentate patients should receive topical fluoride and be offered an artificial saliva.

Effects on patient management
Use of goserelin is associated with an increased risk of osteoporosis. The latter is now regarded as a significant risk factor for periodontal disease.

Drug interactions
None of any dental significance.

Granisetron (Kytril)

Description
A serotonin antagonist.

Indications
Used in the treatment of nausea, especially that caused by cytotoxic chemotherapy and radiotherapy.

Effects on oral and dental structures
None specific to this drug.

Effects on patient management
The patient is probably undergoing chemotherapy or radiotherapy; this will affect the timing of treatments and can interfere with surgical healing. Ideally a preventive regimen should be in place.

Drug interactions
None of importance in dentistry.

Grepafloxacin (Raxar)

Description
A quinolone antibiotic.

Indications
Used to treat urinary tract infections.

Effects on oral and dental structures
This drug can cause xerostomia, taste disturbance, and Stevens–Johnson syndrome.

Effects on patient management
As the drug is only used short term xerostomia should not produce significant problems, however a preventive regimen may be considered. This drug may cause thrombocytopenia, leucopenia and anaemia. Thrombocytopenia may cause postoperative bleeding. If the platelet count is low (<100,000) then the socket should be packed and sutured. Persistent bleeding may require platelet transfusion. Leucopenia and anaemia may result in poor healing. Any anaemia will need correction prior to elective general anaesthesia and sedation.

Drug interactions
Combined therapy with non-steroidal anti-inflammatory drugs increases the risk of convulsions.

Griseofulvin (Fulcin, Grisovin)

Description
An antifungal drug.

Indications
Used in the treatment of intractable dermatophyte infections.

Effects on oral and dental structures
Erythema multiforme, lupus erythematosus, stomatitis, xerostomia, taste disturbance, and lichenoid reactions may be produced.

Effects on patient management
This drug can interfere with co-ordination and cause confusion which may interfere with dental treatment. Impaired healing may occur due to leucopenia and agranulocytosis. Griseofulvin may reduce the efficacy of aspirin. Xerostomia may increase caries incidence and thus a preventive regimen is important. If the xerostomia is severe artificial saliva may be indicated.

Drug interactions
The effect of warfarin is reduced during combined therapy, oral contraceptive efficacy is also reduced.

Haloperidol (Dozic, Haldol, Serenace)

Description
A butyrophenone antipsychotic drug.

Indications
Used in the treatment of hyperactive psychoses, motor tics and Gilles de la Tourette syndrome and as an anti-emetic in chemotherapy-induced nausea.

Effects on oral and dental structures
Dry and painful mouth and involuntary movements of oro-facial musculature may be produced.

Effects on patient management
Xerostomia may increase caries incidence and thus a preventive regimen is important. If the xerostomia is severe artificial saliva may be indicated. The underlying psychosis may also cause problems in management. Involuntary muscle movements e.g. of the tongue will interfere with operative dentistry. Postural hypotension may occur with this drug, therefore rapid changes in patient position should be avoided.

Drug interactions

Enhanced sedative effects may occur with any central nervous system depressant, including opioid analgesics and alcohol. Indomethacin causes severe drowsiness. Carbamazepine reduces the effects of haloperidol. There is a theoretical risk of hypotension with epinephrine in dental local anaesthetics. Combined therapy with tricyclic antidepressants increases the chances of cardiac arrhythmias and exacerbates antimuscarinic effects such as xerostomia. The photosensitive effect of tetracyclines may be increased during combined therapy.

Haloperidol decanoate (Haldol decanoate)

Description

A butyrophenone antipsychotic drug.

Indications

Used as a depot injection in the treatment of schizophrenia and other psychoses.

Effects on oral and dental structures

Dry and painful mouth and involuntary movements of oro-facial musculature may be produced.

Effects on patient management

Xerostomia may increase caries incidence and thus a preventive regimen is important. If the xerostomia is severe artificial saliva may be indicated. The underlying psychosis may also cause problems in management. Involuntary muscle movements e.g. of the tongue will interfere with operative dentistry. Postural hypotension may occur with this drug, therefore rapid changes in patient position should be avoided.

Drug interactions

Enhanced sedative effects may occur with any central nervous system depressant, including opioid analgesics and alcohol. Indomethacin causes severe drowsiness. Carbamazepine reduces the effects of haloperidol. There is a theoretical risk of hypotension with epinephrine in dental local anaesthetics. Combined therapy with tricyclic antidepressants increases the chances of cardiac arrhythmias and exacerbates antimuscarinic effects such as xerostomia. The photosensitive effect of tetracyclines may be increased during combined therapy.

Heparin

Description

An anticoagulant drug.

Indications

Initial treatment and prevention of deep vein thrombosis and pulmonary embolism. Used to prevent blood coagulation in patients on haemodialysis.

Effects on oral and dental structures

No direct effect, although patients who are repeatedly heparinized are susceptible to osteoporosis. This latter condition may make such patients susceptible to periodontal breakdown.

Effects on patient management

Heparin can only be given parenterally which reduces the impact of the drug in dental practice. However dentists, especially those working in a hospital environment, will encounter patients who are heparinized on a regular basis (e.g. renal dialysis patients). Bleeding is the main problem with treating such patients. This can arise as a direct effect on the blood coagulation system or from a drug-induced immune-mediated thrombocytopenia. From the coagulation perspective, it is the best to treat heparinized patients between treatments since the half-life of the drug is approximately 4 hours. If urgent treatment is required, then the anticoagulation effect of heparin can be reversed with protamine sulphate 10 mg IV. If bleeding is due to thrombocytopenia then a platelet transfusion may be required and patients transferred to a heparinoid such as danaparoid.

Drug interactions

Aspirin and parenteral NSAIDs (e.g. diclofenac and ketorolac) should be avoided in patients who are taking heparin or who are heparinized on a regular basis. Such analgesics cause impairment of platelet aggregation which would compound a heparin-induced thrombocytopenia and likewise cause serious problems with obtaining haemostasis.

Hexetidine (Oraldene)

Description

An antiseptic mouthwash.

Indications

Used as an aid to oral hygiene.

Presentations

As a 0.1% solution.

Dose

15 ml twice daily as a rinse.

Contraindications

Allergy.

Precautions
None significant.

Unwanted effects
None significant.

Drug interactions
None of importance in dentistry.

Hydralazine (Apresoline)

Description
A vasodilator antihypertensive drug.

Indications
Used in conjunction with beta-blockers or thiazide diuretics to treat severe hypertension. Used singularly to treat a hypertensive crisis.

Effects on oral and dental structures
Rarely a cause of numbness, tingling (paraesthesia) or burning sensation in the face or mouth.

Effect on patient management
Very rarely causes haemolytic anaemia.

Drug interactions
NSAIDs such as ibuprofen may enhance the hypotensive actions of hydralazine.

Hydrocortisone (Efcortesol, Hydrocortone, Solu-cortel)

Description
A corticosteroid.

Indications
Suppression of inflammation and allergic disorders. Used in the management of inflammatory bowel diseases, asthma, immunosuppression and in various rheumatic diseases.

Effects on oral and dental structures
Although systemic corticosteroids can induce cleft lip and palate formation in mice, there is little evidence that this unwanted effect occurs in humans. The main impact of systemic corticosteroids on the mouth is to cause an increased susceptibility to opportunistic infections. These include candidiasis and those due to herpes viruses. The anti-inflammatory and immunosuppressant properties of corticosteroids may afford the patient some degree of protection against periodontal

breakdown. Paradoxically long-term systemic use can precipitate osteoporosis. The latter is now regarded as a risk factor for periodontal disease.

Effects on patient management

The main unwanted effect of corticosteroid treatment is the suppression of the adrenal cortex and the possibility of an adrenal crisis when such patients are subjected to 'stressful events'. Whilst such suppression does occur physiologically, its clinical significance does appear to be over-stated. As far as dentistry is concerned, there is increasing evidence that supplementary corticosteroids are not required. This would apply to all restorative procedures, periodontal surgery and the uncomplicated dental extraction. For more complicated dento-alveolar surgery, each case must be judged on its merit. An apprehensive patient may well require cover. It is important to monitor the patient's blood pressure before, during, and for 30 minutes after the procedure. If diastolic pressure drops by more than 25%, hydrocortisone 100 mg IV should be administered and the patient's blood pressure should continue to be monitored.

Patients should be screened regularly for oral infections such as fungal or viral infections. When these occur, they should be treated promptly with the appropriate chemotherapeutic agent. Likewise, any patient on corticosteroids that presents with an acute dental infection should be treated urgently as such infections can readily spread.

Drug interactions

Aspirin and NSAIDs should not be prescribed to patients on long-term corticosteroids. Both drugs are ulcerogenic and hence increase the risk of gastrointestinal bleeding and ulceration. The antifungal agent amphotericin increases the risk of corticosteroid-induced hypokalaemia, whilst ketoconazole inhibits corticosteroid hepatic metabolism.

Hydrogen peroxide mouthwash (Peroxyl)

Description

An oxidizing agent.

Indications

Used as an aid to oral hygiene.

Presentations

As 1.5% and 6% solutions.

Dose

10–15 mL as a rinse 2–4 times daily.

Contraindications
Allergy.

Precautions
None.

Unwanted effects
None.

Drug interactions
Avoid concurrent use with povidone–iodine rinses.

Hydromorphone hydrochloride (Palladone)

Description
An opioid analgesic.

Indications
Severe cancer pain.

Effects on oral and dental structures
Can cause xerostomia leading to an increased risk of root caries, candidal infections and poor denture retention. If the xerostomia is severe, dentate patients should receive topical fluoride and be offered an artificial saliva.

Effects on patient management
Hydromorphone hydrochloride is a drug of dependence and can thus cause withdrawal symptoms if the medication is stopped abruptly. Such cessation of hydromorphone hydrochloride may account for unusual behavioural changes and poor compliance with dental treatment. The drug also depresses respiration and causes postural hypotension.

Drug interactions
Hydromorphone hydrochloride will enhance the sedative properties of midazolam and diazepam. Reduce the dose of these sedative agents.

Hydrotalcite

Description
An antacid (aluminium magnesium carbonate hydroxide hydrate).

Indications
Used to treat dyspepsia.

Effects on oral and dental structures
Patients may complain of a chalky taste. The underlying condition of reflux can lead to erosion of the teeth, especially the palatal surfaces.

Effects on patient management
Patients may not be comfortable in the fully supine position due to
gastric reflux. Any drug with which there is an interaction (such as
tetracycline) should be taken a few hours in advance of antacid dose.

Drug interactions
Reduced absorption of phenytoin, tetracyclines, the non-steroidal
analgesic diflunisal, and the antifungal drugs ketoconazole and itraconazole. Antacids can increase the excretion of aspirin and reduce
plasma concentration to non-therapeutic levels.

Hydroxocobalamin

Description
A derivative of Vitamin B_{12}.

Indications
Pernicious anaemia and other macrocytic anaemias.

Effects on oral and dental structures
None reported.

Effects on patient management
Nothing of significance.

Drug interactions
None of any dental significance.

Hydroxyzine hydrochloride (Atarax, Ucerax)

Description
An antihistamine.

Indications
Used to manage short term anxiety and in the treatment of pruritus.

Effects on oral and dental structures
Can produce xerostomia.

Effects on patient management
The patient may be drowsy which may interfere with co-operation.
Xerostomia may increase caries incidence and thus a preventive
regimen is important. If the xerostomia is severe artificial saliva may
be indicated.

Drug interactions
Enhanced sedative effects occur with anxiolytic and hypnotic drugs.
Tricyclic and monoamine oxidase inhibitor antidepressants increase
antimuscarinic effects such as xerostomia.

Hyoscine butylbromide (Buscopan)

Description
An antimuscarinic drug.

Indications
Used for symptomatic relief in gastrointestinal disorders such as dyspepsia, diverticular disease, and irritable bowel syndrome. Also used in dysmenorrhoea.

Effects on oral and dental structures
Xerostomia may occur.

Effects on patient management
If use is prolonged xerostomia may increase caries incidence and thus a preventive regimen is important. If the xerostomia is severe artificial saliva may be indicated. Patients may not be comfortable in fully supine condition due to underlying gastrointestinal disorder.

Drug interactions
Absorption of ketoconazole is decreased. Side effects increased with concurrent medication with tricyclic and monoamine oxidase inhibitor antidepressants.

Hyoscine hydrobromide (Scopoderm)

Description
An antimuscarinic drug.

Indications
Used as a premedicament and in the management of motion sickness.

Effects on oral and dental structures
Xerostomia may be produced.

Effects on patient management
As this drug is only for short term use xerostomia should not be a persistent problem.

Drug interactions
Absorption of ketoconazole is decreased. Side effects increased with concurrent medication with tricyclic and monoamine oxidase inhibitor antidepressants.

Ibuprofen (Brufen, Nurofen, Fenbid)

Description
A peripherally acting, non-steroidal anti-inflammatory analgesic that is derived from propionic acid.

Indications
Pain with a significant inflammatory component (e.g. postoperative pain after dental surgical procedures). Also used in the management of musculoskeletal pain, dysmenorrhoea, and to reduce fever.

Presentations
A 200, 400 and 600 mg tablet.
As a suspension (Ibuprofen 100 mg/5 ml).
Effervescent granules (Ibuprofen 600 mg).

Dose
Analgesia for adults, Ibuprofen 1.2–1.8 g daily in divided doses. For children, 20–40 mg/kg.

Contraindications
Ibuprofen is contraindicated in patients with a history of allergy to aspirin or any other NSAID. The drug should not be prescribed to asthmatics (can precipitate bronchoconstriction) or patients with a history of angioedema and urticaria. Ibuprofen should not be prescribed to patients with active peptic ulceration (ibuprofen is ulcerogenic) or to patients with haemorrhagic disorders since it will affect platelet aggregation. Ibuprofen should be used with caution in patients who exhibit renal, cardiac or hepatic impairment since the repeated use of the drug can result in a deterioration in renal function.

Precautions
Elderly, pregnancy, and breastfeeding mothers.

Unwanted effects
Ibuprofen is ulcerogenic although of all the NSAIDs, it has one of the lowest risk of gastrointestinal irritation. This unwanted effect can be further reduced by taking the drug with food or milk. Other rare unwanted effects include blood disorders, fluid retention, renal damage, eye changes, and the precipitation of Stevens–Johnson syndrome. Patients who suffer from systemic lupus erythematosus may be susceptible to a NSAID-induced aseptic meningitis. Excessive high doses of ibuprofen can cause a metabolic acidosis; if untreated, this can lead to coma.

Drug interactions
Ibuprofen should not be given with other NSAIDs or aspirin since using such combinations will increase the risk of unwanted effects. The anticoagulant effects of both warfarin and heparin are enhanced by ibuprofen and could increase the risk of haemorrhage. Ibuprofen

can antagonize the hypotensive effects of the ACE inhibitors (e.g. captopril, lisinopril). There is the additional increased risk of renal impairment and hyperkalaemia with these drugs and ibuprofen. Antidiabetic drugs such as the sulphonylureas are extensively protein bound and can be displaced by ibuprofen leading to hypoglycaemia. Ibuprofen can increase the risk of gastrointestinal haemorrhage if given to patients taking antiplatelet drugs such as clopidogrel. Ibuprofen should be avoided in patients taking beta-adrenoceptor blockers as there will be an antagonism of their hypotensive effect. Ibuprofen may exacerbate heart failure, reduce glomerular filtration rate and increase plasma concentration of digoxin. Both ibuprofen and corticosteroids (systemic) cause peptic ulceration, therefore avoid the combination. The excretion of methotrexate is reduced by ibuprofen which can lead to increased toxicity. Ibuprofen reduces the excretion of the muscle relaxant baclofen. The excretion of lithium is reduced by ibuprofen, thus increasing the risk of lithium toxicity.

Idarubicin hydrochloride (Zavedos)

Description
A cytotoxic antibiotic.

Indications
Advanced breast cancer, acute leukaemias.

Effects on oral and dental structures
Idarubicin hydrochloride causes bone marrow suppression with an accompanying thrombocytopenia and agranulocytosis. Bone marrow suppression can lead to troublesome oral ulceration, exacerbation of an existing periodontal condition and rapid spread of any residual (e.g. periapical) infections.

Effects on patient management
The effect of idarubicin hydrochloride on the bone marrow is transient and routine dental treatment is best avoided until the white blood cells and platelet counts start to recover. If emergency dental treatment is required such as an extraction then antibiotic cover may be required depending on the degree of myelosuppression. If the platelet count is low (<100,000) then the socket should be packed and sutured. Persistent bleeding may require a platelet transfusion.

Patients on chemotherapeutic agents such as idarubicin hydrochloride often neglect their oral hygiene and thus there could be an increase in both caries and periodontal disease. If time permits, patients about to go on chemotherapy should have a dental check up and any potential areas of infection should be treated. Similarly, to reduce the mucosal irritation (sensitivity) that often accompanies chemotherapy, it is advisable to remove any ill-fitting dentures and smooth over rough cusps or restorations.

Drug interactions
None of any dental significance.

Ifosfamide (Mitoxana)

Description
An alkylating agent.

Indications
Chronic lymphocytic leukaemia, lymphomas, and solid tumour.

Effects on oral and dental structures
Ifosfamide causes bone marrow suppression with an accompanying thrombocytopenia and agranulocytosis. Bone marrow suppression can lead to troublesome oral ulceration, exacerbation of an existing periodontal condition and rapid spread of any residual (e.g. periapical) infections.

Effects on patient management
The effect of ifosfamide on the bone marrow is transient and routine dental treatment is best avoided until the white blood cells and platelet counts start to recover. If emergency dental treatment such as an extraction is required then antibiotic cover may be necessary depending on the degree of myelosuppression. If the platelet count is low (<100,000) then the socket should be packed and sutured. Persistent bleeding may require a platelet transfusion.

Patients on chemotherapeutic agents such as ifosfamide often neglect their oral hygiene and thus there could be an increase in both caries and periodontal disease. If time permits, patients about to go on chemotherapy should have a dental check up and any potential areas of infection should be treated. Similarly, to reduce the mucosal irritation (sensitivity) that often accompanies chemotherapy, it is advisable to remove any ill-fitting dentures and smooth over rough cusps or restorations.

Drug interactions
None of any dental significance.

Imidapril (Tanatril)

Description
Imidapril is an ACE inhibitor, that is it inhibits the renal angiotensin converting enzyme which is necessary to convert angiotensin I to the more potent angiotensin II.

Indications

Mild to moderate hypertension, congestive heart failure, and post myocardial infarction where there is left ventricular dysfunction.

Effects on oral and dental structures

Imidapril can cause taste disturbances, angioedema, dry mouth, glossitis, and lichenoid drug reactions. Many of these unwanted effects are dose related and compounded if there is an impairment of renal function. Imidapril-induced xerostomia increases the risk of fungal infections (candidiasis) and caries, especially root caries. Antifungal treatment should be used when appropriate and topical fluoride (e.g. Duraphat) will reduce the risk of root surface caries.

Effects on patient management

Imidapril-induced angioedema is perhaps the most significant unwanted effect that impacts upon dental management, since dental procedures can induce the angioedema. Management of imidapril-induced angioedema is problematic because the underlying mechanisms are poorly understood. Standard anti-anaphylactic treatment is of little value (epinephrine and hydrocortisone) since the angioedema is not mediated via mast cells or antibody/antigen interactions. Usually the angioedema subsides and patients on these drugs should be questioned as to whether they have experienced any problems with breathing or swallowing. This will alert the dental practitioner to the possible risk of this unwanted effect arising during dental treatment.

Imidapril is also associated with suppression of bone marrow activity giving rise to possible neutropenia, agranulocytosis, thrombocytopenia and aplastic anaemia. Patients on imidapril who present with excessive bleeding of their gums, sore throats or oral ulceration should have a full haematological investigation.

Drug interactions

Non-steroidal anti-inflammatory drugs (NSAIDs) such as ibuprofen may reduce the antihypertensive effect of imidapril.

Imipenem (Primaxin)

Description

A beta-lactam antibiotic (imipenem) combined with an enzyme inhibitor which prevents renal metabolism of the antibiotic (ciastatin).

Indications

Treatment of multi-drug resistant infection and surgical prophylaxis.

Effects on oral and dental structures

This is a broad spectrum antibiotic and thus oral candidiasis may be produced. Taste disturbance may occur.

Effects on patient management
Antifungal treatment may be required. This drug may cause neutropenia which may affect healing adversely.

Drug interactions
Convulsions may occur if used in combination with the antiviral drug ganciclovir.

Imipramine hydrochloride (Tofranil)

Description
A tricyclic antidepressant.

Indications
Used in the management of depressive illness and for the treatment of nocturnal enuresis in children.

Effects on oral and dental structures
Xerostomia, taste disturbance and stomatitis may occur.

Effects on patient management
Xerostomia may increase caries incidence and thus a preventive regimen is important. If the xerostomia is severe artificial saliva may be indicated. Postural hypotension may occur with this drug, therefore rapid changes in patient position should be avoided. This drug may cause thrombocytopenia, agranulocytosis, and leucopenia. Thrombocytopenia may cause postoperative bleeding. If the platelet count is low (<100,000) then the socket should be packed and sutured. Persistent bleeding may require platelet transfusion. Agranulocytosis and leucopenia may affect healing adversely.

Drug interactions
Increased sedation occurs with alcohol and sedative drugs such as benzodiazepines. This drug may antagonize the action of anticonvulsants such as carbamazepine and phenytoin. This drug increases the pressor effects of epinephrine. Nevertheless, the use of epinephrine-containing local anaesthetics is not contraindicated; however, epinephrine dose limitation is recommended. Normal anticoagulant control by warfarin may be upset, both increases and decreases in INR have been noted during combined therapy with tricyclic antidepressants. Combined therapy with other antidepressants should be avoided and if prescribing another class of antidepressant a period of one to two weeks should elapse between changeover. Antimuscarinic effects such as xerostomia are increased when used in combination with other anticholinergic drugs such as antipsychotics.

Indapamide (Natrillix)

Description
A thiazide diuretic.

Indications
Essential hypertension.

Effects on oral and dental structures
Thiazide diuretics can cause lichenoid eruptions in the mouth, xerostomia, and taste disturbances due to hyperzincuria.

Effects on patient management
Less likely to cause postural hypotension when compared to other thiazide diuretics. Rarely causes blood disorders including agranulocytosis, neutropenia, and thrombocytopenia. The latter may have an effect on haemostasis after various dental surgical procedures.

Drug interactions
Indapamide can cause hypokalaemia which can be further exacerbated by systemic amphotericin and epinephrine containing local anaesthetic solutions. No more than 3 cartridges should be administered per adult patient.

Indinavir (Crixivan)

Description
A protease inhibitor.

Indications
Used in the management of HIV infection.

Effects on oral and dental structures
Taste disturbance, xerostomia, oral ulceration, and Stevens–Johnson syndrome may occur. Paraesthesia may be produced.

Effects on patient management
Sensitive handling of the underlying disease state is essential. Excellent preventive dentistry and regular examinations are important in patients suffering from HIV, as dental infections are best avoided. HIV will interfere with postoperative healing and antibiotic prophylaxis prior to oral surgery may be advisable.

Sedation with midazolam should be avoided (see below), dose limitation with lidocaine local anaesthetics is wise (see below). Indinavir can produce anaemia and leucopenia. Neutropenia will affect healing adversely and if severe prophylactic antibiotics should be prescribed to cover surgical procedures. Anaemia may result in poor healing. Any anaemia will need correction prior to elective general anaesthesia and sedation. Xerostomia may increase caries incidence and thus a preventive regimen is important. If the xerostomia is severe artificial saliva may be indicated.

Drug interactions
Concurrent use with midazolam will produce prolonged sedation and this combination should be avoided. Protease inhibitors appear to increase the plasma levels of lidocaine and increase cardiotoxicity of the latter drug. The anticonvulsants carbamazepine and phenytoin and the steroid dexamethasone reduce the plasma levels of indinavir. The antifungals ketoconazole and itraconazole inhibit the metabolism of indinavir and the latter antifungal should be avoided. Erythromycin may increase indinavir levels in plasma.

Indomethacin (Rimacid, Indocid)

Description
A peripherally acting, non-steroidal anti-inflammatory analgesic.

Indications
Pain and inflammation associated with musculoskeletal disorders, e.g. rheumatoid arthritis, osteoarthritis, and ankylosing spondylitis. Postoperative analgesia.

Effects on oral and dental structures
Patients on long-term NSAIDs such as indomethacin may be afforded some degree of protection against periodontal breakdown. This arises from the drug's inhibitory action on prostaglandin synthesis. The latter is an important inflammatory mediator in the pathogenesis of periodontal breakdown.

Indomethacin has also been implicated for inducing oral lichenoid eruptions and oral ulceration. The drug does have a higher incidence of bone marrow suppression when compared to other NSAIDs. This can cause agranulocytosis, leucopenia, aplastic anaemia and/or thrombocytopenia. Such depression of bone marrow function will affect the oral mucosa (high risk of ulceration), the periodontal tissue (high risk of gingival bleeding and periodontal breakdown) and healing after any dental surgical procedure.

Effects on patient management
The risk of thrombocytopenia will cause an increased bleeding tendency following dental surgical procedures. If the platelet count is low (<100,000) then the socket should be packed and sutured. Persistent bleeding may require a platelet transfusion.

Drug interactions
Ibuprofen, aspirin, and diflunisal should be avoided in patients taking indomethacin due to an increase in unwanted effects, especially

gastrointestinal ulceration, renal, and liver damage. Systemic corticosteroids increase the risk of peptic ulceration and gastrointestinal bleeding.

Indoramin (Baratol)

Description
An alpha-adrenoceptor blocking drug.

Indications
Hypertension and benign prostatic hyperplasia.

Effects on oral and dental structures
Xerostomia can occur leading to an increased risk of caries (especially root caries), candidal infections and poor denture retention. Indoramin can also produce extrapyramidal effects resulting facial grimacing, protruding and rolling of the tongue and involuntary chewing movements.

Effects on patient management
Extrapyramidal effects could make it difficult to carry out various aspects of dentistry, in particular denture construction. If the xerostomia is severe, dentate patients should receive topical fluoride and be offered an artificial saliva.

Drug interactions
NSAIDs such as ibuprofen and systemic corticosteroids may antagonize the hypotensive actions of indoramin.

Inosine pranobex (Imunovir)

Description
An antiviral drug.

Indications
Used in the management of herpetic infections but less suitable than other anti-herpetic drugs.

Effects on oral and dental structures
None reported.

Effects on patient management
Elective treatment should be postponed during an acute viral infection.

Drug interactions
None reported.

Ipratropium bromide (Atrovent, Respontin)

Description
An antimuscarinic drug.

Indications
Used in the management of asthma, and chronic obstructive airway disease.

Effects on oral and dental structures
Xerostomia, taste disturbance, and stomatitis may be produced.

Effects on patient management
Patients may not be comfortable in the supine position if they have respiratory problems. If the patient suffers from asthma then aspirin-like compounds should not be prescribed as many asthmatic patients are allergic to these analgesics. Similarly, sulphite-containing compounds (such as preservatives in epinephrine-containing local anaesthetics) can produce allergy in asthmatic patients. Xerostomia may increase caries incidence and thus a preventive regimen is important. If the xerostomia is severe artificial saliva may be indicated. The use of a rubber dam in patients with obstructive airway disease may further embarrass the airway. If a rubber dam is essential then supplemental oxygen via a nasal cannula may be required.

Drug interactions
The absorption of ketoconazole is decreased during combined therapy. Antimuscarinic effects (such as xerostomia) are increased with concurrent use of tricyclic and monoamine oxidase inhibitor antidepressant drugs.

Insulin zinc suspension (Human Monotard, Humulin Lente)

Description
Intermediate and long acting insulin.

Indications
Diabetes mellitus.

Effects on oral and dental structures
Soluble insulin can cause pain and swelling of the salivary glands.

Effects on patient management
The main concern with treating diabetic patients on insulin zinc suspension is to avoid hypoglycaemia. Thus it is important to ensure that patients have taken their normal food and insulin prior to their dental appointment. Wherever possible treat diabetic patients in the

first half of the morning and ensure that any treatment does not preclude them from eating. If an insulin-dependant diabetic requires a general anaesthetic, then patients should be referred to hospital.

Drug interactions

Aspirin and the NSAIDs can cause hypoglycaemia which could be a problem in a poorly-controlled insulin dependent diabetic. These analgesics should be used with caution in such patients. Systemic corticosteroids will antagonize the hypoglycaemic properties of insulin. If these drugs are required in an insulin-dependent diabetic, then consult the patient's physician before prescribing.

Irbesartan (Aprovel)

Description

An angiotensin II receptor antagonist.

Indications

Used as an alternative to ACE inhibitors where the latter cannot be tolerated.

Effects on oral and dental structures

Angioedema has been reported, but the incidence of this unwanted effect is much less than when compared to ACE inhibitors.

Effects on patient management

None of any significance.

Drug interactions

NSAIDs such as ibuprofen may reduce the antihypertensive action of irbesartan.

Irinotecan hydrochloride (Campto)

Description

A topoisomerase I inhibitor.

Indications

Metastatic colorectal cancer.

Effects on oral and dental structures

Irinotecan hydrochloride causes bone marrow suppression with an accompanying thrombocytopenia and agranulocytosis. Bone marrow suppression can lead to troublesome oral ulceration, exacerbation of an existing periodontal condition, and rapid spread of any residual (e.g. periapical) infections.

Effects on patient management

The effect of irinotecan hydrochloride on the bone marrow is transient and routine dental treatment is best avoided until the white blood cells and platelet counts start to recover. If emergency dental treatment such as an extraction is required then antibiotic cover may be necessary depending on the degree of myelosuppression. If the platelet count is low (<100,000) then the socket should be packed and sutured. Persistent bleeding may require a platelet transfusion.

Patients on chemotherapeutic agents such as irinotecan hydrochloride often neglect their oral hygiene and thus there could be an increase in both caries and periodontal disease. If time permits, patients about to go on chemotherapy should have a dental check up and any potential areas of infection should be treated. Similarly, to reduce the mucosal irritation (sensitivity) that often accompanies chemotherapy, it is advisable to remove any ill-fitting dentures and smooth over rough cusps or restorations.

Drug interactions

None of any dental significance.

Isocarboxazid

Description

A monoamine oxidase inhibitor.

Indications

Used in the management of depression.

Effects on oral and dental structures

Xerostomia may be produced.

Effects on patient management

Xerostomia may increase caries incidence and thus a preventive regimen is important. If the xerostomia is severe artificial saliva may be indicated. This drug may cause postural hypotension, thus the patient should not be changed from the supine to the standing position too rapidly.

Drug interactions

Combined therapy with opioid analgesics can create serious shifts in blood pressure (both elevation and depression) and thus opioids such as pethidine must be avoided for up to two weeks after monoamine oxidase inhibitor therapy. Similarly, change to another antidepressant group such as tricyclics or selective serotonin uptake inhibitors should only take place after a gap of two weeks from the end of monoamine oxidase inhibitor therapy. The anticonvulsant effects of anti-epileptic drugs is antagonized by monoamine oxidase inhibitors. Carbamazepine should not be administered within two weeks of monoamine oxidase inhibitor therapy. Hypertensive crisis can occur if administered with ephedrine. Epinephrine in dental local anaesthetics is not a concern as this is metabolized by a route independent of monoamine oxidase.

Isometheptene mucate (Midrid)

Description
A sympathomimetic drug.

Indications
Used in the treatment of acute migraine.

Effects on oral and dental structures
None specific to this drug.

Effects on patient management
Dose reduction of epinephrine-containing local anaesthetics is advised (see drug interaction below). Any factor which precipitates a migrainous attack such as a sudden bright light or noise should be avoided in the surgery.

Drug interactions
Combined therapy with monoamine oxidase inhibitors can produce hypertensive crisis. As this drug is a sympathomimetic agent any adverse effect of epinephrine in dental local anaesthetics may be exacerbated.

Isoniazid

Description
An antituberculous drug.

Indications
Used in the treatment of tuberculosis.

Effects on oral and dental structures
Stevens–Johnson syndrome and lupus erythematosus-like syndromes may occur. This drug may cause oro-facial dysaesthesia.

Effects on patient management
Only emergency dental treatment should be performed during active tuberculosis and care must be exercised to eliminate spread of tuberculosis between the patient and dental personnel, e.g. masks and glasses should be worn and where possible treatment should be performed under a rubber dam to reduce aerosol spread. This drug may cause thrombocytopenia, agranulocytosis, and anaemia. Thrombocytopenia may cause postoperative bleeding. If the platelet count is low

(<100,000) then the socket should be packed and sutured. Persistent bleeding may require platelet transfusion. Agranulocytosis and anaemia may affect healing adversely. Any anaemia will need correction prior to elective general anaesthesia and sedation.

Drug interactions
Isoniazid increases the toxicity of paracetamol and intake of the latter drug should be limited. Isoniazid decreases the metabolism of carbamazepine, and phenytoin. In addition carbamazepine increases the toxicity of isoniazid. Isoniazid inhibits the metabolism of diazepam and decreases the efficacy of ketoconazole. Isoniazid may increase the anticoagulant effect of warfarin and increase hypotension with pethidine. Corticosteroids may decrease the plasma levels of isoniazid but this is not thought to be of clinical importance.

Isophane insulin

Description
Intermediate and long acting insulin.

Indications
Diabetes mellitus.

Effects on oral and dental structures
Soluble insulin can cause pain and swelling of the salivary glands.

Effects on patient management
The main concern with treating diabetic patients on isophane insulin suspension is to avoid hypoglycaemia. Thus it is important to ensure that patients have taken their normal food and insulin prior to their dental appointment. Wherever possible treat diabetic patients in the first half of the morning and ensure that any treatment does not preclude them from eating. If an insulin-dependent diabetic requires a general anaesthetic, then patients should be referred to hospital.

Drug interactions
Aspirin and the NSAIDs can cause hypoglycaemia which could be a problem in a poorly-controlled insulin dependent diabetic. These analgesics should be used with caution in such patients. Systemic corticosteroids will antagonize the hypoglycaemic properties of insulin. If these drugs are required in an insulin dependent diabetic, then consult the patient's physician before prescribing.

Isosorbide mononitrate

Description
A nitrate.

Indications
Angina prophylaxis and adjunctive treatment in congestive heart failure.

Effects on oral and dental structures
The sublingual preparation has been associated with halitosis.

Effects on patient management
Dry mouth may reduce the sublingual absorption of isosorbide mononitrate. Postural hypotension may occur and patient may feel dizzy when the dental chair is restored to upright after they have been treated in the supine position.

Drug interactions
None of any dental significance.

Ispaghula husk (Fybogel, Konsyl, Isogel, Regulan)

Description
A bulk-forming laxative.

Indications
Used to treat constipation and in the management of hypercholesterolaemia.

Effects on oral and dental structures
None specific.

Effects on patient management
Avoid the use of codeine and other opioid compounds as they exacerbate constipation.

Drug interactions
None of importance in dentistry.

Isradipine (Prescal)

Description
A calcium-channel blocker.

Indications
Hypertension and angina prophylaxis.

Effects on oral and dental structures
Isradipine can cause gingival overgrowth, especially in the anterior part of the mouth. It also causes taste disturbances by inhibiting calcium-channel activity that is necessary for normal function of taste and smell receptors.

Effects on patient management
None of any significance.

Drug interactions
None of any dental significance.

Itraconazole (Sporanox)

Description
A triazole antifungal agent.

Indications
The treatment of oral fungal infections.

Presentations
(i) A 100 mg capsule.
(ii) A liquid (10 mg/mL).

Dose
100 mg daily for 15 days.

Contraindications
Previous hypersensitivity (plus see important drug interactions below).
Pregnancy, breastfeeding, children, and the elderly.

Precautions
Use with caution in patients with renal and hepatic disease. Discontinue if peripheral neuropathy occurs.

Unwanted effects
Hypersensitivity reactions.
Gastrointestinal problems.
Hypokalaemia.

Drug interactions
There are a number of important drug interactions with itraconazole. It inhibits the metabolism of the antihistamines terfenadine and astemizole which may cause cardiac dysryhthmias. Itraconazole enhances the anticoagulant effect of warfarin. The anticonvulsants phenytoin and carbamazepine and H_2 blockers such as cimetidine reduce the plasma concentrations of itraconazole. Itraconazole increases the plasma concentration of midazolam, ciclosporin, and cardiac glycosides such as digoxin. Itraconazole also inhibits the metabolism of the anti-spasmodic drug cisapride, and this can lead to ventricular arrhythmias. Itraconazole may reduce the efficacy of oral contraceptives. Itraconazole increases the risk of myopathy when administered concurrently with the anti-cholesterol drug simvastatin. The plasma concentration of calcium-channel blocking drugs such as felodipine

and nifedipine are raised by itraconazole and this increases the side effects (such as limb oedema) of the former drugs.

The pharmacokinetics of itraconazole are interfered with by cytotoxic drugs used in the treatment of leukaemia. These effects are variable with no pattern. However such effects are not seen with fluconazole, and this alternative antifungal is recommended in the presence of cytotoxic medication. Rifampicin increases the metabolism and elimination of itraconazole and this might lead to a reduction in antifungal action. When itraconazole is used concurrently with amphotericin combined activity is less than when amphotericin is used alone.

Kanamycin (Kannasyn)

Description
An aminoglycoside antibiotic.

Indications
Used to treat serious Gram-negative infections resistant to other antibiotics, but it has generally been superseded by other aminoglycosides.

Effects on oral and dental structures
None specific.

Effects on patient management
This drug can produce disturbances of hearing and balance, thus rapid movements of the dental chair should be avoided and care taken when the patient leaves the chair.

Drug interactions
The ototoxic effect of this drug is exacerbated by vancomycin. Nephrotoxicity is increased when used in combination with amphotericin B and clindamycin. The risk of hypocalcaemia produced by bisphophonates, which are used in the management of Paget's disease of bone, is increased by kanamycin.

Kaolin (Kaolin mixture)

Description
An adsorbent.

Indications
Used in the treatment of some diarrhoeas.

Effects on oral and dental structures
None specific.

Effects on patient management

Prolonged treatment sessions should be avoided during therapy with this drug due to the fact that it is used to treat diarrhoea.

Drug interactions

Kaolin reduces the absorption of aspirin and tetracyclines.

Ketoconazole (Nizoral)

Description

An imidazole antifungal agent.

Indications

The treatment of systemic fungal infections and severe resistant muco-cutaneous candidiasis.

Presentations

(i) A 200 mg tablet.

(ii) A suspension (100 mg/5 mL).

Dose

200 mg once daily for 14 days.
In children 3 mg/kg daily.

Contraindications

Previous hypersensitivity (plus see important drug interactions below).
History of porphyria.
Best avoided in pregnancy.

Precautions

Ketoconazole is more readily absorbed than miconazole and can lead to nephrotoxicity. It is not advised for superficial fungal infections.

Unwanted effects

Hypersensitivity reactions.
Gastrointestinal disturbances.

Drug interactions

Ketoconazole should not be prescribed to patients receiving the anti-histamines astemizole and terfenadine as cardiac dysrhythmias may occur. Ketoconazole inhibits the metabolism of the anti-spasmodic drug cisapride and this can lead to ventricular arrhythmias; thus concurrent use should be avoided. Ketoconazole enhances the anticoagulant effect of warfarin even after topical use. Ketoconazole increases the plasma concentrations of benzodiazepines (including midazolam) and ciclosporin. Ketoconazole increases the hypoglycaemic effect of tolbutamide. Phenytoin reduces the plasma concentration of ketoconazole. Ketoconazole and amphotericin antagonize each others' antifungal action. Anti-ulcer medications (including cimetidine, omeprazole, and sucralfate), and antimuscarinic drugs decrease the absorption of keto-conazole. Other drugs which decrease the plasma concentration of ketoconazole include rifampicin and isoniazid.

Ketoconazole reduces the metabolism and excretion of methyl pred-nisolone. Ketoconazole can lead to oral contraceptive failure. A disul-firam-like (antabuse) reaction can occur with alcohol consumption and thus alcohol intake is best avoided during ketoconazole therapy.

Ketoprofen (Orudis)

Description
A peripherally acting, non-steroidal anti-inflammatory analgesic.

Indications
Pain and inflammation associated with musculoskeletal disorders, e.g. rheumatoid arthritis, osteoarthritis, and ankylosing spondylitis.

Effects on oral and dental structures
Patients on long-term NSAIDs such as ketoprofen may be afforded some degree of protection against periodontal breakdown. This arises from the drug's inhibitory action on prostaglandin synthesis. The latter is an important inflammatory mediator in the pathogene-sis of periodontal breakdown.

Effects on patient management
Rare unwanted effects of ketoprofen include angioedema and throm-bocytopenia. The latter may cause an increased bleeding tendency following any dental surgical procedure.

Drug interactions
Ibuprofen, aspirin, and diflunisal should be avoided in patients taking ketoprofen due to an increase in unwanted effects, especially gastroin-testinal ulceration, renal, and liver damage. Systemic corticosteroids increase the risk of peptic ulceration and gastrointestinal bleeding.

Ketotifen (Zaditen)

Description
An antihistamine.

Indications
Used in the treatment of asthma.

Effects on oral and dental structures
Xerostomia may be produced.

Effects on patient management
The patient may be drowsy which may interfere with co-operation during treatment. Patients may not be comfortable in the supine

position if they have respiratory problems. If the patient suffers from asthma then aspirin-like compounds should not be prescribed as many asthmatic patients are allergic to these analgesics. Similarly, sulphite-containing compounds (such as preservatives in epinephrine-containing local anaesthetics) can produce allergy in asthmatic patients.

Xerostomia may increase caries incidence and thus a preventive regimen is important. If the xerostomia is severe artificial saliva may be indicated.

Drug interactions
Increased sedative effects with sedation agents and antimuscarinic effects (such as xerostomia) are increased during combined therapy with tricyclic and monoamine oxidase inhibitor antidepressant drugs.

Labetalol (Trandate)

Description
An alpha and beta-adrenoceptor blocking drug.

Indications
Hypertension, including hypertension in pregnancy.

Effects on oral and dental structures
Rarely causes lichenoid eruptions.

Effects on patient management
Postural hypotension may occur and the patient may feel dizzy when the dental chair is restored to upright after they have been treated in the supine position.

Drug interactions
NSAIDs such as ibuprofen may antagonize the hypotensive action of labetalol. Possible interaction between epinephrine and labetalol which might cause a slight transient increase in blood pressure. Do not exceed more than 3 cartridges of epinephrine containing local anaesthetic solution per patient.

Lacidipine (Motens)

Description
A calcium-channel blocker.

Indications
Hypertension and angina prophylaxis.

Effects on oral and dental structures
Lacidipine can cause gingival overgrowth, especially in the anterior part of the mouth. It also causes taste disturbances by inhibiting

calcium-channel activity that is necessary for normal function of taste and smell receptors.

Effects on patient management
None of any significance.

Drug interactions
None of any dental significance.

Lactitol

Description
An osmotic laxative.

Indications
Used to treat constipation.

Effects on oral and dental structures
None specific.

Effects on patient management
See interactions below.

Drug interactions
Avoid the use of codeine and other opioid compounds as they exacerbate constipation.

Lactulose

Description
An osmotic laxative.

Indications
Used to treat constipation.

Effects on oral and dental structures
None specific.

Effects on patient management
See interactions below.

Drug interactions
Avoid the use of codeine and other opioid compounds as they exacerbate constipation.

Lamivudine (Epivir)

Description
A nucleoside reverse transcriptase inhibitor.

Indications
Used in the management of HIV infection.

Effects on oral and dental structures
This drug may produce paraesthesia.

Effects on patient management
Sensitive handling of the underlying disease state is essential. Excellent preventive dentistry and regular examinations are important in patients suffering from HIV, as dental infections are best avoided. HIV will interfere with postoperative healing and antibiotic prophylaxis prior to oral surgery may be advisable. This drug may produce anaemia, neutropenia, and thrombocytopenia. Anaemia may result in poor healing. Any anaemia will need correction prior to elective general anaesthesia and sedation. Thrombocytopenia may cause postoperative bleeding. If the platelet count is low (<100,000) then the socket should be packed and sutured. Persistent bleeding may require platelet transfusion.

Drug interactions
Avoid high doses of co-trimoxazole as this increases toxicity of lamivudine.

Lamotrigine (Lamictal)

Description
An anticonvulsant drug.

Indications
Used in the management of epilepsy.

Effects on oral and dental structures
Xerostomia, halitosis, gingival overgrowth, stomatitis, and Stevens–Johnson syndrome may occur.

Effects on patient management
Xerostomia may increase caries incidence and thus a preventive regimen is important. If the xerostomia is severe artificial saliva may be indicated. Epileptic fits are possible especially if the patient is stressed, therefore sympathetic handling and perhaps sedation should be considered for stressful procedures. Emergency anticonvulsant medication (diazepam or midazolam) must be available.

Drug interactions

Lamotrigine toxicity is increased by other anticonvulsants. Paracetamol increases lamotrigine loss but the importance of this is
uncertain.

Lansoprazole (HeliClear, Zoton)

Description

A proton-pump inhibitor.

Indications

Used in the management of gastrointestinal ulceration and oesophagitis.

Effects on oral and dental structures

Xerostomia, taste disturbance, halitosis, candidiasis, stomatitis and
bullae may be produced, Stevens–Johnson syndrome may occur. The
underlying con-dition of reflux can lead to erosion of the teeth,
especially the palatal surfaces.

Effects on patient management

Xerostomia may increase caries incidence and thus a preventive regimen is important. If the xerostomia is severe artificial saliva may be
indicated. Non-steroidal anti-inflammatory drugs should be avoided
due to gastrointestinal irritation. Similarly, high dose systemic steroids should not be prescribed in patients with gastrointestinal ulceration. Patients may be uncomfortable in the fully supine position as a
result of their underlying gastrointestinal disorder. Lansoprazole can
cause a pancytopenia. Leucopenia will affect healing adversely and if
severe prophylactic antibiotics should be prescribed to cover surgical
procedures. Thrombocytopenia may cause postoperative bleeding. If
the platelet count is low (<100,000) then the socket should be packed
and sutured. Persistent bleeding may require platelet transfusion.

Drug interactions

The absorption of the antifungals ketoconazole and itraconazole is
reduced. See comments on non-steroidals and steroids above.

Lercanidipine (Zandip)

Description

A calcium-channel blocker.

Indications

Hypertension and angina prophylaxis.

Effects on oral and dental structures

Lercanidipine can cause gingival overgrowth, especially in the anterior part of the mouth. It also causes taste disturbances by inhibiting

calcium-channel activity that is necessary for normal function of taste and smell receptors.

Effects on patient management
None of any significance.

Drug interactions
None of any dental significance.

Letrozole (Femara)

Description
A non-steroidal aromatase inhibitor.

Indications
Advanced postmenopausal breast cancer.

Effects on oral and dental structures
Nothing reported.

Effects on patient management
Nothing of any significance.

Drug interactions
None of any dental significance.

Leuprorelin acetate

Description
A gonadorelin analogue.

Indications
Endometriosis, prostate cancer.

Effects on oral and dental structures
Rare unwanted effects of leuprorelin acetate include paraesthesia of the lips and oedema of the lips and tongue. The drug is also associated with dry mouth which increases the risk of dental caries, especially root caries, poor denture retention, and an increased susceptibility to candidal infection.

Effects on patient management
Use of leuprorelin acetate is associated with an increased risk of osteoporosis. The latter is now regarded as a significant risk factor for periodontal disease.

Drug interactions
None of any dental significance.

Levacetylmethadol hydrochloride (OrLAAM)

Description
An opioid.

Indications
Used in the maintenance of opioid withdrawal therapy.

Effects on oral and dental structures
This drug is used following stabilization on methadone and the former drug may have produced caries.

Effects on patient management
The use of opioid analgesics must be avoided as patients receiving this medication are undergoing withdrawal from this group of drugs.

Drug interactions
Erythromycin and the antidepressants amitryptiline, doxepine, imipramine and maprotiline should not be prescribed to patients taking levacetylmethadol as ventricular arrhythmias can occur. Monoamine oxidase inhibitors should also be avoided as CNS excitation or depression can occur with concurrent use. This drug enhances the sedative effects of anxiolytic and sedative drugs including alcohol and benzodiazepines.

Levobupivacaine (Chirocain)

Description
An amide local anaesthetic; an isomer of bupivacaine.

Indications
Local anaesthesia, especially long-lasting anaesthesia after regional block injection.

Presentations
10 mL vials of 0.25%, 0.5% or 0.75% levobupivacaine for injection (containing 25, 50 and 75 mg bupivacaine respectively).

Dose
Recommended maximum dose is 1.3 mg/kg with an absolute ceiling of 90 mg.

Contraindications
Allergy to amide local anaesthetics.

Precautions
Reduce dose in hepatic disease.

Unwanted effects
Levo-bupivacaine is more cardiotoxic than lidocaine.

Drug interactions
The success of levobupivacaine when used as a regional (spinal) anaesthetic is reduced by concomitant administration of the anti-rheumatic drug indomethacin and in individuals who abuse alcohol (the mechanism is not understood). The depressant effect on the heart produced by levobupivacaine is exacerbated by calcium-channel blockers, but this is probably only important if accidental intravascular injection of the local anaesthetic occurs. As with lidocaine, beta-blocking drugs, especially propranolol, increase the plasma concentration of bupivacaine. Serum levels of levobupivacaine are also increased by diazepam. The toxicity of levobupivacaine has been reported to be increased when used in combination with mepivacaine (probably due to displacement of levobupivacaine from its binding sites).

Levodopa

Description
A dopaminergic drug.

Indications
Used in the treatment of Parkinsonism.

Effects on oral and dental structures
Xerostomia and taste disturbance may be produced. Long term combined use with carbidopa leads to Meige's syndrome (blepherospasm-oromandibular dystonia).

Effects on patient management
General anaesthesia and sedation are affected (see drug interactions below). Xerostomia may increase caries incidence and thus a preventive regimen is important. If the xerostomia is severe artificial saliva may be indicated. This drug may cause postural hypotension, thus the patient should not be changed from the supine to the standing position too rapidly. Parkinsonism can lead to management problems as the patient may have uncontrollable movement. Short appointments are recommended.

Drug interactions
Combined use with volatile anaesthetics such as halothane increase the risk of cardiac arrhythmias. The effect of levodopa is antagonized by some benzodiazepines including diazepam and by Vitamin B6 (pyridoxine). Monoamine oxidase inhibitors should not be used concurrently as life-threatening hypertension can occur.

Levofloxacin (Tavanic)

Description
A quinolone antibiotic.

Indications
Used to treat respiratory and urinary tract infections.

Effects on oral and dental structures
This drug can cause taste disturbance, xerostomia and Stevens–Johnson syndrome.

Effects on patient management
This drug may cause thrombocytopenia, leucopenia and anaemia. Thrombocytopenia may cause postoperative bleeding. If the platelet count is low (<100,000) then the socket should be packed and sutured. Persistent bleeding may require platelet transfusion. Leucopenia and anaemia may result in poor healing. Any anaemia will need correction prior to elective general anaesthesia and sedation.

Drug interactions
Combined therapy with non-steroidal anti-inflammatory drugs increases the risk of convulsions.

Levomepromazine/Methotrimeprazine (Nozinan)

Description
A phenothiazine antipsychotic medication.

Indications
Used in the treatment of psychoses such as schizophrenia and occasionally as an anti-emetic drug.

Effects on oral and dental structures
Xerostomia and uncontrollable oro-facial muscle activity (tardive dyskenesia) may be produced. The oral mucosa may be discoloured and have a bluish-grey appearance. Stevens–Johnson syndrome and lichenoid reactions may occur with this drug.

Effects on patient management
Xerostomia may increase caries incidence and thus a preventive regimen is important. If the xerostomia is severe artificial saliva may be indicated. Uncontrollable muscle movement of jaws and tongue as well as the underlying psychotic condition may interfere with management as satisfactory co-operation may not be achieved readily. There may be problems with denture retention and certain stages of denture construction (e.g. jaw registration) can be difficult. Postural

hypotension often occurs with this drug, therefore rapid changes in patient position should be avoided. This drug can produce leucocytosis, agranluocytosis and anaemia which may interfere with postoperative healing.

Drug interactions
There is increased sedation when used in combination with CNS depressant drugs such as alcohol, opioid analgesics and sedatives. Combined therapy with tricyclic antidepressants increases the chances of cardiac arrhythmias and exacerbates antimuscarinic effects such as xerostomia. The photosensitive effect of tetracyclines is increased during combined therapy. There is a theoretical risk of hypotension being exacerbated by the epinephrine in dental local anaesthetics.

Lidocaine/Lignocaine dental preparations (Lignostab, Lignospan, Xylocaine, Xylotox)

Description
An amide local anaesthetic.

Indications
Local anaesthesia (topical and by injection). Lidocaine with epinephrine is the 'gold standard' local anaesthetic for dental anaesthesia.

Presentations
  (i) 2.0 mL or 2.2 mL cartridges for injection of a 2% solution (containing 40 and 44 mg lidocaine respectively).
 (ii) 1.8 mL, 2.0 mL or 2.2 mL cartridges for injection of a 2% solution with 1 : 80,000 epinephrine [adrenaline] (containing 36, 40 and 44 mg lidocaine and 22.5, 25 and 27.5 μg epinephrine respectively).
(iii) Topical preparations containing 1%, 4%, 5% and 10% lidocaine for intra-oral use.
 (iv) As a component of EMLA cream which is a topical anaesthetic for skin use (EMLA is a 5% mixture of lidocaine and prilocaine).

Dose
Recommended maximum dose is 4.4 mg/kg with an absolute ceiling of 300 mg.

Contraindications
Allergy to amide local anaesthetics.
Acute porphyria.
EMLA should not be used in infants under one year of age.

Precautions

Reduce dose in hepatic disease.

Epinephrine-containing solutions have additional precautions (see epinephrine).

Unwanted effects

Central nervous and cardiovascular system depression at high dose.

Drug interactions

Lidocaine prolongs the period of apnoea produced by succinylcholine. Beta-adrenergic blocking drugs, especially propranolol, increase the toxicity of lidocaine by inhibiting the liver enzymes that metabolize the local anaesthetic. Similarly, the calcium channel blocker verapamil increases the toxicity of lidocaine. Midazolam reduces the central nervous system toxicity of lidocaine. Lidocaine and phenytoin both have depressant effects on the heart, the clinical relevance of this is probably only important at high doses. The protease inhibitor drugs used in the management of HIV appear to increase the plasma levels of lidocaine and potentially increase cardiotoxicity. Thus the use of alternative local anaesthetics or administration of minimal doses of lidocaine appears wise.

Lignocaine/Lidocaine dental preparations (Lignostab, Lignospan, Xylocaine, Xylotox)

Description

An amide local anaesthetic.

Indications

Local anaesthesia (topical and by injection). Lidocaine with epinephrine is the 'gold standard' local anaesthetic for dental anaesthesia.

Presentations

(i) 2.0 mL or 2.2 mL cartridges for injection of a 2% solution (containing 40 and 44 mg lidocaine respectively).

(ii) 1.8 mL, 2.0 mL or 2.2 mL cartridges for injection of a 2% solution with 1 : 80,000 epinephrine [adrenaline] (containing 36, 40, and 44 mg lidocaine and 22.5, 25 and 27.5 μg epinephrine respectively).

(iii) Topical preparations containing 1%, 4%, 5% and 10% lidocaine for intra-oral use.

(iv) As a component of EMLA cream which is a topical anaesthetic for skin use (EMLA is a 5% mixture of lidocaine and prilocaine).

Dose
Recommended maximum dose is 4.4 mg/kg with an absolute ceiling of 300 mg.

Contraindications
Allergy to amide local anaesthetics.

Acute porphyria.

EMLA should not be used in infants under one year of age.

Precautions
Reduce dose in hepatic disease.

Epinephrine-containing solutions have additional precautions (see epinephrine).

Unwanted effects
Central nervous and cardiovascular system depression at high dose.

Drug interactions
Lidocaine prolongs the period of apnoea produced by succinylcholine. Beta-adrenergic blocking drugs, especially propranolol, increase the toxicity of lidocaine by inhibiting the liver enzymes that metabolize the local anaesthetic. Similarly, the calcium-channel blocker verapamil increases the toxicity of lidocaine. Midazolam reduces the central nervous system toxicity of lidocaine. Lidocaine and phenytoin both have depressant effects on the heart, the clinical relevance of this is probably only important at high doses. The protease inhibitor drugs used in the management of HIV appear to increase the plasma levels of lidocaine and potentially increase cardiotoxicity. Thus the use of alternative local anaesthetics or administration of minimal doses of lidocaine appears wise.

Liothyronine sodium (Tertroxin)

Description
A thyroid hormone.

Indications
Hypothyroidism.

Effects on oral and dental structures
None reported.

Effects on patient management
High or excessive doses of liothyronine can induce a thyrotoxic state. The patient will be restless, agitated and excitable. In such circumstances, dental treatment will be difficult to complete.

Drug interactions
None of any dental significance.

Lisinopril (Zestril)

Description
Lisinopril is an ACE inhibitor, that is it inhibits the renal angiotensin converting enzyme which is necessary to convert angiotensin I to the more potent angiotensin II.

Indications
Mild to moderate hypertension, congestive heart failure, and post myocardial infarction where there is left ventricular dysfunction.

Effects on oral and dental structures
Lisinopril can cause taste disturbances, angioedema, dry mouth, glossitis, and lichenoid drug reactions. Many of these unwanted effects are dose related and compounded if there is an impairment of renal function.

Lisinopril-induced xerostomia increases the risk of fungal infections (candidiasis) and caries, especially root caries. Antifungal treatment should be used when appropriate and topical fluoride (e.g. Duraphat) will reduce the risk of root surface caries.

Effects on patient management
Lisinopril-induced angioedema is perhaps the most significant unwanted effect that impacts upon dental management, because dental procedures can induce the angioedema. Management of lisinopril-induced angioedema is problematic because the underlying mechanisms are poorly understood. Standard anti-anaphylactic treatment is of little value (epinephrine and hydrocortisone) because the angioedema is not mediated via mast cells or antibody/antigen interactions. Usually the angioedema subsides and patients on these drugs should be questioned as to whether they have experienced any problems with breathing or swallowing. This will alert the dental practitioner to the possible risk of this unwanted effect arising during dental treatment.

Lisinopril is also associated with suppression of bone marrow activity giving rise to possible neutropenia, agranulocytosis, thrombocytopenia, and aplastic anaemia. Patients on lisinopril who present with excessive bleeding of their gums, sore throats, or oral ulceration should have a full haematological investigation.

Drug interactions
Non-steroidal anti-inflammatory drugs (NSAIDs) such as ibuprofen may reduce the antihypertensive effect of lisinopril.

Lisuride maleaten (Revanil)

Description
A dopaminergic drug (an ergot derivative).

Indications
Used in the management of Parkinsonism.

Effects on oral and dental structures
None reported, but as other ergot derivatives can produce xerostomia this is a possibility.

Effects on patient management
This drug may cause postural hypotension, thus the patient should not be changed from the supine to the standing position too rapidly. Parkinsonism can lead to management problems as the patient may have uncontrollable movement. Short appointments are recommended.

Drug interactions
None of importance in dentistry.

Lithium salts [carbonate:citrate] (Camcolit, Liskonum, Priadel: Li-Liquid, Litarex, Priadel)

Description
An antimanic medication.

Indications
Used in the treatment of mania, depression, and manic depression.

Effects on oral and dental structures
Xerostomia, taste disturbance and lichenoid eruptions may be produced.

Effects on patient management
Xerostomia may increase caries incidence and thus a preventive regimen is important. If the xerostomia is severe artificial saliva may be indicated. These drugs can produce postural hypotension, thus the patient should be allowed time to equilibrate after alteration in position of the dental chair.

Drug interactions
Toxicity of lithium is increased by carbamazepine, phenytoin, metronidazole, and non-steroidal anti-inflammatory drugs (ketoralac should not be used concurrently).

Lofepramine (Gamanil)

Description
A tricyclic antidepressant.

Indications
Used in the management of depressive illness.

Effects on oral and dental structures
Xerostomia and taste disturbance may occur.

Effects on patient management
Xerostomia may increase caries incidence and thus a preventive regimen is important. If the xerostomia is severe artificial saliva may be indicated. Postural hypotension may occur with this drug, therefore rapid changes in patient position should be avoided. This drug may cause thrombocytopenia, agranulocytosis and leucopenia. Thrombocytopenia may cause postoperative bleeding. If the platelet count is low (<100,000) then the socket should be packed and sutured. Persistent bleeding may require platelet transfusion. Agranulocytosis and leucopenia may affect healing adversely.

Drug interactions
Increased sedation occurs with alcohol and sedative drugs such as benzodiazepines. This drug may antagonize the action of anticonvulsants such as carbamazepine and phenytoin. This drug increases the pressor effects of epinephrine. Nevertheless, the use of epinephrine-containing local anaesthetics is not contraindicated. However, epinephrine dose limitation is recommended.

Normal anticoagulant control by warfarin may be upset, both increases and decreases in INR have been noted during combined therapy with tricyclic antidepressants. Combined therapy with other antidepressants should be avoided and if prescribing another class of antidepressant a period of one to two weeks should elapse between changeover. Antimuscarinic effects such as xerostomia are increased when used in combination with other anticholinergic drugs such as antipsychotics.

Lofexadine hydrochloride (BritLofex)

Description
An anti-dependence drug.

Indications
Used during withdrawal from opioid dependence.

Effects on oral and dental structures
This drug produces a xerostomia.

Effects on patient management

The use of opioid analgesics must be avoided as patients receiving this medication are undergoing withdrawal from this group of drugs. Xerostomia may increase caries incidence and thus a preventive regimen is important. If the xerostomia is severe artificial saliva may be indicated. This drug may cause hypotension, thus the patient should not be changed from the supine to the standing position too rapidly.

Drug interactions

This drug enhances the sedative effects of anxiolytic and sedative drugs including alcohol and benzodiazepines.

Lomustine

Description

An alkylating agent.

Indications

Hodgkin's disease and certain solid tumours.

Effects on oral and dental structures

Lomustine causes bone marrow suppression with an accompanying thrombocytopenia and agranulocytosis. Bone marrow suppression can lead to troublesome oral ulceration, exacerbation of an existing periodontal condition, and rapid spread of any residual (e.g. periapical) infections.

Effects on patient management

The effect of lomustine on the bone marrow is transient and routine dental treatment is best avoided until the white blood cells and platelet counts start to recover. If emergency dental treatment such as an extraction is required then antibiotic cover may be necessary depending on the degree of myelosuppression. If the platelet count is low (<100,000) then the socket should be packed and sutured. Persistent bleeding may require a platelet transfusion.

Patients on chemotherapeutic agents such as lomustine often neglect their oral hygiene and thus there could be an increase in both caries and periodontal disease. If time permits, patients about to go on chemotherapy should have a dental check up and any potential areas of infection should be treated. Similarly, to reduce the mucosal irritation (sensitivity) that often accompanies chemotherapy, it is advisable to remove any ill-fitting dentures and smooth over rough cusps or restorations.

Drug interactions

None of any dental significance.

Loperamide hydrochloride (Imodium, Imodium plus)

Description
An antimotility drug.

Indications
Used in the management of acute diarrhoea.

Effects on oral and dental structures
Xerostomia can be produced.

Effects on patient management
As the drug is only used short term xerostomia should not produce significant problems, however a preventive regimen may be considered.

Drug interactions
The toxicity of central nervous system depressants such as opioid analgesics may be increased.

Loprazolam

Description
A benzodiazepine hypnotic.

Indications
Used as a short term treatment of insomnia.

Effects on oral and dental structures
Xerostomia is a side effect.

Effects on patient management
The main interaction in the management of patients receiving any benzodiazepine therapy is the use of benzodiazepine sedation. During short term use an additive effect will be noted, after long term benzodiazepine therapy tolerance occurs and large doses of benzodiazepines may be needed to achieve sedation. Also the confusion and amnesia that benzodiazepines produce may necessitate the presence of an escort.

Drug interactions
As with all benzodiazepines enhanced effects occur with combined therapy with other CNS depressants such as alcohol, other hypnotic or sedative agents, and opioid analgesics.

Loratadine (Clarityn)

Description
An antihistamine.

Indications
Used in the treatment of allergies such as hay fever.

Effects on oral and dental structures
May produce xerostomia, but this is less common compared to older antihistamines.

Effects on patient management
The patient may be drowsy and dizzy which may interfere with co-operation. Xerostomia may increase caries incidence and thus a preventive regimen is important. If the xerostomia is severe artificial saliva may be indicated.

Drug interactions
Erythromycin, ketoconazole and probably fluconazole increase the plasma concentration of loratidine. There is an enhanced sedative effect with anxiolytic and hypnotic drugs. Tricyclic and monoamine oxidase inhibitor antidepressants increase antimuscarinic effects such as xerostomia.

Lorazepam (Dalmane)

Description
A benzodiazepine anxiolytic.

Indications
Used in the short term treatment of anxiety, insomnia, and as a preoperative sedative.

Effects on oral and dental structures
Xerostomia can occur.

Effects on patient management
The main interaction in the management of patients receiving any benzodiazepine therapy is the use of benzodiazepine sedation. During short term use an additive effect will be noted, after long term benzodiazepine therapy tolerance occurs and large doses of benzodiazepines may be needed to achieve sedation. Also the confusion and amnesia that benzodiazepines produce may necessitate the presence of an escort. As the drug is only used short term xerostomia should not produce significant problems, however a preventive regimen may be considered.

Drug interactions
As with all benzodiazepines enhanced effects occur with combined therapy with other CNS depressants such as alcohol, other hypnotic or sedative agents, and opioid analgesics. Sodium valproate may raise the serum levels of lorazepam, leading to increased drowsiness.

Lormetazepam

Description
A benzodiazepine hypnotic.

Indications
Used in the short term treatment of insomnia.

Effects on oral and dental structures
Xerostomia may occur.

Effects on patient management
The main interaction in the management of patients receiving any benzodiazepine therapy is the use of benzodiazepine sedation. During short term use an additive effect will be noted, after long term benzodiazepine therapy tolerance occurs and large doses of benzodiazepines may be needed to achieve sedation. Also the confusion and amnesia that benzodiazepines produce may necessitate the presence of an escort. As the drug is only used short term xerostomia should not produce significant problems, however a preventive regimen may be considered.

Drug interactions
As with all benzodiazepines enhanced effects occur with combined therapy with other CNS depressants such as alcohol, other hypnotic or sedative agents and opioid analgesics.

Losartan (Cozaar)

Description
An angiotensin II receptor antagonist.

Indications
Used as an alternative to ACE inhibitors where the latter cannot be tolerated.

Effects on oral and dental structures
Angioedema has been reported, but the incidence of this unwanted effect is much less than when compared to ACE inhibitors.

Effects on patient management
None of any significance.

Drug interactions
NSAIDs such as ibuprofen may reduce the antihypertensive action of losartan.

Loxapine (Loxapac)

Description
A substituted benzamide antipsychotic medication.

Indications
Used in the treatment of psychoses.

Effects on oral and dental structures
Xerostomia and uncontrollable oro-facial muscle activity (tardive dyskenesia) may be produced.

Effects on patient management
Xerostomia may increase caries incidence and thus a preventive regimen is important. If the xerostomia is severe artificial saliva may be indicated. Uncontrollable muscle movement of jaws and tongue as well as the underlying psychotic condition may interfere with management as satisfactory co-operation may not be achieved readily. There may be problems with denture retention and certain stages of denture construction (e.g. jaw registration) can be difficult. Postural hypotension may occur with this drug, therefore rapid changes in patient position should be avoided. This drug can produce leucocytosis, agranluocytosis, and anaemia which may interfere with postoperative healing.

Drug interactions
There is increased sedation when used in combination with CNS depressant drugs such as alcohol, opioid analgesics, and sedatives. Combined therapy with tricyclic antidepressants increases the chances of cardiac arrhythmias and exacerbates antimuscarinic effects such as xerostomia. This drug may decrease the activity of phenytoin. Carbamazepine toxicity may be increased by loxapine. Carbamazepine and loxapine in combination may increase the incidence of Stevens–Johnson syndrome. There is a theoretical risk of hypotension being exacerbated by the epinephrine in dental local anaesthetics.

Lymecycline (Terasyl 300)

Description
A tetracycline antibiotic.

Indications
Used to treat bacterial infection.

Effects on oral and dental structures

Can produce oral candidiasis, lichenoid reactions, fixed drug eruptions, tooth staining, and discolouration of the tongue.

Effects on patient management

Antifungal therapy may be needed.

Drug interactions

Iron and zinc inhibit the absorption of tetracyclines. Tetracyclines reduce the efficacy of penicillins and cephalosporins. Tetracyclines may enhance the anticoagulant effect of warfarin and the other coumarin anticoagulants.

Macrogols (Movicol)

Description

A polyethylene glycol osmotic laxative.

Indications

Used to treat constipation.

Effects on oral and dental structures

None specific.

Effects on patient management

See drug interactions below.

Drug interactions

Avoid the use of codeine and other opioid compounds as they exacerbate constipation.

Magnesium carbonate (Algicon, Topal)

Description

An antacid.

Indications

Used to treat dyspepsia.

Effects on oral and dental structures

Patients may complain of a chalky taste. The underlying condition of reflux can lead to erosion of the teeth especially the palatal surfaces.

Effects on patient management

Patients may not be comfortable in the fully supine position due to gastric reflux. Any drug with which there is an interaction (such as tetracycline) should be taken a few hours in advance of antacid dose.

Drug interactions

There is a reduced absorption of phenytoin, tetracyclines, the non-steroidal analgesic diflunisal and the antifungal drugs ketoconazole and itraconazole. Antacids can increase the excretion of aspirin and reduce plasma concentration to non-therapeutic levels. The neuromuscular blocking activity of aminoglycoside antibiotics such as gentamycin is exacerbated by magnesium salts. There is a theoretical risk of respiratory arrest with combined therapy but this may only be of relevance with very young patients.

Magnesium hydroxide

Description

An osmotic laxative and used in combination with aluminium hydroxide in antacids.

Indications

Used to treat constipation.

Effects on oral and dental structures

Antacid preparations may produce a chalky taste.

Effects on patient management

Avoid the use of codeine and other opioid compounds as they exacerbate constipation.

Drug interactions

Decreased absorption of tetracyclines can occur. In antacid preparations there is reduced absorption of phenytoin, tetracyclines, the non-steroidal analgesic diflunisal, and the antifungal drugs ketoconazole and itraconazole. Antacids can increase the excretion of aspirin and reduce plasma concentration to non-therapeutic levels. The neuromuscular blocking activity of aminoglycoside antibiotics such as gentamycin is exacerbated by magnesium salts. There is a theoretical risk of respiratory arrest with combined therapy but this may only be of relevance with very young patients.

Magnesium sulphate

Description

An osmotic laxative.

Indications

Used to treat constipation.

Effects on oral and dental structures

None specific.

Effects on patient management

Avoid the use of codeine and other opioid compounds as they exacerbate constipation.

Drug interactions

Decreased absorption of tetracyclines can occur. The neuromuscular blocking activity of aminoglycoside antibiotics such as gentamycin is exacerbated by magnesium salts. There is a theoretical risk of respiratory arrest with combined therapy but this may only be of relevance with very young patients.

Magnesium trisilicate (Gastrocote, Gaviscon)

Description

An antacid.

Indications

Used to treat dyspepsia.

Effects on oral and dental structures

Patients may complain of a chalky taste. The underlying condition of reflux can lead to erosion of the teeth, especially the palatal surfaces.

Effects on patient management

Patients may not be comfortable in the fully supine position due to gastric reflux. Any drug with which there is an interaction (such as tetracycline) should be taken a few hours in advance of antacid dose.

Drug interactions

Combined therapy reduces absorption of phenytoin, tetracyclines, the non-steroidal analgesic diflunisal, and the antifungal drugs ketoconazole and itraconazole. Antacids can increase the excretion of aspirin and reduce plasma concentration to non-therapeutic levels. The neuromuscular blocking activity of aminoglycoside antibiotics such as gentamycin is exacerbated by magnesium salts. There is a theoretical risk of respiratory arrest with combined therapy but this may only be of relevance with very young patients.

Maprotiline hydrochloride (Ludiomil)

Description

A tetracyclic antidepressant drug.

Indications

Used in the management of depressive illness.

Effects on oral and dental structures

Xerostomia may occur but this is less troublesome than with traditional tricyclics.

Effects on patient management
Xerostomia may increase caries incidence and thus a preventive regimen is important. If the xerostomia is severe artificial saliva may be indicated. Postural hypotension may occur with this drug, therefore rapid changes in patient position should be avoided. This drug may cause thrombocytopenia, agranulocytosis and leucopenia. Thrombocytopenia may cause postoperative bleeding. If the platelet count is low (<100,000) then the socket should be packed and sutured. Persistent bleeding may require platelet transfusion. Agranulocytosis and leucopenia may affect healing adversely.

Drug interactions
Increased sedation with alcohol and sedative drugs such as benzodiazepines may occur. This drug increases the pressor effects of epinephrine. Nevertheless, the use of epinephrine-containing local anaesthetics is not contraindicated. However, epinephrine dose limitation is recommended. Combined therapy with other antidepressants should be avoided and if prescribing another class of antidepressant a period of one to two weeks should elapse between changeover. Antimuscarinic effects such as xerostomia are increased when used in combination with other anticholinergic drugs such as antipsychotics.

Mebendazole (Vermox)

Description
An antihelminthic drug.

Indications
Used in the management of threadworms.

Effects on oral and dental structures
None known.

Effects on patient management
None specific.

Drug interactions
Carbamazepine and phenytoin reduce serum mebendezole levels.

Mebeverine hydrochloride (Colofac, Fybogel)

Description
An antispasmodic drug.

Indications
Used for symptomatic relief in gastrointestinal disorders such as dyspepsia, diverticular disease, and irritable bowel syndrome.

Effects on oral and dental structures
None specific.

Effects on patient management
Patients may not be comfortable in fully supine condition due to underlying gastrointestinal disorder.

Drug interactions
None of importance in dentistry.

Meclozine hydrochloride

Description
An antihistamine.

Indications
Used in the treatment of motion sickness.

Effects on oral and dental structures
This drug can produce xerostomia.

Effects on patient management
As the drug is only used short term xerostomia should not produce significant problems, however a preventive regimen may be considered.

Drug interactions
Xerostomia is exacerbated by other antimuscarinic agents such as antidepressants.

Mecysteine hydrochloride (Visclair)

Description
A mucolytic drug.

Indications
Used in chronic bronchitis and asthma.

Effects on oral and dental structures
None specific.

Effects on patient management
Patients may not be comfortable in the supine position if they have respiratory problems. If the patient suffers from asthma then aspirin-like compounds should not be prescribed as many asthmatic patients are allergic to these analgesics. Similarly, sulphite-containing compounds (such as preservatives in epinephrine-containing local anaesthetics) can produce allergy in asthmatic patients. The use of a rubber dam in patients with obstructive airway disease may further embarrass

the airway. If a rubber dam is essential then supplemental oxygen via a nasal cannula may be required.

Drug interactions
None of importance in dentistry.

Mefenamic acid (Ponstan)

Description
A peripherally acting, non-steroidal anti-inflammatory analgesic.

Indications
Pain and inflammation associated with musculoskeletal disorders, e.g. rheumatoid arthritis, osteoarthritis, and ankylosing spondylitis. Dysmenorrhoea and menorrhagia.

Effects on oral and dental structures
Patients on long-term NSAIDs such as mefenamic acid may be afforded some degree of protection against periodontal breakdown. This arises from the drug's inhibitory action on prostaglandin synthesis. The latter is an important inflammatory mediator in the pathogenesis of periodontal breakdown.

Effects on patient management
Rare unwanted effects of mefenamic acid include angioedema and thrombocytopenia. The latter may cause an increased bleeding tendency following any dental surgical procedure. If the platelet count is low (<100,000) then the socket should be packed and sutured. Persistent bleeding may require a platelet transfusion.

Drug interactions
Ibuprofen, aspirin and diflunisal should be avoided in patients taking mefenamic acid due to an increase in unwanted effects, especially gastrointestinal ulceration, renal, and liver damage. Systemic corticosteroids increase the risk of peptic ulceration and gastrointestinal bleeding.

Mefloquine (Lariam)

Description
An antimalarial drug.

Indications
Used in the prophylaxis and treatment of malaria.

Effects on oral and dental structures
This drug may cause Stevens–Johnson syndrome.

Effects on patient management

This drug can cause leucopenia and thrombocytopenia. Leucopenia may affect healing adversely. Thrombocytopenia may cause postoperative bleeding. If the platelet count is low (<100,000) then the socket should be packed and sutured. Persistent bleeding may require platelet transfusion.

Drug interactions

Mefloquine antagonizes the effects of anticonvulsant drugs. Mefloquine levels in serum are increased by tetracycline but concurrent use may still be employed. Concurrent use with tricyclic anti depressants may cause bradycardia.

Meloxicam (Mobic)

Description

A peripherally acting, non-steroidal anti-inflammatory analgesic.

Indications

Pain and inflammation associated with musculoskeletal disorders, e.g. rheumatoid arthritis, osteoarthritis, and ankylosing spondylitis. Dysmenorrhoea and menorrhagia.

Effects on oral and dental structures

Patients on long-term NSAIDs such as meloxicam may be afforded some degree of protection against periodontal breakdown. This arises from the drug's inhibitory action on prostaglandin synthesis. The latter is an important inflammatory mediator in the pathogenesis of periodontal breakdown.

Effects on patient management

Rare unwanted effects of meloxicam include angioedema and thrombocytopenia. The latter may cause an increased bleeding tendency following any dental surgical procedure. If the platelet count is low (<100,000) then the socket should be packed and sutured. Persistent bleeding may require a platelet transfusion.

Drug interactions

Ibuprofen, aspirin, and diflunisal should be avoided in patients taking meloxicam due to an increase in unwanted effects, especially gastrointestinal ulceration, renal, and liver damage. Systemic corticosteroids increase the risk of peptic ulceration and gastrointestinal bleeding.

Melphalan (Alkeran)

Description
An alkylating agent.

Indications
Myelomatosis.

Effects on oral and dental structures
Melphalan causes bone marrow suppression with an accompanying thrombocytopenia and agranulocytosis. Bone marrow suppression can lead to troublesome oral ulceration, exacerbation of an existing periodontal condition, and rapid spread of any residual (e.g. periapical) infections.

Effects on patient management
The effect of melphalan on the bone marrow is transient and routine dental treatment is best avoided until the white blood cells and platelet counts start to recover. If emergency dental treatment such as an extraction is required then antibiotic cover may be necessary depending on the degree of myelosuppression. If the platelet count is low (<100,000) then the socket should be packed and sutured. Persistent bleeding may require a platelet transfusion.

Patients on chemotherapeutic agents such as melphalan often neglect their oral hygiene and thus there could be an increase in both caries and periodontal disease. If time permits, patients about to go on chemotherapy should have a dental check up and any potential areas of infection should be treated. Similarly, to reduce the mucosal irritation (sensitivity) that often accompanies chemotherapy, it is advisable to remove any ill-fitting dentures and smooth over rough cusps or restorations.

Drug interactions
None of any dental significance.

Mepacrine hydrochloride

Description
An antiprotozoal drug.

Indications
Used in the management of giardiasis and in the treatment of discoid lupus erythematosus.

Effects on oral and dental structures
Discolouration of oral mucosa (blue-black palate and yellowish mucosa) and lichenoid eruptions may occur.

Effects on patient management
This drug can produce anaemia and this may result in poor healing. Any anaemia will need correction prior to elective general anaesthesia and sedation.

Drug interactions
None of importance in dentistry.

Mepivacaine (Scandonest)

Description
An amide local anaesthetic.

Indications
Local anaesthesia by injection. Similar properties to lidocaine but with a slightly longer action of duration. The plain solution is more effective than plain lidocaine.

Presentations
(i) In 2.0 mL dental local anaesthetic cartridges as a 3% solution containing 60 mg mepivacaine.
(ii) In 2.0 mL dental local anaesthetic cartridges as a 2% solution with 1 : 100,000 epinephrine (adrenaline) containing 40 mg mepivacaine and 20 μg epinephrine.

Dose
The maximum recommended dose is 4.4 mg/kg with an absolute ceiling of 300 mg.

Contraindications
Allergy to amide local anaesthetics.

Precautions
Reduce dose in patients with liver disease.
Epinephrine-containing solutions have additional precautions (see epinephrine).

Unwanted effects
Central nervous and cardiovascular system depression at high dose.

Drug interactions
Mepivacaine increases the toxicity of bupivacaine, probably by displacing the latter drug from its binding sites.

Meprobamate (Equagesic)

Description
An anxiolytic drug.

Indications
Occasionally used in the short-term management of anxiety and as a muscle relaxant, but is not used much these days.

Effects on oral and dental structures
Xerostomia, stomatitis, purpura, lichenoid reactions, and Stevens–Johnson syndrome may occur.

Effects on patient management
The patient is anxious, therefore short appointments are best. Thrombocytopenia and agranulocytosis may be produced by meprobamate. Thrombocytopenia may cause postoperative bleeding. If the platelet count is low (<100,000) then the socket should be packed and sutured. Persistent bleeding may require platelet transfusion. Agranulocytosis may result in poor healing.

Drug interactions
Increased effects of other CNS depressants, including alcohol can occur.

Meptazinol (Meptid)

Description
As opioid analgesic.

Indications
Moderate to severe pain.

Effects on oral and dental structures
Can cause xerostomia leading to an increased risk of root caries, candidal infections, and poor denture retention.

Effects on patient management
Meptazinol is a drug of dependence and can thus cause withdrawal symptoms if the medication is stopped abruptly. Such cessation of meptazinol may account for unusual behavioural changes and poor compliance with dental treatment. The drug also depresses respiration and causes postural hypotension. If the xerostomia is severe, dentate patients should receive topical fluoride and be offered an artificial saliva.

Drug interactions
Meptazinol will enhance the sedative properties of midazolam and diazepam. Reduce the dose of both sedative agents.

Mercaptopurine (Puri-Nethol)

Description
An antimetabolic drug.

Indications

Acute leukaemias, inflammatory bowel disease.

Effects on oral and dental structures

Mercaptopurine causes bone marrow suppression with an accompanying thrombocytopenia and agranulocytosis. Bone marrow suppression can lead to troublesome oral ulceration, exacerbation of an existing periodontal condition and rapid spread of any residual (e.g. periapical) infections.

Effects on patient management

The effect of mercaptopurine on the bone marrow is transient and routine dental treatment is best avoided until the white blood cells and platelet counts start to recover. If emergency dental treatment such as an extraction is required then antibiotic cover may be necessary depending on the degree of myelosuppression. If the platelet count is low (<100,000) then the socket should be packed and sutured. Persistent bleeding may require a platelet transfusion.

Patients on chemotherapeutic agents such as mercaptopurine often neglect their oral hygiene and thus there could be an increase in both caries and periodontal disease. If time permits, patients about to go on chemotherapy should have a dental check up and any potential areas of infection should be treated. Similarly, to reduce the mucosal irritation (sensitivity) that often accompanies chemotherapy, it is advisable to remove any ill-fitting dentures and smooth over rough cusps or restorations.

Drug interactions

None of any dental significance.

Meropenem (Meronem)

Description

A beta-lactam antibiotic.

Indications

Used to treat multi-drug resistant infections.

Effects on oral and dental structures

This is a broad spectrum antibiotic and thus oral candidiasis and glossitis may be produced.

Effects on patient management

Antifungal therapy may be required. This drug may cause thrombocytopenia, neutropenia, and anaemia. Thrombocytopenia may cause postoperative bleeding. If the platelet count is low (<100,000) then the socket should be packed and sutured. Persistent bleeding may require platelet transfusion. Neutropenia and anaemia may result in poor healing. Any anaemia will need correction prior to elective general anaesthesia and sedation.

Drug interactions
Probenecid interferes with the excretion of meropenem.

Mesalazine (Asacol, Pentasa, Salofalk)

Description
An aminosalicylate.

Indications
Used in the management of ulcerative colitis.

Effects on oral and dental structures
May produce lupus erythematosus.

Effects on patient management
Non-steroidal inflammatory drugs are best avoided. In order to avoid pseudomembranous ulcerative colitis discussion with the supervising physician is advised prior to prescription of an antibiotic.

The aminosalicylates can produce blood dyscrasias including anaemia, leucopenia, and thrombocytopenia. Anaemia may result in poor healing. Any anaemia will need correction prior to elective general anaesthesia and sedation. Leucopenia will affect healing adversely, if severe prophylactic antibiotics should be prescribed to cover surgical procedures. Thrombocytopenia may cause postoperative bleeding. If the platelet count is low (<100,000) then the socket should be packed and sutured. Persistent bleeding may require platelet transfusion. Patients may be receiving steroids in addition to aminosalicylates and thus the occurrence of adrenal crisis should be borne in mind.

Drug interactions
See comment on non-steroidals above.

Mesterolone (Pro-Viron)

Description
An ester of testosterone.

Indications
Androgen deficiency and male infertility associated hypogonadism.

Effects on oral and dental structures
None reported.

Effects on patient management
Mesterolone can cause significant behavioural changes, especially if misused. Patients may become aggressive, depressed or more anxious.

All changes can have an impact on the delivery and acceptance of dental care.

Drug interactions
None of any dental significance.

Metformin hydrochloride (Glucophage)

Description
A biguanide oral antidiabetic drug.

Indications
Diabetes mellitus.

Effects on oral and dental structures
Metformin does cause taste disorders and patients on the drug may complain of a metallic taste. The drug also interferes with the absorption of Vitamin B_{12}. Such a deficiency could lead to a glossitis and paraesthesis of the lips.

Effects on patient management
Although hypoglycaemia is less of a problem with the biguanides than the sulphonylureas, it is always wise to check that patients have both taken their medication and eaten prior to dental treatment. If there is any doubt, give the patient a glucose drink. As with any diabetic patient, try and treat in the first half of the morning and always ensure that any dental treatment does not prevent the patient from eating. If a patient on metformin requires a general anaesthetic then refer to hospital.

Drug interactions
Systemic corticosteroids antagonize the hypoglycaemic actions of metformin. If these drugs required, then consult the patient's physician before prescribing.

Methadone hydrochloride (Methadose, Physeptone)

Description
An opioid analgesic.

Indications
Severe pain, cough suppressant in terminal illness; used extensively in the treatment of opioid dependence.

Effects on oral and dental structures
Can cause xerostomia leading to an increased risk of root caries, candidal infections, and poor denture retention. When methadone is

used as substitution therapy in opioid dependence it is administered in the form of a thick syrup with a high sugar content. This is to prevent the drug from being injected and to allow the dosage to be titrated to each individual's need with ease. Although sugar-free preparations are available, they do not have the advantages of the syrup. There is a significant risk of 'methadone-induced caries' and patients undergoing this treatment should be aware of the risk and afforded the appropriate anti-caries treatment.

Effects on patient management

Methadone is a drug of dependence and can thus cause withdrawal symptoms if the medication is stopped abruptly. Such cessation of methadone may account for unusual behavioural changes and poor compliance with dental treatment. The drug also depresses respiration and causes postural hypotension. Patients on methadone substitution therapy must be regularly screened for increased susceptibility to caries. Opioids should not be prescribed.

Drug interactions

Methadone will enhance the sedative properties of midazolam and diazepam. Reduce the dose of both sedative agents. Carbamazepine and phenytoin decrease the efficacy of methadone by increasing its metabolism. Methadone increases the concentration of the antiviral drug zidovudine. Conversely the antiviral agent ritonavir decreases the plasma concentration of methadone. Concurrent use of monoamine oxidase inhibitors should be avoided.

Methenamine hippurate [Hexamine hippurate] (Hiprex)

Description

An antibiotic.

Indications

Used in the treatment of urinary tract infections.

Effects on oral and dental structures

This drug may cause stomatitis.

Effects on patient management

This drug causes gastrointestinal discomfort including nausea and vomiting, thus the patient may be uncomfortable in the fully supine position.

Drug interactions

None of importance in dentistry.

Methotrexate

Description
An antimetabolic drug.

Indications
Maintenance therapy for childhood acute leukaemias, choriocarcinoma, non-Hodgkin's lymphoma, meningeal cancer, rheumatoid arthritis, and psoriasis.

Effects on oral and dental structures
Methotrexate causes bone marrow suppression with an accompanying thrombocytopenia and agranulocytosis. Bone marrow suppression can lead to troublesome oral ulceration, exacerbation of an existing periodontal condition, and rapid spread of any residual (e.g. periapical) infections.

Effect on patient management
The effect of methotrexate on the bone marrow is transient and routine dental treatment is best avoided until the white blood cells and platelet counts start to recover. If emergency dental treatment such as an extraction is required then antibiotic cover may be necessary depending on the degree of myelosuppression. If the platelet count is low (<100,000) then the socket should be packed and sutured. Persistent bleeding may require a platelet transfusion.

Patients on chemotherapeutic agents such as methotrexate often neglect their oral hygiene and thus there could be an increase in both caries and periodontal disease. If time permits, patients about to go on chemotherapy should have a dental check up and any potential areas of infection should be treated. Similarly, to reduce the mucosal irritation (sensitivity) that often accompanies chemotherapy, it is advisable to remove any ill-fitting dentures and smooth over rough cusps or restorations.

Drug interactions
Aspirin and NSAIDs such as ibuprofen reduce the excretion of methotrexate and thus increase toxicity. These drugs should be avoided in patients medicated with methotrexate. Systemic corticosteroids increase the risk of methotrexate-induced haematological toxicity and should also be avoided. Penicillins reduce the renal excretion of methotrexate and thus significantly increase the risk of toxicity. These antibiotics are contraindicated.

Methotrimeprazine/Levomepromazine (Nozinan)

Description
A phenothiazine antipsychotic medication.

Indications
Used in the treatment of psychoses such as schizophrenia and occasionally as an anti-emetic drug.

Effects on oral and dental structures
Xerostomia and uncontrollable oro-facial muscle activity (tardive dyskenesia) may be produced. The oral mucosa may be discoloured and have a bluish-grey appearance. Stevens–Johnson syndrome and lichenoid reactions may occur with this drug.

Effects on patient management
Xerostomia may increase caries incidence and thus a preventive regimen is important. If the xerostomia is severe artificial saliva may be indicated. Uncontrollable muscle movement of jaws and tongue as well as the underlying psychotic condition may interfere with management as satisfactory co-operation may not be achieved readily. There may be problems with denture retention and certain stages of denture construction (e.g. jaw registration) can be difficult. Postural hypotension often occurs with this drug, therefore rapid changes in patient position should be avoided. This drug can produce leucocytosis, agranluocytosis, and anaemia which may interfere with postoperative healing.

Drug interactions
There is increased sedation when used in combination with CNS depressant drugs such as alcohol, opioid analgesics, and sedatives. Combined therapy with tricyclic antidepressants increases the chances of cardiac arrhythmias and exacerbates antimuscarinic effects such as xerostomia. The photosensitive effect of tetracyclines is increased during combined therapy. There is a theoretical risk of hypotension being exacerbated by the epinephrine in dental local anaesthetics.

Methylcellulose (Celevac)

Description
A bulk-forming laxative.

Indications
Used to treat constipation and in the management of obesity.

Effects on oral and dental structures
None specific.

Effects on patient management
See drug interactions below.

Drug interactions
Avoid the use of codeine and other opioid compounds as they exacerbate constipation.

Methyldopa (Aldomet)

Description
A centrally acting anti-hypertensive drug.

Indications
Hypertension (used in conjunction with a diuretic in hypertensive crisis).

Effects on oral and dental structure
Xerostomia can occur leading to an increased risk of root caries, candidal infections, and poor denture retention. Lichenoid eruptions and discolouration of the tongue (rare) may be produced. Nasal obstruction can occur giving rise to an increased tendency to mouth breath. Rarely causes Vitamin B_{12} and folate deficiency which can cause sore tongue.

Effects on patient management
Can cause depression of the bone marrow leading to agranulocytosis and thrombocytopenia. The latter will result in impaired haemostasis. If the platelet count is low (<100,000) then the socket should be packed and sutured. Persistent bleeding may require a platelet transfusion. If the xerostomia is severe, dentate patients should receive topical fluoride and be offered an artificial saliva.

Drug interactions
NSAIDs such as ibuprofen and systemic corticosteroids may antagonize hypotensive actions of methyldopa.

Methylphenidate hydrochloride (Equasym, Ritalin)

Description
A central nervous stimulant.

Indications
Used in the management of attention deficit disorder in children and in the treatment of narcolepsy.

Effects on oral and dental structures
This drug may produce xerostomia. Stevens–Johnson syndrome may occur.

Effects on patient management

Dose reduction of epinephrine in dental local anaesthetics is advisable (see drug interaction below). The underlying condition may make compliance for prolonged procedures under local anaesthesia difficult. Xerostomia may increase caries incidence and thus a preventive regimen is important. If the xerostomia is severe, artificial saliva may be indicated. This drug may cause thrombocytopenia, and leucopenia. Thrombocytopenia may cause postoperative bleeding. If the platelet count is low (<100,000) then the socket should be packed and sutured. Persistent bleeding may require platelet transfusion. Leucopenia may affect healing adversely.

Drug interactions

Combined therapy with monoamine oxidase inhibitors can produce a hypertensive crisis. Methylphenidate inhibits the metabolism of tricyclic antidepressants. The unwanted effects of epinephrine in dental local anaesthetics will be enhanced during combined therapy. Methylphenidate increases the analgesic effect of morphine while reducing the sedative action of the opioid. Methylphenidate occasionally increases the toxicity of phenytoin.

Methylphenobarbital (Prominal)

Description

An anticonvulsant drug.

Indications

Used in the management of epilepsy.

Effects on oral and dental structures

Xerostomia, fixed drug eruptions and Stevens–Johnson syndrome can be produced.

Effects on patient management

Xerostomia may increase caries incidence and thus a preventive regimen is important. If the xerostomia is severe, artificial saliva may be indicated. Epileptic fits are possible especially if the patient is stressed, therefore sympathetic handling and perhaps sedation should be considered for stressful procedures. Emergency anticonvulsant medication (diazepam or midazolam) must be available.

Drug interactions

The effects of barbiturates are increased by alcohol and other central nervous system depressants. The effects of barbiturates are decreased by folic acid. Barbiturates decrease the effects of the antimicrobials chloramphenicol, doxycycline, griseofulvin, indinavir, metronidazole, nelfiavir and saquinavir, anticoagulants including warfarin, corticosteroids, and oral contraceptives. They possibly reduce the effectiveness of paracetamol.

Methylprednisolone (Medrone)

Description
A corticosteroid.

Indications
Suppression of inflammation and allergic disorders. Used in the management of inflammatory bowel diseases, asthma, immunosuppression, and in various rheumatic diseases.

Effects on oral and dental structures
Although systemic corticosteroids can induce cleft lip and palate formation in mice, there is little evidence that this unwanted effect occurs in humans. The main impact of systemic corticosteroids on the mouth is to cause an increased susceptibility to opportunistic infections. These include candidiasis and those due to herpes viruses. The anti-inflammatory and immunosuppressant properties of corticosteroids may afford the patient some degree of protection against periodontal breakdown. Paradoxically long-term systemic use can precipitate osteoporosis. The latter is now regarded as a risk factor for periodontal disease.

Effects on patient management
The main unwanted effect of corticosteroid treatment is the suppression of the adrenal cortex and the possibility of an adrenal crisis when such patients are subjected to 'stressful events'. Whilst such suppression does occur physiologically, its clinical significance does appear to be overstated. As far as dentistry is concerned, there is increasing evidence that supplementary corticosteroids are not required. This would apply to all restorative procedures, periodontal surgery and uncomplicated dental extractions. For more complicated dento-alveolar surgery, each case must be judged on its merit. An apprehensive patient may well require cover. It is important to monitor the patient's blood pressure before, during and for 30 minutes after the procedure. If diastolic pressure drops by more than 25%, then hydrocortisone 100 mg IV should be administered and the patient's blood should continue to be monitored.

Patients should be screened regularly for oral infections such as fungal or viral infections. When these occur, they should be treated promptly with the appropriate chemotherapeutic agent. Likewise, any patient on corticosteroids that presents with an acute dental infection should be treated urgently as such infections can readily spread.

Drug interactions

Aspirin and NSAIDs should not be prescribed to patients on long-term corticosteroids. Both drugs are ulcerogenic and hence increase the risk of gastrointestinal bleeding and ulceration. The antifungal agent amphotericin increases the risk of corticosteroid-induced hypokalaemia, whilst ketoconazole inhibits corticosteroid hepatic metabolism.

Methysergide (Deseril)

Description
A serotonin antagonist.

Indications
Used in the prophylaxis of vascular headache such as migraine and cluster headache.

Effects on oral and dental structures
None specific.

Effects on patient management
This drug may cause postural hypotension, thus the patient should not be changed from the supine to the standing position too rapidly. Avoid stimuli which may induce migraine, such as directly shining the dental light in the patient's eyes. The use of dark glasses may be of benefit to the patient.

Drug interactions
None of importance in dentistry.

Metoclopramide hydrochloride (Gastrobid Continus, Gastromax, Maxolon) [Also found in combination with analgesics in Migraleve, MigraMax, Paramax]

Description
An anti-emetic drug.

Indications
Used in the management of nausea and vomiting; also used in combination with analgesics in anti-migraine drugs.

Effects on oral and dental structures
This drug can produce xerostomia and uncontrollable movement of the oro-facial musculature (the latter is most commonly seen in children).

Effects on patient management

Xerostomia may increase caries incidence and thus a preventive regimen is important. If the xerostomia is severe, artificial saliva may be indicated. The underlying condition may increase the incidence of dental erosion, especially of the palatal surfaces of teeth. Patients may be uncomfortable in the fully supine position as a result of their underlying gastrointestinal disorder.

Drug interactions

This drug accelerates the absorption of aspirin, paracetamol, and diazepam, enhancing their effects. Metoclopramide increase the absorption of tetracyclines but this is of little clinical importance. Opioids antagonize the gastrointestinal effects of metoclopramide.

Metoprolol (Betaloc, Lopressor)

Description

A selective β adrenoceptor blocking drug.

Indications

Hypertension, angina, arrhythmias, migraine prophylaxis, and adjunctive treatment in thyrotoxicosis.

Effects on oral and dental structures

Xerostomia and lichenoid eruptions may be produced.

Effects on patient management

Xerostomia will make the dentate patient more susceptible to dental caries (especially root caries) and will cause problems with denture retention. If the xerostomia is severe, dentate patients should receive topical fluoride and be offered an artificial saliva. Postural hypotension may occur and patients may feel dizzy when the dental chair is restored to upright after they have been treated in the supine position.

Drug interactions

NSAIDs such as ibuprofen may antagonize the hypotensive action of metoprolol: there is a possible interaction between epinephrine and metoprolol which may cause a slight transient increase in blood pressure. Do not exceed more than 3 cartridges of epinephrine-containing local anaesthetic solution per adult patient.

Metronidazole (Anabact, Elyzol Flagyl, Metrogel, Metrolyl, Metrotop, Rozex, Zadstat)

Description

A nitroimidazole antimicrobial drug.

Indications
Anaerobic bacterial infections such as dental abscesses, acute pericoronitis and acute ulcerative gingivitis.

Presentations
(i) 200 mg and 400 mg tablets.

(ii) An oral suspension (200 mg/5 mL).

(iii) An intravenous infusion (5 mg/mL).

(iv) A topical preparation for application in the gingival sulcus.

(v) 500 mg suppositories.

Dose
400 mg orally three times daily for 7 days, or 500 mg twice daily intravenously.

Contraindications
Hypersensitivity.

High doses contraindicated in pregnancy and during breastfeeding.

Precautions
Avoid alcohol as severe side effects occur (disulfiram-like [antabuse] reaction).

Liver disease.

Unwanted effects
Hypersensitivity reactions.

Blackening of tongue.

Altered (metallic) taste.

Gastrointestinal upset.

Headache, dizziness, and ataxia.

Dark urine.

Prolonged therapy can produce seizures, neuropathy, and leucopenia.

Drug interactions
The disulfiram reaction with alcohol is very unpleasant. This is caused by metronidazole inhibiting the metabolism of alcohol, leading to a build-up of aldehydes which produce nausea and vomitting. Similarly, metronidazole interacts with disulfiram and can cause psychosis and confusion. In addition a disulfiram-like reaction may occur during concurrent therapy with the antiviral agent ritinovir. Ritinovir increases the serum level of metronidazole.

The anticoagulant effect of warfarin is significantly increased by metronidazole. The anti-cholesterol drug cholestyramine and the antacid aluminium hydroxide reduce the absorption of metronidazole and thus dosing of these agents should be separated. Corticosteroids and barbiturates increase metronidazole loss and increased dosing of the antimicrobial is necessary. Similarly rifampicin increases the loss of metronidazole but the importance of this is unknown.

Metronidazole may increase the serum levels of carbamazepine and increase the toxicity of the latter drug. Similarly, plasma levels of phenytoin rise with combined therapy with metronidazole. Metronidazole may decrease the efficacy of oral contraceptives and other means of contraception are advised during antibiotic therapy. Metronidazole may increase serum ciclosporin levels and combined therapy should be closely monitored. Metronidazole increases the toxicity of lithium carbonate and the cytotoxic drug 5-fluorouracil.

Mequitazine (Primalan)

Description
An antihistamine.

Indications
Used in the treatment of allergies such as hay fever and urticaria.

Effects on oral and dental structures
This drug can produce xerostomia.

Effects on patient management
Patient may be drowsy which may interfere with co-operation. Xerostomia may increase caries incidence and thus a preventive regimen is important. If the xerostomia is severe, artificial saliva may be indicated.

Drug interactions
Enhanced sedative effect with anxiolytic and hypnotic drugs. Tricyclic and monoamine oxidase inhibitor antidepressants increase antimuscarinic effects such as xerostomia.

Mianserin hydrochloride

Description
An antidepressant drug related to the tricyclic group.

Indications
Used in the management of depressive illness.

Effects on oral and dental structures
Xerostomia may occur but this is less troublesome than with traditional tricyclics. Facial oedema and glossitis may be produced.

Effects on patient management
Xerostomia may increase caries incidence and thus a preventive regimen is important. If the xerostomia is severe, artificial saliva may be indicated. Postural hypotension may occur with this drug, therefore rapid changes in patient position should be avoided. This drug

may cause anaemia, thrombocytopenia, agranulocytosis, and leuco-penia. Any anaemia will need correction prior to elective general anaesthesia and sedation. Thrombocytopenia may cause postopera-tive bleeding. If the platelet count is low (<100,000) then the socket should be packed and sutured. Persistent bleeding may require plate-let transfusion. Anaemia, agranulocytosis, and leucopenia may affect healing adversely.

Drug interactions
Increased sedation occurs with alcohol and sedative drugs such as benzodiazepines. This drug increases the pressor effects of epinephrine. Nevertheless, the use of epinephrine-containing local anaesthetics is not contraindicated. However, epinephrine dose limitation is recom-mended. Combined therapy with other antidepressants should be avoided and if prescribing another class of antidepressant a period of one to two weeks should elapse between changeover. Antimuscarinic effects such as xerostomia are increased when used in combination with other anticholinergic drugs such as antipsychotics. Mianserin may upset the anticoagulant effect of warfarin, both increases and decreases in INR have been noted. Carbamazepine and phenytoin accelerate the metabolism of mianserin and the antidepressant antagonizes the effects of the anticonvulsants.

Miconazole (Daktarin, Dumicoat)

Description
An imidazole antifungal agent.

Indications
The treatment of oral fungal infections. It is also active against some bacteria including streptococci and staphylococci.

Presentations
(i) An oral gel (25 mg/mL).
(ii) In a cream at a concentration of 2% in combination with 1% hydrocortisone.
(iii) A 250 mg tablet.
(iv) A denture lacquer (50 mg/g).

Dose
5–10 mL of the gel held over the lesion four times daily (alternatively suck a 250 mg tablet four times daily).

Contraindications
Previous hypersensitivity (plus see important drug interactions below).
History of porphyria.
Best avoided in pregnancy.

Unwanted effects

Hypersensitivity reactions may occur.
Gastrointestinal disturbances.

Drug interactions

Miconazole should not be prescribed to patients receiving the anti-histamines astemizole and terfenadine as cardiac dysryhthmias may occur. Miconazole enhances the anticoagulant effect of warfarin even after topical use. Miconazole increases the anti-epileptic effects of phenytoin and increases the plasma concentrations of the sulphony-lurea oral hypoglycaemics and the benzodiazepine midazolam. Miconazole also increases the plasma concentration of ciclosporin by inhibiting the metabolism of this immunosuppressant. Miconazole inhibits the metabolism of the anti-spasmodic drug cisapride and this can lead to ventricular arrhythmias. Miconazole and ampho-tericin antagonize each others' antifungal action.

Midazolam (Hypnovel)

Description

A benzodiazepine sedative.

Indications

Used in dental sedation.

Presentations

(i) 2 mL vial containing 5 mg/mL.

(ii) 5 mL vial containing 2 mg/mL.

Dose

Injection of 1 mg increments until satisfactory sedation obtained. The dose must be titrated to the individual patient (usual dose is in range 0.05–0.1 mg/kg).

Contraindications

Respiratory depression.

Precautions

Respiratory disease.
Children.

Unwanted effects

Respiratory depression.

Drug interactions

Drugs which produces CNS depression, including alcohol and opioid analgesics, will exacerbate the CNS depressant properties of mida-zolam and combined administration should be avoided. Erythromy-cin inhibits the metabolism of midazolam and combined therapy can result in profound sedation. The effect of midazolam is also increased by the antifungal drugs itraconazole, ketoconazole, and fluconazole, the antiviral drugs efavirenz, indinavir, nelfinavir, ritonavir and saquinavir, the calcium-channel blockers diltiezam and verapamil, aspirin, baclofen, cimetidine, diclofenac, disulfiram, the cannibinoid nabilone, probenecid, and possibly by the ulcer-healing drug omeprazole. The interaction with the antiviral drugs efavirenz, indinavir, nelfinavir, ritonavir, and saquinavir is such that concurrent use should be avoided.

The sedative effects of midazolam and propofol when administered concurrently are more than additive. Flumazenil antagonizes the action of midazolam and is used in dental practice to reverse the effects of the latter drug as an emergency measure. The effect of midazolam may be antagonized by aminophylline. Midazolam reduces the serum concentration of lidocaine (this effect does not occur with all local anaesthetics). Midazolam may increase recovery from the effects of the neuromuscular blocking drugs atracurium and vecuronium. Profound hypotension is a risk if midazolam is administered with sufentanil.

Milrinone (Primacor)

Description
A selective phosphodiesterase inhibitor.

Indications
Severe congestive heart failure – usually prescribed to patients awaiting heart transplantation.

Effects on oral and dental structures
None known.

Effect on patient management
Patients on milrinone will be severely compromised from their cardiac condition and will only seek emergency dental treatment. In such instances there should be a limitation on the use of epinephrine containing local anaesthetic solution (no more than 3 cartridges per adult patient).

Drug interactions
None of any dental significance.

Minocycline (Minocin MR)

Description
A tetracycline antibiotic.

Indications

Used to treat bacterial infections.

Effects on oral and dental structures

Can produce oral candidiasis, lichenoid reactions, fixed drug eruptions, lupus erythematosus, tooth staining, and discolouration of the tongue.

Effects on patient management

Antifungal therapy may be needed.

Drug interactions

Iron and zinc inhibit the absorption of tetracyclines. Tetracyclines reduce the efficacy of penicillins and cephalosporins. Tetracyclines may enhance the anticoagulant effect of warfarin and the other coumarin anticoagulants.

Minoxidil (Loniten)

Description

A vasodilator antihypertensive drug.

Indications

Used in conjunction with diuretics and beta-blockers in the management of severe hypertension.

Effects on oral and dental structures

This drug is a rare cause of erythema multiforme.

Effects on patient management

Can cause a thrombocytopenia leading to impaired haemostasis after dental surgical procedures.

Drug interactions

NSAIDs such as ibuprofen may enhance the hypotensive actions of minoxidil.

Mirtazapine (Zispin)

Description

A tetracyclic antidepressant drug.

Indications

Used in the management of depression.

Effects on oral and dental structures

Stomatitis, aphthous ulceration, candidiasis, gingival bleeding, lingual oedema, xerostomia, and salivary gland swelling may all occur.

Effects on patient management

Xerostomia may increase caries incidence and thus a preventive regimen is important. If the xerostomia is severe, artificial saliva may be indicated. Local measures for the ease of ulceration, stomatitis, and candidiasis may be required. Postural hypotension may occur with this drug, therefore rapid changes in patient position should be avoided. This drug causes a degree of sedation and this might interfere with compliance during treatment. Dose reduction of dental sedatives is required (see drug interactions below). This drug may cause thrombocytopenia, agranulocytosis, and leucopenia. Thrombocytopenia may cause postoperative bleeding. If the platelet count is low (<100,000) then the socket should be packed and sutured. Persistent bleeding may require platelet transfusion. Agranulocytosis and leucopenia may affect healing adversely.

Drug interactions

Combined therapy with other antidepressants should be avoided and if prescribing another class of antidepressant a period of one to two weeks should elapse between changeover. This drug enhances the sedative effects of hypnotics and anxiolytics such as benzodiazepines.

Misoprostol (Cytotec)

Description
A synthetic prostaglandin.

Indications
Used in the management of gastrointestinal ulceration.

Effects on oral and dental structures
If the underlying condition is associated with gastric reflux erosion of the teeth may be a problem.

Effects on patient management
Although this drug can protect against ulceration produced by non-steroidal anti-inflammatory drugs the use of the latter is best avoided. High dose systemic steroids should not be prescribed in patients with gastrointestinal ulceration.

Drug interactions
Misoprostol increases the gastrointestinal side effects (such as pain and nausea) produced by both diclofenac and indomethacin.

Mitomycin

Description
A cytotoxic antibiotic.

Indications
Upper gastrointestinal tract cancers, breast cancer, and bladder cancer.

Effects on oral and dental structures
Mitomycin causes bone marrow suppression with an accompanying thrombocytopenia and agranulocytosis. Bone marrow suppression can lead to troublesome oral ulceration, exacerbation of an existing periodontal condition, and rapid spread of any residual (e.g. periapical) infections.

Effects on patient management
The effect of mitomycin on the bone marrow is transient and routine dental treatment is best avoided until the white blood cells and platelet counts start to recover. If emergency dental treatment such as an extraction is required then antibiotic cover may be necessary depending on the degree of myelosuppression. If the platelet count is low (<100,000) then the socket should be packed and sutured. Persistent bleeding may require a platelet transfusion.

Patients on chemotherapeutic agents such as mitomycin often neglect their oral hygiene and thus there could be an increase in both caries and periodontal disease. If time permits, patients about to go on chemotherapy should have a dental check up and any potential areas of infection should be treated. Similarly, to reduce the mucosal irritation (sensitivity) that often accompanies chemotherapy, it is advisable to remove any ill-fitting dentures and smooth over rough cusps or restorations.

Drug interactions
None of any dental significance.

Mitoxantrone (Novantrone)

Description
A cytotoxic antibiotic.

Indications
Breast cancer.

Effects on oral and dental structures
Mitoxantrone causes bone marrow suppression with an accompanying thrombocytopenia and agranulocytosis. Bone marrow suppression can lead to troublesome oral ulceration, exacerbation of an existing periodontal condition, and rapid spread of any residual (e.g. periapical) infections.

Effects on patient management
The effect of mitoxantrone on the bone marrow is transient and routine dental treatment is best avoided until the white blood cells

and platelet counts start to recover. If emergency dental treatment such as an extraction is required then antibiotic cover may be necessary depending on the degree of myelosuppression. If the platelet count is low (<100,000) then the socket should be packed and sutured. Persistent bleeding may require a platelet transfusion.

Patients on chemotherapeutic agents such as mitoxantrone often neglect their oral hygiene and thus there could be an increase in both caries and periodontal disease. If time permits, patients about to go on chemotherapy should have a dental check up and any potential areas of infection should be treated. Similarly, to reduce the mucosal irritation (sensitivity) that often accompanies chemotherapy, it is advisable to remove any ill-fitting dentures and smooth over rough cusps or restorations.

Drug interactions
None of any dental significance.

Mizolastine (Mistamine, Mizollen)

Description
An antihistamine.

Indications
Used in the treatment of allergies such as hay fever.

Effects on oral and dental structures
May produce xerostomia, but this is less common compared to older antihistamines.

Effects on patient management
The patient may be drowsy which may interfere with co-operation. Xerostomia may increase caries incidence and thus a preventive regimen is important. If the xerostomia is severe, artificial saliva may be indicated.

Drug interactions
There may be an enhanced sedative effect with anxiolytic and hypnotic drugs. Tricyclic and monoamine oxidase inhibitor antidepressants increase anti-muscarinic effects such as xerostomia.

Moclobemide (Manerix)

Description
A reversible monoamine oxidase inhibitor.

Indications
Used in the management of depression.

Effects on oral and dental structures

Xerostomia may be produced.

Effects on patient management

Xerostomia may increase caries incidence and thus a preventive regimen is important. If the xerostomia is severe artificial saliva may be indicated.

Drug interactions

Combined therapy with opioid analgesics can create serious shifts in blood pressure (both elevation and depression) and thus opioids such as pethidine must be avoided for up to two weeks after monoamine oxidase inhibitor therapy. The effects of ibuprofen and perhaps other non steroidal analgesics may be enhanced by moclobemide. Moclobemide should not be used with other antidepressants. Therapy with this drug should not begin until one week following the discontinuation of tricyclic or selective serotonin reuptake inhibitor therapy. Hypertensive crisis can occur if administered with ephedrine. Epinephrine in dental local anaesthetics is not a concern as this is metabolized by a route independent of monoamine oxidase.

Modafinil (Provigil)

Description

A central nervous system stimulant.

Indications

Used in the management of narcolepsy.

Effects on oral and dental structures

Xerostomia and uncontrollable movements of the oro-facial musculature may be produced.

Effects on patient management

Xerostomia may increase caries incidence and thus a preventive regimen is important. If the xerostomia is severe, artificial saliva may be indicated. Involuntary muscle movements e.g. of the tongue will interfere with operative dentistry. The underlying condition of narcolepsy may interfere with co-operation during treatment.

Drug interactions

None of importance in dentistry.

Moexipril (Perdix)

Description

Moexipril is an ACE inhibitor, that is it inhibits the renal angiotensin converting enzyme which is necessary to convert angiotensin I to the more potent angiotensin II.

Indications
Mild to moderate hypertension, congestive heart failure, and post myocardial infarction where there is left ventricular dysfunction.

Effects on oral and dental structures
Moexipril can cause taste disturbances, angioedema, dry mouth, glossitis, and lichenoid drug reactions. Many of these unwanted effects are dose related and compounded if there is an impairment of renal function. Moexipril-induced xerostomia increases the risk of fungal infections (candidiasis) and caries, especially root caries. Antifungal treatment should be used when appropriate and topical fluoride (e.g. Duraphat) will reduce the risk of root surface caries.

Effects on patient management
Moexipril-induced angioedema is perhaps the most significant unwanted effect that impacts upon dental management, since dental procedures can induce the angioedema. Management of moexipril-induced angioedema is problematic since the underlying mechanism is poorly understood. Standard anti-anaphylactic treatment is of little value (epinephrine and hydrocortisone) since the angioedema is not mediated via mast cells or antibody/antigen interactions. Usually the angioedema subsides and patients on these drugs should be questioned as to whether they have experienced any problems with breathing or swallowing. This will alert the dental practitioner to the possible risk of this unwanted effect arising during dental treatment.

Moexipril is also associated with suppression of bone marrow activity giving rise to possible neutropenia, agranulocytosis, thrombocytopenia, and aplastic anaemia. Patients on moexipril who present with excessive bleeding of their gums, sore throats or oral ulceration should have a full haematological investigation.

Drug interactions
Non-steroidal anti-inflammatory drugs (NSAIDs) such as ibuprofen may reduce the antihypertensive effect of moexipril.

Montelukast (Singulair)

Description
A leukotriene receptor antagonist.

Indications
Used in the treatment of asthma.

Effects on oral and dental structures
None specific.

Effects on patient management
Patients may not be comfortable in the supine position if they have respiratory problems. Aspirin-like compounds should not be prescribed

as many asthmatic patients are allergic to these analgesics. Similarly, sulphite-containing compounds (such as preservatives in epinephrine-containing local anaesthetics) can produce allergy in asthmatic patients.

Drug interactions
None of importance in dentistry.

Morphine (Oramorph, MST)

Description
An opioid analgesic.

Indications
Moderate to severe pain.

Effects on oral and dental structures
Can cause xerostomia leading to an increased risk of root caries, candidial infections, and poor denture retention.

Effects on patient management
Morphine is a drug of dependence and can thus cause withdrawal symptoms if the medication is stopped abruptly. Such cessation of morphine may account for unusual behavioural changes and poor compliance with dental treatment. The drug also depresses respiration and causes postural hypotension. If the xerostomia is severe, dentate patients should receive topical fluoride and be offered an artificial saliva.

Drug interactions
Morphine will enhance the sedative properties of midazolam and diazepam. Reduce the dose of both sedative agents.

Moxonidine (Physiotens)

Description
A centrally acting antihypertensive study.

Indications
Mild to moderate essential hypertension.

Effects on oral and dental structures
Xerostomia leading to an increased risk of caries (especially root caries), candidial infections, and poor denture retention.

Effects on patient management
If the xerostomia is severe, dentate patients should receive topical fluoride and be offered an artificial saliva.

Drug interactions

Moxonidine may enhance the sedative effects of benzodiazepines.

Mycophenolate mofetil (Cellcept)

Description

An immunosuppressant.

Indications

Prophylaxis of acute renal transplant rejection.

Effects on oral and dental structures

The immunosuppressant properties of mycophenolate mofetil could impact upon expression of periodontal disease (reduce breakdown), cause delayed healing, and make the patient more susceptible to opportunist oral infections such as candida or herpetic infections. Organ transplant patients on mycophenolate mofetil are more prone to malignancy and lesions which can affect the mouth, including Kaposi's sarcoma and lip cancer. Hairy leukoplakia can also develop in these patients and again this is attributed to the immunosuppressant properties of mycophenolate mofetil.

Mycophenolate does have a significant affect on the bone marrow leading to agranulocytosis, aplastic anaemia, and thrombocytopenia. Any suppression of bone marrow activity can cause an exacerbation of periodontal disease, oral ulceration and an increased propensity to spontaneous gingival bleeding. If the platelet count is low ($<100,000$) then the socket should be packed and sutured following dental extraction. Persistent bleeding may require a platelet transfusion.

Effects on patient management

All patients on immunosuppressant therapy should receive a regular oral screening because of the increased propensity to 'oral' and lip malignancies. Any suspicious lesion must be biopsied. Likewise signs of opportunistic oral infections must be treated promptly to avoid systemic complications. The delayed healing and increased susceptibility to infection does not warrant the use of prophylactic antibiotic cover before specific dental procedures.

Drug interactions

Aciclovir interacts with mycophenolate and the interaction results in high plasma concentrations of both compounds. Such rises in plasma concentration increase the risk of unwanted effects.

Nabilone

Description

A synthetic cannabinoid drug.

Indications

Used in the management of nausea and vomiting due to cytotoxic chemotherapy.

Effects on oral and dental structures

This drug can produce xerostomia.

Effects on patient management

The patient is probably undergoing chemotherapy which will influence the timing of treatment and can affect postoperative healing. The xerostomia produced by the drug is a short term problem, however this will be exacerbated by chemotherapy and a preventive regimen should be instigated. Dose reduction of benzodiazepines during sedation may be required (see drug interaction below).

Drug interactions

The effects of sedative agents are enhanced by nabilone.

Nabumetone (Relifex)

Description

A peripherally acting, non-steroidal anti-inflammatory analgesic.

Indications

Pain and inflammation associated with musculoskeletal disorders, e.g. rheumatoid arthritis, osteoarthritis, and ankylosing spondylitis. Dysmenorrhoea and menorrhagia.

Effects on oral and dental structures

Patients on long-term NSAIDs such as nabumetone may be afforded some degree of protection against periodontal breakdown. This arises from the drug's inhibitory action on prostaglandin synthesis. The latter is an important inflammatory mediator in the pathogenesis of periodontal breakdown.

Effects on patient management

Rare unwanted effects of nabumetone include angioedema and thrombocytopenia. The latter may cause an increased bleeding tendency following any dental surgical procedure. If the platelet count is low (<100,000) then the socket should be packed and sutured. Persistent bleeding may require a platelet transfusion.

Drug interactions

Ibuprofen, aspirin, and diflunisal should be avoided in patients taking nabumetone due to an increase in unwanted effects, especially gastrointestinal ulceration, renal, and liver damage. Systemic corticosteroids increase the risk of peptic ulceration and gastrointestinal bleeding.

Nadolol (Corfaretic)

Description
A beta-adrenoceptor blocking drug.

Indications
Hypertension, angina prophylaxis, arrhythmias, and migraine prophylaxis.

Effects on oral and dental structures
Nadolol can cause xerostomia and lichenoid eruptions. Xerostomia will make the dentate patient more susceptible to dental caries (especially root caries) and will cause problems with denture retention.

Effects on patient management
Postural hypotension may occur and patients may feel dizzy when the dental chair is restored to upright after they have been treated in the supine position. If the xerostomia is severe, dentate patients should receive topical fluoride and be offered an artificial saliva.

Drug interactions
NSAIDs such as ibuprofen may antagonize the hypotensive action of nadolol: possible interaction between epinephrine and nadolol which may cause a slight transient increase in blood pressure. Do not exceed more than 3 cartridges of epinephrine containing local anaesthetic solution per adult patient.

Nafarelin

Description
A gonadorelin analogue.

Indications
Endometriosis, prostate cancer.

Effects on oral and dental structures
Rare unwanted effects of nafarelin include paraesthesia of the lips and oedema of the lips and tongue. The drug is also associated with dry mouth which increases the risk of dental caries, especially root caries, poor denture retention and an increased susceptibility to candidial infection.

Effects on patient management
Use of nafarelin is associated with an increased risk of osteoporosis. The latter is now regarded as a significant risk factor for periodontal disease.

Drug interactions
None of any dental significance.

Nalidixic acid (Mictral, Negram, Uriben)

Description
A quinolone antibiotic.

Indications
Used to treat urinary tract infections.

Effects on oral and dental structures
This drug can cause taste disturbance and Stevens–Johnson syndrome. It may occasionally cause cranial nerve palsy and orofacial dysaesthesia.

Effects on patient management
This drug may cause thrombocytopenia, leucopenia, and anaemia. Thrombocytopenia may cause postoperative bleeding. If the platelet count is low (<100,000) then the socket should be packed and sutured. Persistent bleeding may require platelet transfusion. Leucopenia and anaemia may result in poor healing. Any anaemia will need correction prior to elective general anaesthesia and sedation.

Drug interactions
Nalidixic acid increases the anticoagulant effect of warfarin and nicoumalone. Combined therapy with non-steroidal anti-inflammatory drugs increases the risk of convulsions.

Naltrexone hydrochloride (Nalorex)

Description
An opioid antagonist.

Indications
Used to avoid relapse in those who are withdrawing from opioid dependence.

Effects on oral and dental structures
This drug increases thirst and if this is satisfied with drinks that are high in carbohydrate caries may increase.

Effects on patient management
The use of opioid analgesics must be avoided as patients receiving this medication are undergoing withdrawal from this group of drugs. This drug may occasionally produce a thrombocytopenia, agranulocytosis, and anaemia. Thrombocytopenia may cause postoperative bleeding. If the platelet count is low (<100,000) then the socket should be packed and sutured. Persistent bleeding may require platelet transfusion. Agranulocytosis may affect healing adversely. Anaemia may

result in poor healing. Any anaemia will need correction prior to elective general anaesthesia and sedation.

Drug interactions
None of importance in dentistry.

Nandrolone (Deca-Durabolin)

Description
An anabolic steroid.

Indications
Osteoporosis in postmenopausal women. NB Also used (abused) by athletes and sportsmen to enhance performance.

Effects on oral and dental structures
None reported.

Effects on patient management
Cessation of nandrolone can cause severe depression, including suicidal tendencies. Such mood changes can have an impact on the delivery and acceptance of dental care.

Drug interactions
None of any dental significance.

Naproxen (Naprosyn)

Description
A peripherally acting, non-steroidal anti-inflammatory analgesic.

Indications
Pain and inflammation associated with musculoskeletal disorders, e.g. rheumatoid arthritis, osteoarthritis, and ankylosing spondylitis.

Effects on oral and dental structures
Patients on long-term NSAIDs such as naproxen may be afforded some degree of protection against periodontal breakdown. This arises from the drug's inhibitory action on prostaglandin synthesis. The latter is an important inflammatory mediator in the pathogenesis of periodontal breakdown. Case reports have also implicated naproxen as a cause of parotid swelling and oral ulceration.

Effects on patient management
Rare unwanted effects of naproxen include angioedema and thrombocytopenia. The latter may cause an increased bleeding tendency following any dental surgical procedure. If the platelet count is low (<100,000) then the socket should be packed and sutured. Persistent bleeding may require a platelet transfusion.

Drug interactions

Ibuprofen, aspirin and diflunisal should be avoided in patients taking naproxen due to an increase in unwanted effects, especially gastro-intestinal ulceration, renal, and liver damage. Systemic corticosteroids increase the risk of peptic ulceration and gastrointestinal bleeding.

Naratriptan (Naramig)

Description
A 5HT$_1$ agonist.

Indications
Used in the treatment of acute migraine.

Effects on oral and dental structures
None specific.

Effects on patient management
Avoid stimuli which may induce migraine, such as directly shining the dental light in the patient's eyes. The use of dark glasses may be of benefit to the patient.

Drug interactions
None of importance in dentistry.

Nedocromil sodium (Rapitil, Tilade)

Description
A mast cell stabilizing drug.

Indications
Used in the management of asthma and allergic conjunctivitis.

Effects on oral and dental structures
Xerostomia, burning mouth and taste disturbance may occur.

Effects on patient management
Xerostomia may increase caries incidence and thus a preventive regi-men is important. If the xerostomia is severe, artificial saliva may be indicated. Patients may not be comfortable in the supine position if they have respiratory problems. If the patient is asthmatic, aspirin-like compounds should not be prescribed. Similarly sulphite-containing compounds (such as preservatives in epinephrine-containing local anaesthetics) can produce allergy in asthmatic patients.

Drug interactions
None of importance in dentistry.

Nefazodone hydrochloride (Dutonin)

Description
A serotonin reuptake inhibitor.

Indications
Used in the management of depression.

Effects on oral and dental structures
This drug causes xerostomia, stomatitis and candidiasis.

Effects on patient management
Xerostomia may increase caries incidence and thus a preventive regimen is important. If the xerostomia is severe, artificial saliva may be indicated. Local therapy for stomatitis and candidiasis may be required. This drug may cause postural hypotension, thus the patient should not be changed from the supine to the standing position too rapidly. Dose reduction of benzodiazepines is required during dental sedation (see drug interaction below).

Drug interactions
Combined therapy with other antidepressants should be avoided and if prescribing another class of antidepressant a period of one to two weeks should elapse between changeover. During combined therapy with carbamazepine the concentration of the anticonvulsant is increased and the plasma levels of nefazodone decreased. Nefazodone increases the sedative effects of benzodiazepines.

Nefopam hydrochloride (Acupan)

Description
A non-opioid analgesic.

Indications
Moderate pain.

Effects on oral and dental structures
Can cause xerostomia lending to an increased risk of root caries, candidial infections, and poor denture retention. If the xerostomia is severe, dentate patients should receive topical fluoride and be offered an artificial saliva.

Effects on patient management
Nefopam can cause patients to become confused, which could impact upon their compliance with dental treatment.

Drug interactions
None of any dental significance.

Nelfinavir (Viracept)

Description
A protease inhibitor antiviral drug.

Indications
Used in the management of HIV infection.

Effects on oral and dental structures
Oral ulceration may be produced.

Effects on patient management
Sedation with midazolam should be avoided (see below). Dose limitation with lidocaine local anaesthetics is wise (see below). Sensitive handling of the underlying disease state is essential. Excellent preventive dentistry and regular examinations are important in patients suffering from HIV, as dental infections are best avoided. HIV will interfere with postoperative healing and antibiotic prophylaxis prior to oral surgery may be advisable. Nelfinavir can produce anaemia, leucopenia and thrombocytopenia. Anaemia may result in poor healing. Any anaemia will need correction prior to elective general anaesthesia and sedation. Leucopenia will affect healing adversely and if severe prophylactic antibiotics should be prescribed to cover surgical procedures. Thrombocytopenia may cause postoperative bleeding. If the platelet count is low (<100,000) then the socket should be packed and sutured. Persistent bleeding may require platelet transfusion.

Drug interactions
Concurrent use with midazolam produces prolonged sedation and this combination should be avoided. Protease inhibitors appear to increase the plasma levels of lidocaine and increase cardiotoxicity of the latter drug; thus excessive doses of local anaesthetics should be avoided. Carbamazepine and phenytoin reduce the plasma concentration of nelfinavir. In addition protease inhibitors may increase the serum levels of carbamazepine and phenytoin. Dexamethasone decreases the plasma levels of protease inhibitors and serum concentrations of the steroid may be increased during concurrent therapy.

Neomycin sulphate (Nivemycin)

Description
An aminoglycoside antibiotic.

Indications
Used to sterilize the bowel preoperatively.

Effects on oral and dental structures
This drug may cause increased salivation and stomatitis.

Effects on patient management
As this drug is used preoperatively in hospital it will not interfere with routine management.

Drug interactions
The ototoxic effect of this drug is exacerbated by vancomycin. Nephrotoxicity is increased when used in combination with amphotericin B and clindamycin. The risk of hypocalcaemia produced by bisphosphonates, which are used in the management of Paget's disease of bone, is increased by neomycin. Neomycin reduces the absorption of phenoxymethylpenicillin.

Netilmicin (Netillin)

Description
An aminoglycoside antibiotic.

Indications
Used to treat serious Gram-negative infections resistant to gentamicin.

Effects on oral and dental structures
None specific.

Effects on patient management
This drug can produce disturbances of hearing and balance, thus rapid movements of the dental chair should be avoided and care taken when the patient leaves the chair. This drug may cause thrombocytopenia and agranulocytosis. Thrombocytopenia may cause postoperative bleeding. If the platelet count is low (<100,000) then the socket should be packed and sutured. Persistent bleeding may require platelet transfusion. Agranulocytosis may affect healing adversely.

Drug interactions
The ototoxic effect of this drug is exacerbated by vancomycin. Nephrotoxicity is increased when used in combination with amphotericin B and clindamycin. The risk of hypocalcaemia produced by bisphophonates, which are used in the management of Paget's disease of bone, is increased by netilmicin.

Nevirapine (Viramune)

Description
A non-nucleoside reverse transcriptase inhibitor antiviral drug.

Indications
Used in the management of HIV infection.

Effects on oral and dental structures
This drug may produce Stevens–Johnson syndrome.

Effects on patient management
Sensitive handling of the underlying disease state is essential. Excellent preventive dentistry and regular examinations are important in patients suffering from HIV infection as dental infections are best avoided. HIV will interfere with postoperative healing and antibiotic prophylaxis prior to oral surgery may be advisable.

Drug interactions
Nevirapine reduces the plasma concentration of ketoconazole and concurrent use should be avoided.

Nicardipine (Cardene)

Description
A calcium-channel blocker.

Indications
Hypertension and angina prophylaxis.

Effects on oral and dental structures
Nicardipine can cause gingival overgrowth, especially in the anterior part of the mouth. It can also causes taste disturbances by inhibiting calcium-channel activity that is necessary for normal function of taste and smell receptors.

Effect on patient management
None of any significance.

Drug interactions
None of any dental significance.

Niclosamide (Yomesan)

Description
An antihelminthic drug.

Indications
Used in the management of tapeworms.

Effects on oral and dental structures
Taste disturbance can occur.

Effects on patient management
Sparing use of alcohol-containing mouthwashes is advised – patients should avoid swallowing alcohol-containing mouthwashes (see drug interaction below).

Drug interactions
Alcohol increases the side effects (such as nausea, vomiting, abdominal pain and light-headedness) of niclosamide.

Nicorandil (Ikorel)

Description
A potassium-channel activator.

Indications
Prophylaxis and treatment of angina.

Effects on oral and dental structures
None reported.

Effects on patient management
None of any significance.

Drug interactions
None of any dental significance.

Nicotine (Nicorette, Nicotinell, NiQuitin CQ)

Description
An alkaloid which stimulates autonomic ganglia.

Indications
Used in anti-smoking therapy.

Effects on oral and dental structures
Oral preparations and inhalators can cause oral ulceration, xerostomia (although the chewing gum form can produce excess saliva), stomatitis, lingual swelling, and taste disturbance.

Effects on patient management
Xerostomia may increase caries incidence and thus a preventive regimen is important. If the xerostomia is severe, artificial saliva may be indicated. Use of the chewing gum formulation may lead to aching jaw muscles and TMJ (temporomanidbular joint) dysfunction. See drug interaction below.

Drug interactions
Nicotine patches should be removed the night before a general anaesthetic as coronary vasospasm is a possibility.

Nicotinic acid (Hexopal)

Description
A vitamin with lipid-lowering and vasodilatory properties.

Indications
Used in the treatment of hyperlipidemia and as a vasodilator.

Effects on oral and dental structures
This drug may produce xerostomia.

Effects on patient management
Xerostomia may increase caries incidence and thus a preventive regimen is important. If the xerostomia is severe, artificial saliva may be indicated.

Drug interactions
None of importance in dentistry.

Nifedipine (Adalat, Angiopine, Coracten, Corday, Fortipine, Solfedipine, Tensipine)

Description
A calcium-channel blocker.

Indications
Hypertension and angina prophylaxis.

Effects on oral and dental structures
Nifedipine can cause gingival overgrowth, especially in the anterior part of the mouth; taste disturbances can occur through inhibition of calcium-channel activity that is necessary for normal function of taste and smell receptors.

Effects on patient management
None of any significance.

Drug interactions
None of any dental significance.

Nimodipine (Nimotop)

Description
A calcium-channel blocker.

Indications
Hypertension and angina prophylaxis.

Effects on oral and dental structures
Nimodipine can cause gingival overgrowth, especially in the anterior part of the mouth: taste disturbances can occur through inhibition of calcium-channel activity that is necessary for normal function of taste and smell receptors.

Effects on patient management
None of any significance.

Drug interactions
None of any dental significance.

Nisoldipine (Syscor)

Description
A calcium-channel blocker.

Indications
Hypertension and angina prophylaxis.

Effects on oral and dental structures
Nisoldipine can cause gingival overgrowth, especially in the anterior part of the mouth: taste disturbance can occur through inhibition of calcium-channel activity that is necessary for normal function of taste and smell receptors.

Effects on patient management
None of any significance.

Drug interactions
None of any dental significance.

Nitrazepam (Remnos, Mogadon, Unisomnia)

Description
A benzodiazepine hypnotic.

Indications
Used in the short term treatment of insomnia.

Presentations
(i) 5 mg tablet.

(ii) Oral suspension (2.5 mg/mL).

Dose
5–10 mg at bedtime (elderly 2.5–5 mg).
Not recommended for children.

Contraindications
Severe respiratory disease.
Severe liver disease.
Myasthenia gravis.

Precautions
Respiratory disease.
Pregnancy and breastfeeding.
Drug and alcohol abuse.
Psychoses.
Porphyria.

Unwanted effects
Dependence.
Respiratory depression.
Confusion.
Ataxia.

Drug interactions
As with all benzodiazepines, enhanced effects occur during combined
therapy with other CNS depressants such as alcohol and opioid analgesics. Cimetidine raises the plasma concentration of nitrazepam but this
is of little clinical significance. Oral contraceptives increase the effect of
nitrazepam. Probenecid reduces nitrazepam excretion. Rifampicin
markedly increases loss of the benzodiazepine. Nitrazepam may
decrease the efficacy of levodopa. Nitrazepam may increase the toxicity
of the monoamine oxidase inhibitor phenelzine, producing postural
hypotension and sweating.

Nitrofurantoin (Furadantin, Macrobid, Macrodantin)

Description
An antibiotic.

Indications
Used to treat urinary tract infections.

Effects on oral and dental structures
This drug can cause oral dysaesthesia, Stevens–Johnson syndrome, salivary gland pain, and swelling and a brown discolouration of saliva.

Effects on patient management
This drug may cause thrombocytopenia and anaemia. Thrombocytopenia may cause postoperative bleeding. If the platelet count is low (<100,000) then the socket should be packed and sutured. Persistent bleeding may require platelet transfusion. Anaemia may result in poor healing and will need correction prior to elective general anaesthesia and sedation.

Drug interactions
None of importance in dentistry.

Nizatidine (Axid)

Description
An H_2-receptor antagonist.

Indications
Used in the treatment of gastrointestinal ulceration and reflux.

Effects on oral and dental structures
The underlying condition of reflux can lead to erosion of the teeth, especially the palatal surfaces. H_2-receptor antagonists may cause pain and swelling of the salivary glands.

Effects on patient management
Non-steroidal anti-inflammatory drugs should be avoided due to gastrointestinal irritation. Similarly, high dose systemic steroids should not be prescribed in patients with gastrointestinal ulceration. Patients may be uncomfortable in the fully supine position as a result of their underlying gastrointestinal disorder.

Drug interactions
The absorption of the antifungal drug ketoconazole may be reduced. See comments on non-steroidals and steroids above.

Norfloxacin (Utinor)

Description
A quinolone antibiotic.

Indications
Used to treat urinary tract infections.

Effects on oral and dental structures
This drug can cause stomatitis, xerostomia, taste disturbance and Stevens–Johnson syndrome.

Effects on patient management
As the drug is only used short term xerostomia should not produce significant problems, however a preventive regimen may be considered. This drug may cause thrombocytopenia, leucopenia, and anaemia. Thrombocytopenia may cause postoperative bleeding. If the platelet count is low (<100,000) then the socket should be packed and sutured. Persistent bleeding may require platelet transfusion. Leucopenia and anaemia may result in poor healing. Any anaemia will need correction prior to elective general anaesthesia and sedation.

Drug interactions
This drug increases the anticoagulant effect of warfarin and nicoumalone. Combined therapy with NSAIDs increases the risk of convulsions.

Nortriptyline (Allegron, Motipress, Motival)

Description
A tricyclic antidepressant.

Indications
Used in the management of depressive illness and for the treatment of nocturnal enuresis in children.

Effects on oral and dental structures
Xerostomia, taste disturbance, and pain in the salivary glands may occur.

Effects on patient management
Xerostomia may increase caries incidence and thus a preventive regimen is important. If the xerostomia is severe, artificial saliva may be indicated. Postural hypotension may occur with this drug, therefore rapid changes in patient position should be avoided. This drug may cause thrombocytopenia, agranulocytosis, and leucopenia. Thrombocytopenia may cause postoperative bleeding. If the platelet count

is low (<100,000) then the socket should be packed and sutured. Persistent bleeding may require platelet transfusion. Agranulocytosis and leucopenia may affect healing adversely.

Drug interactions

Increased sedation may occur with alcohol and sedative drugs such as benzo-diazepines. This drug may antagonize the action of anticonvulsants such as carbamazepine and phenytoin. This drug increases the pressor effects of epinephrine. Nevertheless, the use of epinephrine-containing local anaesthetics is not contraindicated; however, epinephrine dose limitation is recommended. Normal anticoagulant control by warfarin may be upset, both increases and decreases in INR have been noted during combined therapy with tricyclic antidepressants. Combined therapy with other antidepressants should be avoided and if prescribing another class of antidepressant a period of one to two weeks should elapse between changeover. Antimuscarinic effects such as xerostomia are increased when used in combination with other anticholinergic drugs such as antipsychotics.

Nystatin (Nystan)

Description
A polyene antifungal drug.

Indications
Used in the treatment of candidal infections.

Presentations
(i) A pastille containing 100,000 units.

(ii) A suspension containing 100,000 units/mL.

(iii) An ointment containing 100,000 units/g.

(iv) A tablet containing 500,000 units (not for dental use).

Dose
100,000 units four times daily for 7 days.

Contraindications
Hypersensitivity.

Precautions
None known.

Unwanted effects
Hypersensitivity.
Gastrointestinal upset.

Drug interactions
None known.

Oestrogen (hormone replacement therapy [HRT])

Description
A female sex hormone.

Indications
A constituent of hormone replacement therapy (HRT) that is used in conjunction with progestogen in postmenopausal women with a uterus and used solely for postmenopausal women who have undergone hysterectomy.

Effects on oral and dental structures
Oestrogens can exacerbate an existing gingivitis due to a direct vascular effect of the hormone. Oral pigmentation can also be enhanced by oestrogen, either as a constituent of the oral contraceptive pill or from HRT. Oestrogens can increase production of beta-melano-stimulating hormone. This unwanted effect may be particularly marked in those patients with a high distribution of melanocytes in their gingival tissues.

Effects on patient management
Patients on HRT are very likely to be at risk or suffering from osteoporosis. The latter may be regarded as a significant risk factor for periodontal disease.

Drug interactions
None of any dental significance (but see contraceptive pill).

Ofloxacin (Tarivid)

Description
A quinolone antibiotic.

Indications
Used to treat urinary tract infections and gonorrhoea.

Effects on oral and dental structures
This drug can cause candidiasis, xerostomia, taste disturbance and Stevens–Johnson syndrome.

Effects on patient management
Antifungal therapy may be required if oral candidiasis occurs. As the drug is only used short term xerostomia should not produce significant problems, however a preventive regimen may be considered. This drug

may cause thrombocytopenia, leucopenia, and anaemia. Thrombocytopenia may cause postoperative bleeding. If the platelet count is low (<100,000) then the socket should be packed and sutured. Persistent bleeding may require platelet transfusion. Leucopenia and anaemia may result in poor healing. Any anaemia will need correction prior to elective general anaesthesia and sedation.

Drug interactions
This drug increases the anticoagulant effect of warfarin and nicoumalone. Combined therapy with non-steroidal anti inflammatory drugs increases the risk of convulsions.

Olanzapine (Zyprexa)

Description
An atypical antipsychotic drug.

Indications
Used in the treatment of schizophrenia.

Effects on oral and dental structures
Xerostomia and uncontrollable oro-facial muscle movements (tardive dyskenesia) may be produced.

Effects on patient management
Xerostomia may increase caries incidence and thus a preventive regimen is important. If the xerostomia is severe, artificial saliva may be indicated. Uncontrollable muscle movement of jaws and tongue as well as the underlying psychotic condition may interfere with management, as satisfactory co-operation may not be achieved readily. There may be problems with denture retention and certain stages of denture construction (e.g. jaw registration) can be difficult. Postural hypotension often occurs with this drug, therefore rapid changes in patient position should be avoided. Long-term use can produce blood dyscrasias which may interfere with postoperative healing.

Drug interactions
There is increased sedation when used in combination with CNS depressant drugs such as alcohol, opioid analgesics and sedatives. Combined therapy with tricyclic antidepressants increases the chances of cardiac arrythmias and exacerbates antimuscarinic effects such as xerostomia. Carbamazepine reduces the effects of olanzapine.

Olsalazine sodium (Dipentum)

Description
An aminosalicylate.

Indications
Used to treat ulcerative colitis.

Effects on oral and dental structures
May produce lupus erythematosus.

Effects on patient management
Non-steroidal anti-inflammatory drugs are best avoided. In order to avoid pseudomembranous ulcerative colitis, discussion with the supervising physician is advised prior to prescription of an antibiotic. The aminosalicylates can produce blood dyscrasias including anaemia, leucopenia and thrombocytopenia. Anaemia may result in poor healing. Any anaemia will need correction prior to elective general anaesthesia and sedation. Leucopenia will affect healing adversely, if severe prophylactic antibiotics should be prescribed to cover surgical procedures. Thrombocytopenia may cause postoperative bleeding. If the platelet count is low (<100,000) then the socket should be packed and sutured. Persistent bleeding may require platelet transfusion.

Patients may be receiving steroids in addition to aminosalicylates and thus the occurrence of adrenal crisis should be borne in mind. This is due to adrenal suppression. Whilst such suppression does occur physiologically, its clinical significance does appear to be overstated. As far as dentistry is concerned, there is increasing evidence that supplementary corticosteroids are not required. This would apply to all restorative procedures, periodontal surgery and the uncomplicated dental extraction. For more complicated dentolveolar surgery, each case must be judged on its merits. An apprehensive patient may well require cover. It is important to monitor the patient's blood pressure before, during and for 30 minutes after the procedure. If diastolic pressure drops by more than 25%, then hydrocortisone 100 mg IV should be administered and patient's blood pressure continued to be monitored.

Drug interactions
No interactions of importance in dentistry, however note the comments on non-steroidals and antibiotics above.

Omeprazole (Losec)

Description
A proton-pump inhibitor.

Indications
Used in the management of gastrointestinal ulceration and oesophagitis.

Effects on oral and dental structures

Xerostomia, taste disturbance, candidiasis and stomatitis may be produced. Stevens–Johnson syndrome may occur. The underlying condition of reflux can lead to erosion of the teeth, especially the palatal surfaces.

Effects on patient management

Xerostomia may increase caries incidence and thus a preventive regimen is important. If the xerostomia is severe, artificial saliva may be indicated. Non-steroidal anti-inflammatory drugs should be avoided due to gastrointestinal irritation. Similarly, high dose systemic steroids should not be prescribed in patients with gastrointestinal ulceration. Patients may be uncomfortable in the fully supine position as a result of their underlying gastrointestinal disorder. Omeprazole can cause a pancytopenia. Leucopenia will affect healing adversely and if severe prophylactic antibiotics should be prescribed to cover surgical procedures. Thrombocytopenia may cause postoperative bleeding. If the platelet count is low (<100,000) then the socket should be packed and sutured. Persistent bleeding may require platelet transfusion.

Drug interactions

The absorption of the antifungals ketoconazole and itraconazole is reduced. Omeprazole inhibits the metabolism of diazepam and thus there is an increased sedative effect. Omeprazole increases the anticoagulant effect of warfarin and the anticonvulsant action of phenytoin.

Ondansetron (Zofran)

Description

A serotonin antagonist.

Indications

Used in the treatment of nausea, especially that caused by cytotoxic chemotherapy, radiotherapy, and postoperatively.

Effects on oral and dental structures

This drug rarely produces a xerostomia.

Effects on patient management

As the drug is only used short term, xerostomia should not produce significant problems. However, the patient may be undergoing chemotherapy or radiotherapy and this will affect the timing of treatments and can interfere with surgical healing. Ideally a preventive regimen should be in place.

Drug interactions

None of importance in dentistry.

Orciprenaline sulphate (Alupent)

Description
An adrenoceptor stimulant.

Indications
Used in the treatment of reversible airway obstruction.

Effects on oral and dental structures
May produce xerostomia and taste disturbance.

Effects on patient management
Patients may not be comfortable in the supine position if they have respiratory problems. If the patient is suffering from asthma then aspirin-like compounds should not be prescribed as many asthmatic patients are allergic to these analgesics. Similarly, sulphite-containing compounds (such as preservatives in epinephrine-containing local anaesthetics) can produce allergy in asthmatic patients. Xerostomia may increase caries incidence and thus a preventive regimen is important. If the xerostomia is severe, artificial saliva may be indicated. The use of a rubber dam in patients with obstructive airway disease may further embarrass the airway. If a rubber dam is essential then supplemental oxygen via a nasal cannula may be required.

Drug interactions
The hypokalaemia which may result from large doses of orciprenaline may be exacerbated by a reduction in potassium produced by high doses of steroids, and by epinephrine in dental local anaesthetics.

Orlistat (Xenical)

Description
A pancreatic lipase inhibitor.

Indications
Used in the management of obesity.

Effects on oral and dental structures
None specific.

Effects on patient management
The underlying problem of obesity may interfere with management, especially in relation to general anaesthesia.

Drug interactions
None of importance in dentistry.

Orphenadrine hydrochloride (Biorphen, Disipal)

Description
An antimuscarinic drug.

Indications
Used in the management of Parkinsonism.

Effects on oral and dental structures
Xerostomia may occur.

Effects on patient management
Xerostomia may increase caries incidence and thus a preventive regimen is important. If the xerostomia is severe, artificial saliva may be indicated. Parkinsonism can lead to management problems as the patient may have uncontrollable movement. Short appointments are recommended.

Drug interactions
Absorption of ketoconazole is decreased. Side effects increased with concurrent medication with tricyclic and monoamine oxidase inhibitor antidepressants.

Oxaliplatin (Eloxatin)

Description
A platinum compound.

Indications
Metastatic colorectal cancer in combination with fluorouracil and folinic acid.

Effects on oral and dental structures
Oxaliplatin causes bone marrow suppression with an accompanying thrombocytopenia and agranulocytosis. Bone marrow suppression can lead to troublesome oral ulceration, exacerbation of an existing periodontal condition and rapid spread of any residual (e.g. periapical) infections.

Effects on patient management
The effect of oxaliplatin on the bone marrow is transient and routine dental treatment is best avoided until the white blood cells and platelet counts start to recover. If emergency dental treatment such as an extraction is required then antibiotic cover may be necessary depending on the degree of myelosuppression. If the platelet count is low (<100,000) then the socket should be packed and sutured. Persistent bleeding may require a platelet transfusion.

Patients on chemotherapeutic agents such as oxaliplatin often neglect their oral hygiene and thus there could be an increase in both caries and periodontal disease. If time permits, patients about to go on chemotherapy should have a dental check up and any potential areas of infection should be treated. Similarly, to reduce the mucosal irritation (sensitivity) that often accompanies chemotherapy, it is advisable to remove any ill-fitting dentures and smooth over rough cusps or restorations.

Drug interactions
None of any dental significance.

Oxazepam

Description
A benzodiazepine anxiolytic.

Indications
Used in the short term treatment of anxiety.

Effects on oral and dental structures
Xerostomia may occur.

Effects on patient management
As the drug is only used short term xerostomia should not produce significant problems, however a preventive regimen may be considered. The main interaction in the management of patients receiving any benzodiazepine therapy is the use of benzodiazepine sedation. During short term use an additive effect will be noted, after long term benzodiazepine therapy tolerance occurs and large doses of benzodiazepines may be needed to achieve sedation. Also the confusion and amnesia that benzodiazepines produce may necessitate the presence of an escort.

Drug interactions
As with all benzodiazepines, enhanced effects occur with combined therapy with other CNS depressants such as alcohol, other hypnotic or sedative agents and opioid analgesics. Phenytoin may reduce the serum levels of oxazepam.

Oxcarbazepine (Trileptal)

Description
An anticonvulsant drug.

Indications
Used in the treatment of epilepsy.

Effects on oral and dental structures

Systemic lupus erythematosis and Stevens–Johnson syndrome may occur.

Effects on patient management

Epileptic fits are possible especially if the patient is stressed, therefore sympathetic handling and perhaps sedation should be considered for stressful procedures. Emergency anticonvulsant medication (diazepam or midazolam) must be available. Postoperative haemorrhage is possible due to thrombocytopenia and although not usually severe, local measures such as packing sockets and suturing should be considered.

Drug interactions

Combined use with monoamine oxidase inhibitors should be avoided. There is increased sedative effects when combined with other anti-epileptic drugs.

Oxitropium bromide (Oxivent)

Description

An antimuscarinic drug.

Indications

Used in the management of asthma and chronic obstructive airway disease.

Effects on oral and dental structures

Xerostomia may be produced.

Effects on patient management

Patients may not be comfortable in the supine position if they have respiratory problems. If the patient suffers from asthma then aspirin-like compounds should not be prescribed as many asthmatic patients are allergic to these analgesics. Similarly, sulphite-containing compounds (such as preservatives in epinephrine-containing local anaesthetics) can produce allergy in asthmatic patients. Xerostomia may increase caries incidence and thus a preventive regimen is important. If the xerostomia is severe, artificial saliva may be indicated. The use of a rubber dam in patients with obstructive airway disease may further embarrass the airway. If a rubber dam is essential then supplemental oxygen via a nasal cannula may be required.

Drug interactions

The absorption of ketoconazole is decreased during combined therapy. Antimuscarinic effects (such as xerostomia) are increased with concurrent use of tricyclic and monoamine oxidase inhibitor antidepressant drugs.

Oxprenolol hydrochloride (Trasicor)

Description
A beta-adrenoceptor blocking drug.

Indications
Hypertension, angina prophylaxis, arrhythmias, and reduction of anxiety.

Effects on oral and dental structures
Can produce xerostomia and lichenoid eruptions.

Effect on patient management
Xerostomia will make the dentate patient more susceptible to dental caries (especially root caries) and will cause problems with denture retention. If the xerostomia is severe, dentate patients should receive topical fluoride and be offered an artificial saliva. Postural hypotension may occur and patients may feel dizzy when the dental chair is restored to upright after they have been treated in the supine position.

Drug interactions
NSAIDs such as ibuprofen may antagonize the hypotensive action of oxprenolol: possible interaction between epinephrine and oxprenolol which may cause a slight transient increase in blood pressure. Do not exceed more than 3 cartridges of epinephrine containing local anaesthetic solution per adult patient.

Oxybutynin hydrochloride (Cystrin)

Description
An antimuscarinic drug.

Indications
Urinary frequency, urgency, and incontinence, neurogenic bladder instability, and nocturnal enuresis.

Effects on oral and dental structures
Dry mouth is one of the main unwanted effects of oxybutynin. This will increase the risk of dental caries (especially root caries), impede denture retention, and the patient will be more prone to candidial infections. A rare unwanted effect of oxybutynin is angioedema which can affect the floor of the mouth, tongue, and lips.

Effects on patient management
Patients on oxybutynin may become disorientated and suffer from blurred vision. If the xerostomia is severe, dentate patients should receive topical fluoride and be offered an artificial saliva.

Drug interactions
None of any dental significance.

Oxypertine

Description
A substituted benzamide antipsychotic medication.

Indications
Used in the treatment of psychoses.

Effects on oral and dental structures
Xerostomia and uncontrollable oro-facial muscle activity (tardive dyskenesia) may be produced.

Effects on patient management
Xerostomia may increase caries incidence and thus a preventive regimen is important. If the xerostomia is severe, artificial saliva may be indicated. Uncontrollable muscle movement of jaws and tongue as well as the underlying psychotic condition may interfere with management, as satisfactory co-operation may not be achieved readily. There may be problems with denture retention and certain stages of denture construction (e.g. jaw registration) can be difficult. Postural hypotension may occur with this drug, therefore rapid changes in patient position should be avoided.

Drug interactions
There is increased sedation when used in combination with CNS depressant drugs such as alcohol, opioid analgesics, and sedatives. Combined therapy with tricyclic antidepressants increases the chances of cardiac arrhythmias and exacerbates antimuscarinic effects such as xerostomia. There is a theoretical risk of hypotension being exacerbated by the epinephrine in dental local anaesthetics.

Oxytetracycline (Terramycin)

Description
A bacteriostatic antibiotic.

Indications
Rarely indicated in the management of dental infections but may be used in the treatment of periodontal disease.

Presentations
250 mg tablets.

Dose
250 mg four times daily to treat infections. When used in the management of periodontal disease the duration of therapy is two weeks.

Contraindications
Pregnancy.
Breastfeeding.
Children under 12 years.
Kidney disease.
Systemic lupus erythematosus.

Precautions
Liver disease.

Unwanted effects
Staining of teeth and bones.
Opportunistic fungal infections ('tetracycline sore mouth').
Lichenoid reactions.
Fixed drug eruptions.
Hypersensitivity.
Photosensitivity.
Facial pigmentation.
Headache and visual disturbances.
Anaemia.
Hepatotoxicity.
Pancreatitis.
Gastrointestinal upset including pseudomembranous colitis.

Drug interactions
As tetracycline chelates calcium and other cations a number of drugs (and foodstuffs such as dairy products) which contain cations reduce the absorption of tetracycline. Among the drugs which reduce the absorption of tetracycline are the ACE-inhibitor quinapril, antacids, calcium and zinc salts, ulcer-healing drugs such as sucralfate, and the ion-exchange resin colestipol. Similarly, tetracyclines inhibit the absorption of iron and zinc.

Tetracyclines reduce the efficacy of penicillins and cephalosporins. Tetracyclines raise blood urea levels, and this effect is exacerbated with combined therapy with diuretics. Tetracyclines may enhance the anticoagulant effect of warfarin and the other coumarin anticoagulants. Tetracyclines may interfere with the action of oral contraceptives and alternative methods of contraception should be advised during therapy.

Tetracyclines (especially oxytetracycline) have a hypoglycaemic effect and their administration to patients receiving insulin or oral hypoglycaemics should be avoided. Tetracyclines may increase the serum levels of digoxin, theophylline, and the anti-malarial medication mefloquine. Tetracycline may also increase the risk of methotrexate toxicity.

Combined therapy with ergotamine can produce ergotism (the most dramatic effect of ergotism is vasospasm which can cause gangrene).

Patients who use a contact lens cleaner containing thiomersal have reported ocular irritation during tetracycline therapy. Cranial hypertension leading to headache and dizziness may result with the combined use of tetracycline and retinoids.

Paclitaxel (Taxol)

Description
An antineoplastic drug.

Indications
Primary ovarian cancer, metastatic breast cancer.

Effects on oral and dental structures
Paclitaxel causes bone marrow suppression with an accompanying thrombocytopenia and agranulocytosis. Bone marrow suppression can lead to troublesome oral ulceration, exacerbation of an existing periodontal condition, and rapid spread of any residual (e.g. periapical) infections.

Effects on patient management
The effect of paclitaxel on the bone marrow is transient and routine dental treatment is best avoided until the white blood cells and platelet counts start to recover. If emergency dental treatment such as an extraction is required then antibiotic cover may be necessary depending on the degree of myelosuppression. If the platelet count is low (<100,000) then the socket should be packed and sutured. Persistent bleeding may require a platelet transfusion.

Patients on chemotherapeutic agents such as paclitaxel often neglect their oral hygiene and thus there could be an increase in both caries and periodontal disease. If time permits, patients about to go on chemotherapy should have a dental check up and any potential areas of infection should be treated. Similarly, to reduce the mucosal irritation (sensitivity) that often accompanies chemotherapy, it is advisable to remove any ill-fitting dentures and smooth over rough cusps or restorations.

Drug interactions
None of any dental significance.

Palivizumab (Synagis)

Description
A monoclonal antibody.

Indications
Used in the prevention of respiratory syncytial virus in high-risk infants.

Effects on oral and dental structures
None specific.

Effects on patient management
None specific.

Drug interactions
None of importance in dentistry.

Pancreatin (Creon, Nutrizym, Pancrease, Pancrex)

Description
Porcine pancreatin.

Indications
Used to supplement reduced secretion in cystic fibrosis, reduced pancreatic function or gastrectomy.

Effects on oral and dental structures
Oral mucosal irritation may lead to ulceration.

Effects on patient management
Patients receiving this drug may present many management problems due to their underlying disease. Such issues are beyond the scope of this text. Problems that may be encountered include cystic fibrosis and diabetes.

Drug interactions
None of relevance to dentistry.

Pantoprazole (Protium)

Description
A proton-pump inhibitor.

Indications
Used in the management of gastrointestinal ulceration and oesophagitis.

Effects on oral and dental structures
Xerostomia and taste disturbance may be produced. Stevens–Johnson syndrome may occur. The underlying condition of reflux can lead to erosion of the teeth, especially the palatal surfaces.

Effects on patient management
Xerostomia may increase caries incidence and thus a preventive regimen is important. If the xerostomia is severe, artificial saliva may be indicated. Non-steroidal anti-inflammatory drugs should be avoided due to gastrointestinal irritation. Similarly, high dose systemic steroids

should not be prescribed in patients with gastrointestinal ulceration. Patients may be uncomfortable in the fully supine position as a result of their underlying gastrointestinal disorder.

Drug interactions

The absorption of the antifungals ketoconazole and itraconazole is reduced.

Paracetamol (Acetaminophen, Panadol, Calpol)

Description

A non-opioid analgesic.

Indications

Mild to moderate pain (e.g. headache) and to reduce pyrexia.

Presentations

(i) A 500 mg tablet.

(ii) A 500 mg soluble (dispersible) tablet.

(iii) Oral suspension 120 mg/5 ml and 250 mg/5 ml.

(iv) Suppositories 60 mg, 125 mg and 500 mg.

Doses

Adults: 0.5–1 g every 4–6 hours.
Children: 3 months–1 year 60–120 mg every 4–6 hours.
1–5 years, 120–250 mg every 4–6 hours.
6–12 years, 250–500 mg every 4–6 hours.

Contraindications

Patients with renal failure, since chronic use of paracetamol and overdose can cause both papillary and tubular necrosis. The problem of renal failure is compounded when paracetamol is combined with centrally acting analgesics. Paracetamol can cause bronchoconstriction in asthmatics, although the incidence is much lower than for aspirin or other NSAIDs. Paracetamol is hepatotoxic in overdose (see later) and should be avoided in patients with liver failure.

Precautions

Impaired liver function and asthmatics.

Unwanted effects

The main unwanted effect of paracetamol is hepatotoxicity in overdose. The problem is compounded if there is a history of alcohol abuse. Following overdose with paracetamol, the normal pathways for metabolism (glucuronidation and sulphation) become saturated. As a consequence, metabolism of the drug is directed to the formation of a reactive metabolite, N-acetyl-p-benzoquinoneimine. This metabolite is toxic to hepatocytes leading to necrosis and fulminant liver failure. The problem of paracetamol overdose is further compounded by the lack of obvious signs and symptoms in the early overdose stages. The patient may feel nauseous and vomit, which may reassure them that the paracetamol has been eliminated. This is followed by a period of apparent recovery until signs of hepatic necrosis supervene 48–72 hours after ingestion of the tablet. Hepatic damage almost invariably accompanies ingestion of 15 g or more. Measuring a patient's INR is a good indicator of liver damage. Paracetamol overdose has to be treated promptly to avoid progressive liver damage. The compounds used are methionine 2.5 g orally every 4 hours for 16 hours or N-acetylcysteine 150 mg/kg IV.

Drug interactions
Prolonged use of paracetamol may enhance the anticoagulant action of warfarin. The mechanism of this drug interaction is due to paracetamol (only with prolonged use) causing damage to the hepatic parenchymal cells which will lead to reduced synthesis of the Vitamin K-dependant clotting factors (II, VII, IX and X). Warfarin also exerts its anticoagulant action by inhibiting the synthesis of the Vitamin K clotting factors. Drugs that effect gastric emptying (metoclopramide and domperidone) increase the absorption of paracetamol. This has been used therapeutically to improve the onset of action for paracetamol, e.g. in the treatment of migraine.

Paraldehyde

Description
An aldehyde.

Indications
Used in the management of status epilepticus.

Effects on oral and dental structures
As used only in emergency there are no effects of importance.

Effects on patient management
This drug is for emergency use only and is of little relevance to dental treatment.

Drug interactions
None of importance in dentistry.

Paroxetine (Seroxat)

Description
A selective serotonin reuptake inhibitor.

Indications
Used in the management of depression, panic and obsessive compulsive disorder.

Effects on oral and dental structures
Xerostomia, salivary gland enlargement and taste alteration may occur. Aphthous stomatitis and glossitis may be produced.

Effects on patient management
If the patient suffers from panic disorder then sympathetic handling is required. Xerostomia may increase caries incidence and thus a preventive regimen is important. If the xerostomia is severe, artificial saliva may be indicated. Paroxetine may cause postural hypotension, thus the patient should not be changed from the supine to the standing position too rapidly.

Drug interactions
Combined therapy with other antidepressants should be avoided. Treatment with selective serotonin reuptake inhibitors should not begin until two weeks following cessation of monoamine oxidase inhibitor therapy. Selective serotonin reuptake inhibitors increase the anticoagulant effect of warfarin. Selective serotonin reuptake inhibitors antagonize the anticonvulsant effects of anti-epileptic medication.

Parvastatin (Lipostat)

Description
A cholesterol lowering drug.

Indications
To reduce coronary events by lowering LDL cholesterol.

Effects on oral and dental structures
None reported.

Effects on patient management
None of any significance.

Drug interactions
None of any dental significance.

Penicillamine (Distamine)

Description
A drug which suppresses the rheumatic disease process.

Indications
Severe active rheumatoid arthritis.

Effects on oral and dental structures

Penicillamine is a common cause of taste disturbance. The drug has also been cited as causing lichenoid eruptions, and oral ulceration. Bone marrow suppression is a significant unwanted effect of penicillamine leading to aplastic anaemia, agranulocytosis, and thrombocytopenia. Any suppression of bone marrow activity can cause an exacerbation of periodontal breakdown, oral ulceration, and an increased propensity to spontaneous gingival bleeding. If the platelet count is low (<100,000) then the socket should be packed and sutured after dental extractions. Persistent bleeding may require a platelet transfusion.

Effects on patient management

Penicillamine-induced bone marrow suppression can cause an increased risk of oral infection, especially after dental surgical procedures. The accompanying thrombocytopenia increases the risk of haemorrhage.

Drug interactions

None of dental significance.

Penicillin G [Benzyl penicillin] (Crystapen)/ Penicillin V [Phenoxymethylpenicillin]

Description

A beta-lactam antibacterial drug.

Indications

Used to treat bacterial infections such as dental abscesses.

Presentations

(i) A 250 mg tablet (Penicillin V).

(ii) An oral solution (125 mg/5 mL and 250 mg/5 mL) (Penicillin V).

(iii) A 600 mg vial of powder for reconstitution for intramuscular or intravenous administration (Penicillin G).

Dose

Adult: 500 mg four times a day (Penicillin V).
Child: under 6 years 25% adult dose.
Child: 6 – 12 years 50% adult dose.

Contraindications

Hypersensitivity.

Precautions

Renal disease.

Unwanted effects
Hypersensitivity reactions.
Stevens–Johnson syndrome.
Gastrointestinal upset.

Drug interactions
Penicillin reduces the excretion of the cytotoxic drug methotrexate, leading to increased toxicity of the latter drug which may cause death. There may be a reduced efficacy of oral contraceptives and other methods of contraception are advised during antibiotic therapy. The serum levels of penicillin V are dramatically reduced during combined therapy with neomycin and increased doses (doubling) are needed. Penicillin activity is decreased by tetracyclines. Penicillin G rarely increases the prothrombin time when given to patients receiving warfarin. Probenecid, phenylbutazone, sulphaphenazole, sulphinpyrazone and the anti-inflammatory drugs aspirin and indomethacin significantly increase the half-life of penicillin G.

Pentamidine isethionate (Pentacarinat)

Description
An antiprotozoal drug.

Indications
Used in the management of pneumocystis pneumonia.

Effects on oral and dental structures
Stevens–Johnson syndrome, oral ulceration, abscesses, oro-facial dysaesthesia and taste disturbance may occur.

Effects on patient management
The underlying chest condition will mean that local anaesthesia is the only viable form of anaesthesia. This drug can produce thrombocytopenia, anaemia, and leucopenia. Thrombocytopenia may cause postoperative bleeding. If the platelet count is low (<100,000) then the socket should be packed and sutured. Persistent bleeding may require platelet transfusion. Anaemia and leucopenia will affect healing adversely and if severe prophylactic antibiotics should be prescribed to cover surgical procedures.

Drug interactions
Combined therapy with amphotericin may precipitate acute renal failure.

Pentazocine (Fortral)

Description
An opioid analgesic.

Indications
Moderate to severe pain.

Effects on oral and dental structures
Can cause xerostomia leading to an increased risk of root caries, candidal infections, and poor denture retention.

Effects on patient management
Pentazocine is a drug of dependence and can thus cause withdrawal symptoms if the medication is stopped abruptly. Such cessation of pentazocine may account for unusual behavioural changes and poor compliance with dental treatment. The drug also depresses respiration and causes postural hypotension. Pentazocine is associated with a high incidence of dysphoria and causes hallucinations in approximately 25% of patients. Such unwanted effects may account for unusual behaviour in patients. The drug should not be used to treat pain associated with myocardial infarction since it will cause an increase in pulmonary artery pressure. If the xerostomia is severe, dentate patients should receive topical fluoride and be offered an artificial saliva.

Drug interactions
Pentazocine will enhance the sedative properties of midazolam and diazepam. Reduce the dose of both sedative agents.

Peppermint oil (Colpermin, Mintec)

Description
An antispasmodic drug.

Indications
Used for symptomatic relief in gastrointestinal disorders such as dyspepsia, diverticular disease and irritable bowel syndrome.

Effects on oral and dental structures
If the contents of the capsule escape into the mouth this will cause mucosal irritation.

Effects on patient management
Patients may not be comfortable in the fully supine position due to underlying gastrointestinal disorder.

Drug interactions
None of importance in dentistry.

Pergolide (Celance)

Description
A dopaminergic drug (an ergot derivative).

Indications
Used in the management of Parkinsonism.

Effects on oral and dental structures
Xerostomia, rarely oral ulceration, and sialadenitis may be produced.

Effects on patient management
Xerostomia may increase caries incidence and thus a preventive regimen is important. If the xerostomia is severe, artificial saliva may be indicated. This drug may cause postural hypotension, thus the patient should not be changed from the supine to the standing position too rapidly. Parkinsonism can lead to management problems as the patient may have uncontrollable movement. Short appointments are recommended.

Drug interactions
None of importance in dentistry.

Pericyazine (Neulactil)

Description
A phenothiazine antipsychotic medication.

Indications
Used in the treatment of psychoses such as schizophrenia and in short term management of severe anxiety.

Effects on oral and dental structures
Xerostomia and uncontrollable oro-facial muscle activity (tardive dyskenesia) may be produced. The oral mucosa may be discoloured. Stevens–Johnson syndrome and lichenoid reactions may occur with this drug.

Effects on patient management
Xerostomia may increase caries incidence and thus a preventive regimen is important. If the xerostomia is severe, artificial saliva may be indicated. Uncontrollable muscle movement of jaws and tongue as well as the underlying psychotic condition may interfere with management, as satisfactory co-operation may not be achieved readily. There may be problems with denture retention and certain stages of denture construction (e.g. jaw registration) can be difficult. Postural hypotension often occurs with this drug, therefore rapid changes in patient position should be avoided. This drug can produce leucocytosis, agranluocytosis, and anaemia which may interfere with postoperative healing.

Drug interactions
There is increased sedation when used in combination with CNS depressant drugs such as alcohol, opioid analgesics, and sedatives.

Combined therapy with tricyclic antidepressants increases the chances of cardiac arrhythmias and exacerbates antimuscarinic effects such as xerostomia. There is a theoretical risk of hypotension being exacerbated by the epinephrine in dental local anaesthetics.

Perphenazine (Fentazin)

Description
A phenothiazine antipsychotic medication.

Indications
Used in the treatment of schizophrenia and other psychoses. Occasionally used in the management of alcoholism and as an anti-emetic.

Effects on oral and dental structures
Xerostomia and uncontrollable oro-facial muscle activity (tardive dyskenesia) may be produced. The oral mucosa may be discoloured. Parotid gland enlargement, lichenoid reactions and Stevens–Johnson syndrome may occur.

Effects on patient management
Xerostomia may increase caries incidence and thus a preventive regimen is important. If the xerostomia is severe, artificial saliva may be indicated. Uncontrollable muscle movement of jaws and tongue as well as the underlying psychotic condition may interfere with management, as satisfactory co-operation may not be achieved readily. There may be problems with denture retention and certain stages of denture construction (e.g. jaw registration) can be difficult. Postural hypotension often occurs with this drug, therefore rapid changes in patient position should be avoided. This drug can produce leucocytosis, agranluocytosis, and anaemia which may interfere with postoperative healing.

Drug interactions
There is increased sedation when used in combination with CNS depressant drugs such as alcohol, opioid analgesics, and sedatives. Combined therapy with tricyclic antidepressants increases the chances of cardiac arrhythmias and exacerbates antimuscarinic effects such as xerostomia. The photosensitive effect of tetracyclines is increased during combined therapy. There is a theoretical risk of hypotension being exacerbated by the epinephrine in dental local anaesthetics.

Pethidine hydrochloride

Description
An opioid analgesic.

Indications
Moderate to severe pain.

Presentations
50 mg tablet.
50 mg/ml intramuscular or subcutaneous preparation.

Dose – oral
Adults: 50–150 mg orally every 4 hours.
Children: 0.5–2 mg/kg.

Dose – subcutaneous or intramuscular
Adults: 25–100 mg every 4 hours.
Children: 0.5–2 mg/kg every 4 hours.

Contraindications
All the opioid analgesics are addictive and hence pethidine may be specifically requested by a drug addict, irrespective of their level of pain. Pethidine can precipitate seizures in an epileptic and so should be avoided in these patients.

Precautions
Impaired liver function, elderly, pregnancy and breastfeeding mothers.

Unwanted effects
An intravenous injection of pethidine can cause an alarming increase in heart rate. There are few indications for giving pethidine IV, but if this route of administration is required, then the drug must be diluted with up to 10 ml of water for injection. Pethidine depresses respiration and also reduces gut mobility, which can lead to constipation. Respiratory depression can be a problem with patients prone to asthma or emphysema.

Drug interactions
There is a significant drug interaction between pethidine and monoamine oxidase inhibitors (MAOIs). The latter drugs block the normal hepatic metabolism of pethidine and lead to the production of pethidinic acid which can cause convulsions, hyperpyrexia, and eventually coma. Avoid concomitant use and for 2 weeks after discontinuation of MAOIs. The ulcer healing drug cimetidine inhibits the metabolism of pethidine, thus there is an increase in plasma concentration and increased risk of unwanted effects. Pethidine has a further serious interaction with the dopaminergic drug selegeline. The interaction causes hyperpyrexia and CNS toxicity, thus avoid concomitant use. The combination of pethidine and chlorpromazine is a useful pre-medication regimen. However, both drugs cause depression of the CNS, giving rise to respiratory depression, sedation, and hypotension.

Phenazocine (Narphen)

Description
An opioid analgesic.

Indications
Severe pain.

Effects on oral and dental structures
Can cause xerostomia leading to an increased risk of root caries, candidial infections, and poor denture retention.

Effects on patient management
Phenazocine is a drug of dependence and can thus cause withdrawal symptoms if the medication is stopped abruptly. Such cessation of phenazocine may account for unusual behavioural changes and poor compliance with dental treatment. The drug also depresses respiration and causes postural hypotension. If the xerostomia is severe, dentate patients should receive topical fluoride and be offered an artificial saliva.

Drug interactions
Phenazocine will enhance the sedative properties of midazolam and diazepam. Reduce the dose of both sedative agents.

Phenelzine (Nardil)

Description
A monoamine oxidase inhibitor.

Indications
Used in the management of depression.

Effects on oral and dental structures
Xerostomia and oro-facial dysaesthesia may be produced.

Effects on patient management
Xerostomia may increase caries incidence and thus a preventive regimen is important. If the xerostomia is severe, artificial saliva may be indicated. This drug may cause postural hypotension, thus the patient should not be changed from the supine to the standing position too rapidly.

Drug interactions
Combined therapy with opioid analgesics can create serious shifts in blood pressure (both elevation and depression) and thus opioids such as pethidine must be avoided for up to two weeks after monoamine oxidase inhibitor therapy. Similarly, change to another antidepressant group such as tricyclics or selective serotonin uptake

inhibitors should only take place after a gap of two weeks from the end of monoamine oxidase inhibitor therapy. The anticonvulsant effects of anti-epileptic drugs is antagonized by monoamine oxidase inhibitors. Carbamazepine should not be administered within two weeks of monoamine oxidase inhibitor therapy. Hypertensive crisis can occur if administered with ephedrine. Epinephrine in dental local anaesthetics is not a concern as this is metabolised by a route independent of monoamine oxidase. Chloral hydrate interacts adversely with phenelzine and may cause hyperpyrexia or hypertension.

Pheniramine maleate

Description
An antihistamine.

Indications
Found in cough and decongestant medications.

Effects on oral and dental structures
Can produce xerostomia.

Effects on patient management
The patient may be drowsy which may interfere with co-operation. Xerostomia may increase caries incidence and thus a preventive regimen is important. If the xerostomia is severe, artificial saliva may be indicated.

Drug interactions
An enhanced sedative effect occurs with anxiolytic and hypnotic drugs. Tricyclic and monoamine oxidase inhibitor antidepressants increase antimuscarinic effects such as xerostomia.

Phenobarbital

Description
An anticonvulsant drug.

Indications
Used in the management of epilepsy.

Effects on oral and dental structures
Xerostomia, fixed drug eruptions, purpura, and Stevens–Johnson syndrome may be produced.

Effects on patient management
Xerostomia may increase caries incidence and thus a preventive regimen is important. If the xerostomia is severe, artificial saliva may be indicated. Epileptic fits are possible especially if the patient is

stressed, therefore sympathetic handling and perhaps sedation should be considered for stressful procedures. Emergency anticonvulsant medication (diazepam or midazolam) must be available. Anaemia may result from long-term treatment and cause poor healing. Any anaemia will need correction prior to elective general anaesthesia and sedation.

Drug interactions
The effects of barbiturates are increased by alcohol and other central nervous system depressants. The effects of barbiturates are decreased by folic acid. Barbiturates decrease the effects of the antimicrobials chloramphenicol, doxycycline, griseofulvin, indinavir, metronidazole, nelfiavir, and saquinavir, anticoagulants including warfarin, corticosteroids, and oral contraceptives. They possibly reduce the effectiveness of paracetamol.

Phenoxymethyl penicillin (Penicillin V)

Description
A beta-lactam antibacterial drug.

Indications
Used to treat bacterial infections such as dental abscesses.

Presentations
(i) A 250 mg tablet (Penicillin V).
(ii) An oral solution (125 mg/5 mL and 250 mg/5 mL).

Dose
Adult: 500 mg four times a day.
Child: under 6 years 25% adult dose.
Child: 6–12 years 50% adult dose.

Contraindications
Hypersensitivity.

Precautions
Renal disease.

Unwanted effects
Hypersensitivity reactions.
Gastrointestinal upset.

Drug interactions
Penicillins reduces the excretion of the cytotoxic drug methotrexate, leading to increased toxicity of the latter drug which may cause death.

There may be a reduced efficacy of oral contraceptives and other methods of contraception are advised during antibiotic therapy. The serum levels of phenoxymethylpenicillin are dramatically reduced during combined therapy with neomycin and increased doses (doubling) are needed. Penicillin activity is decreased by tetracyclines.

Phentermine (Duromine, Ionamin)

Description
A sympathomimetic drug.

Indications
Used as an appetite suppressant.

Effects on oral and dental structures
This drug can produce xerostomia and taste disturbance.

Effects on patient management
Dose reduction of epinephrine in dental local anaesthetics is advised (see drug interaction below). This drug can create an agranulocytosis and a leucopenia which may affect healing adversely; if this effect is severe prophylactic antibiotics should be prescribed to cover surgical procedures. As this drug is only used short term xerostomia should not produce significant problems, however a preventive regimen may be considered. The underlying condition of obesity and the increased probability of arrhythmias with hydrocarbon general anaesthetics mediate against general anaesthesia.

Drug interactions
Concurrent use with monoamine oxidase inhibitors can produce a hypertensive crisis. As this drug is a sympathomimetic agent the unwanted effects of epinephrine in dental local anaesthetics may be exacerbated. In addition, the arrhythmia produced by hydrocarbon general anaesthetics is exacerbated by this drug. This drug antagonizes the sedative action of antihistamines and may increase the analgesic effect of pethidine.

Phenylbutazone (Butacote)

Description
A peripherally acting, non-steroidal anti-inflammatory analgesic.

Indications
Phenylbutazone is only used for the treatment of ankylosing spondylitis where other treatment is deemed unsuitable.

Effects on oral and dental structures

Phenylbutazone has been implicated as a cause of salivary gland swelling, oral ulceration, erythema multiforme, and Stevens–Johnson syndrome. The drug has a high prevalence of bone marrow suppression leading to an agranulocytosis, aplastic anaemia, and thrombocytopenia. Any suppression of bone marrow activity can cause an exacerbation of periodontal disease, oral ulceration, and an increased propensity to spontaneous gingival bleeding.

Effects on patient management

Phenylbutazone-induced bone marrow suppression can cause an increased risk of oral infection especially after dental surgical procedures. The accompanying thrombocytopenia increases the risk of haemorrhage. If the platelet count is low (<100,000) then the socket should be packed and sutured. Persistent bleeding may require a platelet transfusion.

Drug interactions

Ibuprofen, aspirin, and diflunisal should be avoided in patients taking phenylbutazone due to an increase in unwanted effects, especially gastrointestinal ulceration, renal, and liver damage. Systemic corticosteroids increase the risk of peptic ulceration and gastrointestinal bleeding.

Phenytoin sodium (Epanutin)

Description

An anticonvulsant drug.

Indications

Indicated in the management of epilepsy and also used to treat neuralgias.

Effects on oral and dental structures

Gingival overgrowth, taste disturbance, Stevens–Johnson syndrome and lupus erythematosus may occur. Dental defects attributed to phenytoin include root shortening, root resorption and hypercementosis. Cervical lymphadenopathy may occur. Rarely salivary gland hypertrophy may be produced. The children of a mother receiving phenytoin are at risk of developing cleft lip and palate.

Effects on patient management

Epileptic fits are possible especially if the patient is stressed, therefore sympathetic handling and perhaps sedation should be considered for stressful procedures. Emergency anticonvulsant medication (diazepam or midazolam) must be available. Phenytoin can produce agranulocytosis, anaemia, and thrombocytopenia. Agranulocytosis and anaemia may result in poor healing. Any anaemia will need correction prior to elective general anaesthesia and sedation. Thrombocytopenia may cause postoperative bleeding. If the platelet count is low (<100,000) then the socket should be packed and sutured. Persistent bleeding may require platelet transfusion. Both lidocaine and phenytoin have a depressant effect on the heart and intravenous lidocaine and phenytoin have been known to cause heart block. The use of high doses of lidocaine should thus be avoided in dental practice in patients taking this anticonvulsant.

Drug interactions
The effects of phenytoin are increased by aspirin (and possibly other non-steroidals including ibuprofen), chloramphenicol, dextropropoxyphene, fluconazole, isoniazid, metronidazole, miconazole, and sulphonamide antimicrobials. The effects of phenytoin are reduced by chronic heavy alcohol consumption, aciclovir and folic acid. Phenytoin has a mixed interaction with benzodiazepines. The effect of the anticonvulsant is increased by chlordiazepoxide, clonazepam and diazepam. Conversely clonazepam and diazepam can also decrease the plasma concentration of phenytoin. Phenytoin reduces effects of anticoagulants including warfarin, corticosteroids, doxycycline, fentanyl, itraconazole, ketoconazole, oral contraceptives, and possibly paracetamol. Phenytoin possibly increases the toxic effects of pethidine.

Pholcodine (Galenphol)

Description
A cough suppressant.

Indications
Used in the management of painful coughs.

Effects on oral and dental structures
None specific.

Effects on patient management
Patients may not be comfortable in the supine position if they have respiratory problems.

Drug interactions
Pholcodine may enhance the sedative properties of midazolam and diazepam. Reduce the dose of the latter drugs.

Pilocarpine hydrochloride (Salagen)

Description
A parasympathomimetic drug.

Indications
Used to increase salivation in patients who have xerostomia secondary to therapeutic irradiation.

Effects on oral and dental structures
Increased salivation is produced as a therapeutic effect; taste alteration may occur.

Effects on patient management
The underlying condition may have produced candidiasis and increased caries incidence and these will require attention. This drug increases frequency of urination and thus long treatment sessions should be avoided. Hypotension may also be a feature of treatment with this drug, thus rapid movement of the dental chair is best avoided.

Drug interactions
None of importance in dentistry.

Pimozide (Orap)

Description
A phenothiazine antipsychotic medication.

Indications
Used in the treatment of psychoses such as schizophrenia.

Effects on oral and dental structures
Xerostomia, altered taste and uncontrollable oro-facial muscle activity (tardive dyskenesia) may be produced. The oral mucosa may be discoloured. Stevens–Johnson syndrome and lichenoid reactions may occur with this drug.

Effects on patient management
Xerostomia may increase caries incidence and thus a preventive regimen is important. If the xerostomia is severe, artificial saliva may be indicated. Uncontrollable muscle movement of jaws and tongue as well as the underlying psychotic condition may interfere with management, as satisfactory co-operation may not be achieved readily. There may be problems with denture retention and certain stages of denture construction (e.g. jaw registration) can be difficult. Postural hypotension often occurs with this drug, therefore rapid changes in patient position should be avoided. This drug can produce leucocytosis, agranluocytosis, and anaemia which may interfere with postoperative healing.

Drug interactions
Erythromycin and related drugs such as clarithromycin and azithromycin should not be prescribed as these can produce fatal

cardiac arrhythmias during combined therapy. There is increased sedation when used in combination with CNS depressant drugs such as alcohol, opioid analgesics, and sedatives. Combined therapy with tricyclic antidepressants must be avoided due to the production of dangerous arrhythmias. There is a theoretical risk of hypotension being exacerbated by the epinephrine in dental local anaesthetics.

Pindolol (Visken)

Description
A beta-adrenoceptor blocking drug.

Indications
Hypertension and angina prophylaxis.

Effects on oral and dental structures
Pindolol can cause xerostomia and lichenoid eruptions. Xerostomia will make the dentate patient more susceptible to dental caries (especially root caries) and will cause problems with denture retention.

Effects on patient management
Postural hypotension may occur and patients may feel dizzy when the dental chair is restored to upright after they have been treated in the supine position. If the xerostomia is severe, dentate patients should receive topical fluoride and be offered an artificial saliva.

Drug interactions
NSAIDs such as ibuprofen may antagonize the hypotensive action of pindolol, there is a possible interaction between epinephrine and pindolol which may cause a slight transient increase in blood pressure. Do not exceed more than 3 cartridges of epinephrine containing local anaesthetic solution per adult patient.

Piperazine (Pripsen)

Description
An antihelminthic drug.

Indications
Used in the management of threadworms.

Effects on oral and dental structures
This drug may cause Stevens–Johnson syndrome.

Effects on patient management
None specific.

Drug interactions
None of importance in dentistry.

Piperacillin (Tazocin)

Description
A beta-lactam antibiotic.

Indications
Used in the treatment of infections caused by *Pseudomonas aeruginosa*.

Effects on oral and dental structures
Oral candidiasis may result from the use of this broad spectrum agent. Stevens–Johnson syndrome may occur.

Effects on patient management
This drug may cause thrombocytopenia, leucopenia and anaemia. Thrombocytopenia may cause postoperative bleeding. If the platelet count is low (<100,000) then the socket should be packed and sutured. Persistent bleeding may require platelet transfusion. Leucopenia and anaemia may result in poor healing. Any anaemia will need correction prior to elective general anaesthesia and sedation.

Drug interactions
Tetracyclines reduce the effectiveness of penicillins. This drug inactivates gentamicin if they are mixed together in the same infusion and this should be avoided.

Pipotiazine palmitate (Piportil Depot)

Description
An antipsychotic depot injection.

Indications
Used in the treatment of schizophrenia.

Effects on oral and dental structures
Xerostomia and uncontrollable oro-facial muscle activity (tardive dyskenesia) may be produced.

Effects on patient management
Xerostomia may increase caries incidence and thus a preventive regimen is important. If the xerostomia is severe, artificial saliva may be indicated. Uncontrollable muscle movement of jaws and tongue as well as the underlying psychotic condition may interfere with management, as satisfactory co-operation may not be achieved readily. There may be problems with denture retention and certain stages of denture construction (e.g. jaw registration) can be difficult. Postural hypotension often occurs with this drug, therefore rapid changes in patient position should be avoided.

Drug interactions
There is increased sedation when used in combination with CNS depressant drugs such as alcohol, opioid analgesics and sedatives. Combined therapy with tricyclic antidepressants increases the chances of cardiac arrythmias and exacerbates antimuscarinic effects such as xerostomia.

Piracetam (Nootropil)

Description
A mild central nervous stimulant.

Indications
Used to treat myoclonus.

Effects on oral and dental structures
May get excessive movement of oral and facial musculature.

Effects on patient management
Involuntary muscle movements, e.g. of the tongue will interfere with operative dentistry.

Drug interactions
Piracetam can increase the anticoagulant effect of warfarin.

Piroxicam (Feldene)

Description
A peripherally acting, non-steroidal anti-inflammatory analgesic.

Indications
Pain and inflammation associated with musculoskeletal disorders, e.g. rheumatoid arthritis, osteoarthritis, and ankylosing spondylitis. Dysmenorrhoea and menorrhagia.

Effects on oral and dental structures
Patients on long-term NSAIDs such as piroxicam may be afforded some degree of protection against periodontal breakdown. This arises from the drug's inhibitory action on prostaglandin synthesis. The latter is an important inflammatory mediator in the pathogenesis of periodontal breakdown.

Effects on patient management
Rare unwanted effects of piroxicam include angioedema and thrombocytopenia. The latter may cause an increased bleeding tendency following any dental surgical procedure. If the platelet count is low (<100,000) then the socket should be packed and sutured. Persistent bleeding may require a platelet transfusion.

Drug interactions
Ibuprofen, aspirin, and diflunisal should be avoided in patients taking piroxicam due to an increase in unwanted effects, especially gastrointestinal ulceration, renal, and liver damage. Systemic corticosteroids increase the risk of peptic ulceration and gastrointestinal bleeding.

Pivmecillinam hydrochloride (Selexid)

Description
A mecillinam antibiotic.

Indications
Used in the treatment of cystitis and salmonellosis.

Effects on oral and dental structures
Prolonged use may lead to oral candidiasis.

Effects on patient management
Prolonged use can cause blood dyscrasias which may lead to excessive bleeding after surgery; local haemostatic measures such as packing and suturing may be required.

Drug interactions
Pivmecillinam activity is decreased by tetracyclines.

Pizotifen (Sanomigran)

Description
An antihistamine serotonin antagonist.

Indications
Used in the prophylaxis of migraine and cluster headache.

Effects on oral and dental structures
This drug can produce xerostomia.

Effects on patient management
Xerostomia may increase caries incidence and thus a preventive regimen is important. If the xerostomia is severe, artificial saliva may be indicated. Avoid stimuli which may induce migraine, such as directly shining the dental light in the patient's eyes. The use of dark glasses may be of benefit to the patient. This drug can cause drowsiness which may interfere with co-operation and co-ordination of the patient.

Drug interactions
None of importance in dentistry.

Polysaccharide–iron complex (Niferex)

Description
An iron salt.

Indications
Iron deficiency anaemia.

Effects on oral and dental structures
Iron salts do stain the tongue and teeth.

Effects on patient management
Nothing of significance.

Drug interactions
Iron salts chelate tetracyclines which in turn prevent their absorption. The two drugs should not be given together.

Povidone-iodine (Betadine)

Description
An iodine containing antiseptic.

Indications
Used as an aid to oral hygiene.

Presentations
As a 1% mouthwash.

Dose
10 mL undiluted or diluted to 20 mL with water as a rinse four times daily.

Contraindications
Allergy.

Precautions
Warn patient of possible mucosal irritation.

Unwanted effects
Mucosal irritation and hypersensitivity.
May interfere with thyroid function tests.
May interfere with tests for faecal occult blood.

Drug interactions
Avoid concurrent use with hydrogen peroxide.

Pramipexole (Mirapexin)

Description
A dopaminergic drug.

Indications
Used as an adjunctive treatment in Parkinsonism.

Effects on oral and dental structures
Xerostomia and taste disturbance can occur.

Effects on patient management
This drug may cause postural hypotension, thus the patient should not be changed from the supine to the standing position too rapidly. Parkinsonism can lead to management problems as the patient may have uncontrollable movement. Short appointments are recommended.

Drug interactions
None of importance in dentistry.

Prazosin (Hypovase)

Description
An alpha-adrenoceptor blocking drug.

Indications
Hypertension, congestive heart failure, and benign prostatic hyperplasia.

Effects on oral and dental structures
None reported.

Effects on patient management
Postural hypotension.

Drug interactions
NSAIDs such as ibuprofen and systemic corticosteroids may antagonize the hypotensive actions of prazosin.

Prednisolone

Description
A corticosteroid.

Indications
Suppression of inflammation and allergic disorders. Used in the management of inflammatory bowel diseases, asthma, immunosuppression and in various rheumatic diseases.

Effects on oral and dental structures
Although systemic corticosteroids can induce cleft lip and palate formation in mice, there is little evidence that this unwanted effect occurs in humans. The main impact of systemic corticosteroids on the mouth is to cause an increased susceptibility to opportunistic infections. These include candidiasis and those due to herpes viruses. The anti-inflammatory and immunosuppressant properties of corticosteroids may afford the patient some degree of protection against periodontal breakdown. Paradoxically long-term systemic use corticosteroids can precipitate osteoporosis. The latter is now regarded as a risk factor for periodontal disease.

Effects on patient management
The main unwanted effect of corticosteroid treatment is the suppression of the adrenal cortex and the possibility of an adrenal crisis when such patients are subjected to 'stressful events'. Whilst such suppression does occur physiologically, its clinical significance does appear to be overstated. As far as dentistry is concerned, there is increasing evidence that supplementary corticosteroids are not required. This would apply to all restorative procedures, periodontal surgery, and uncomplicated dental extractions. For more complicated dentolveolar surgery, each case must be judged on its merits. An apprehensive patient may well require cover. It is important to monitor the patient's blood pressure before, during and for 30 minutes after the procedure. If diastolic pressure drops by more than 25%, then hydrocortisone 100 mg IV should be administered and the patient's blood pressure continued to be monitored.

Patients should be screened regularly for oral infections such as fungal or viral infections. When these occur, they should be treated promptly with the appropriate chemotherapeutic agent. Likewise, any patient on corticosteroids that presents with an acute dental infection should be treated urgently as such infections can readily spread.

Drug interactions
Aspirin and NSAIDs should not be prescribed to patients on long-term corticosteroid. Both drugs are ulcerogenic and hence increase

the risk of gastrointestinal bleeding and ulceration. The antifungal agent amphotericin increases the risk of corticosteroid-induced hypokalaemia, whilst ketoconazole inhibits corticosteroid hepatic metabolism.

Prilocaine (Citanest)

Description
An amide local anaesthetic.

Indications
Used during dental local anaesthesia.

Presentations
(i) 1.8 mL or 2.2 mL cartridges of a 3% solution (containing 54 and 66 mg prilocaine respectively) with 0.03IU/mL felypressin.

(ii) 1.8 mL or 2.2 mL of a 4% plain solution (containing 72 and 88 mg prilocaine respectively).

(iii) As a component of EMLA cream which is a topical anaesthetic for skin use (EMLA is a 5% mixture of prilocaine and lidocaine).

Dose
Recommended maximum dose is 6.0 mg/kg with an absolute ceiling of 400 mg.

Contraindications
Allergy to amide local anaesthetics.
Acute porphyria.
EMLA should not be used in infants under one year of age.

Unwanted effects
Prilocaine can produce methaemoglobinaemia at high dose or as an idiosyncratic reaction. Methaemoglobinaemia presents as cyanosis and is caused by the iron in haemoglobin being present as the ferric, rather than the ferrous, form that reduces oxygen carriage. Central nervous and cardiovascular system depression at high dose. The 4% solution has been implicated in the production of non-surgical paraesthesias after injection.

Drug interactions
There is an additive effect with other drugs that may produce methaemoglobinaemia, e.g. sulphonamide antibacterials. Propranolol increases toxicity of prilocaine by inhibiting the liver enzymes that metabolize the local anaesthetic.

Primaquine

Description
An antiprotozoal drug.

Indications
Used as an adjunct in the management of malarial infection.

Effects on oral and dental structures
None known.

Effects on patient management
This drug may cause anaemia, agranulocytosis, leucopenia, and thrombocytopenia. Anaemia may result in poor healing. Any anaemia will need correction prior to elective general anaesthesia and sedation. Agranulocytosis and leucopenia will affect healing adversely and if severe prophylactic antibiotics should be prescribed to cover surgical procedures. Thrombocytopenia may cause postoperative bleeding. If the platelet count is low (<100,000) then the socket should be packed and sutured. Persistent bleeding may require platelet transfusion.

Drug interactions
None of importance in dentistry.

Primidone (Mysoline)

Description
A barbiturate anticonvulsant drug.

Indications
Used in the management of epilepsy.

Effects on oral and dental structures
Xerostomia, fixed drug eruptions, systemic lupus erythematosus, and Stevens–Johnson syndrome may be produced. Cervical lymphadenopathy may occur.

Effects on patient management
Epileptic fits are possible especially if the patient is stressed, therefore sympathetic handling and perhaps sedation should be considered for stressful procedures. Emergency anticonvulsant medication (diazepam or midazolam) must be available. Postoperative bleeding may be increased due to thrombocytopenia, therefore local measures to control haemorrhage such as packing sockets and suturing should be considered after extractions. Primidone can cause anaemia, which may result in poor healing. Any anaemia will need correction prior to elective general anaesthesia and sedation.

Drug interactions

Primidone possibly reduces the effectiveness of paracetamol and fentanyl. The effects of barbiturates are increased by alcohol and other central nervous system depressants. The effects of barbiturates are decreased by folic acid. Barbiturates decrease the effects of the antimicrobials chloramphenicol, doxycycline, griseofulvin, indinavir, metronidazole, nelfinavir, and saquinavir, anticoagulants including warfarin, corticosteroids, and oral contraceptives.

Probenecid (Benemid)

Indications

Gout prophylaxis and also used to reduce renal excretion of penicillin and the cephalosporins.

Effects on oral and dental structures

Probenecid has been reported to cause painful gingiva. Can affect the bone marrow and cause leucopenia and aplastic anaemia. Leucopenia may exacerbate an existing periodontal condition.

Effects on patient management

If there is bone marrow suppression, then there will be an accompanying thrombocytopenia. This will increase the risk of haemorrhage after dental surgical procedures. If the platelet count is low (<100,000) then the socket should be packed and sutured. Persistent bleeding may require a platelet transfusion.

Drug interactions

Patients on probenecid should not be prescribed aspirin as this will antagonize the uricosuric action of probenecid. The drug also blocks the renal excretion of aciclovir, penicillin, and the cephalosporins. In some instances, this may be desirable therapeutically. However, high plasma concentrations of these antimicrobial/antiviral agents can increase the risk of unwanted effects. It is advisable to reduce the doses.

Procainamide (Pronestyl)

Description

A class Ia antidysrhythmic drug.

Indications

Post myocardial infarction ventricular arrhythmias.

Effects on oral and dental structures

May produce angioedema which can affect the tongue and the floor of the mouth.

Effects on patient management

Rarely causes bone marrow depression resulting in agranulocytosis (high risk of oral ulceration and periodontal breakdown) and thrombocytopenia (impaired haemostasis). If the platelet count is low (<100,000) then the socket should be packed and sutured. Persistent bleeding may require a platelet transfusion.

Drug interactions

None of any dental significance.

Procaine

Description

An ester local anaesthetic.

Indications

Used to provide local anaesthesia by injection. When used intra-orally the addition of epinephrine is advised. The only indication as a dental local anaesthetic is for those extremely rare individuals who are allergic to the amide group of anaesthetics but not hypersensitive to the ester group. Another use for procaine other than for local anaesthesia is as an intra-arterial injection to counter arteriospasm produced by inadvertent intra-arterial injection (procaine is an excellent vasodilator).

Presentations

2 mL ampoules of 2% solution.

Dose

The maximum recommended dose of procaine is 6.0 mg/kg with an absolute ceiling of 400 mg.

Contraindications

Allergy to the ester group of local anaesthetics and allergy to parabens.

Unwanted effects

Allergic reactions to the ester anaesthetics is more common than to the amides such as lidocaine, consequently procaine is seldom used in dentistry.

Drug interactions

Procaine can antagonize the activity of the sulfonamide antibacterials.

Procaine penicillin/Procaine benzylpenicillin (Bicillin)

Description

A beta-lactam antibacterial drug.

Indications
Used to treat bacterial infections such as dental abscesses.

Presentations
(i) A vial containing 1.8 g procaine penicillin and 360 mg benzyl penicillin for reconstitution for intramuscular administration.

Dose
Adult: 300 mg procaine penicillin and 60 mg benzyl penicillin once to twice daily.

Contraindications
Hypersensitivity.

Precautions
Renal disease.

Unwanted effects
Hypersensitivity reactions.
Gastrointestinal upset.

Drug interactions
Penicillins reduce the excretion of the cytotoxic drug methotrexate, leading to increased toxicity of the latter drug which may cause death. There may be a reduced efficacy of oral contraceptives and other methods of contraception are advised during antibiotic therapy. Penicillin activity is decreased by tetracyclines. Benzylpenicillin rarely increases the prothrombin time when given to patients receiving warfarin. Probenecid, phenylbutazone, sulphaphenazole, sulphinpyrazone, and the anti-inflammatory drugs aspirin and indomethacin significantly increase the half-life of benzylpenicillin.

Procarbazine

Description
An antineoplastic drug.

Indications
Hodgkin's disease.

Effects on oral and dental structures
Procarbazine causes bone marrow suppression with an accompanying thrombocytopenia and agranulocytosis. Bone marrow suppression can lead to troublesome oral ulceration, exacerbation of an existing periodontal condition and rapid spread of any residual (e.g. periapical) infections.

Effects on patient management
The effect of procarbazine on the bone marrow is transient and routine dental treatment is best avoided until the white blood cells

and platelet counts start to recover. If emergency dental treatment such as an extraction is required then antibiotic cover may be necessary depending on the degree of myelosuppression. If the platelet count is low (<100,000) then the socket should be packed and sutured. Persistent bleeding may require a platelet transfusion.

Patients on chemotherapeutic agents such as procarbazine often neglect their oral hygiene and thus there could be an increase in both caries and periodontal disease. If time permits, patients about to go on chemotherapy should have a dental check up and any potential areas of infection should be treated. Similarly, to reduce the mucosal irritation (sensitivity) that often accompanies chemotherapy, it is advisable to remove any ill-fitting dentures and smooth over rough cusps or restorations.

Drug interactions
Alcohol produces a disulfiram-type reaction with procarbazine. Many mouthwashes contain alcohol as a solvent and patients should always be advised that they must not swallow any mouthwash.

Prochlorperazine (Buccastem, Stemetil)

Description
A phenothiazine medication.

Indications
Used as an anti-emetic and in the treatment of psychoses such as schizophrenia.

Effects on oral and dental structures
Xerostomia and uncontrollable oro-facial muscle activity (tardive dyskenesia) may be produced. The oral mucosa may be discoloured. Stevens–Johnson syndrome and lichenoid reactions may occur with this drug.

Effects on patient management
Xerostomia may increase caries incidence and thus a preventive regimen is important. If the xerostomia is severe, artificial saliva may be indicated. Uncontrollable muscle movement of jaws and tongue as well as the underlying psychotic condition may interfere with management, as satisfactory cooperation may not be achieved readily. There may be problems with denture retention and certain stages of denture construction (e.g. jaw registration) can be difficult. Postural hypotension often occurs with this drug, therefore rapid changes in patient position should be avoided. This drug can produce leucocytosis, agranluocytosis, and anaemia which may interfere with postoperative healing.

Drug interactions

There is increased sedation when used in combination with CNS depressant drugs such as alcohol, opioid analgesics and sedatives. Combined therapy with tricyclic antidepressants increases the chances of cardiac arrhythmias and exacerbates antimuscarinic effects such as xerostomia. The photosensitive effect of tetracycline may be increased during combined therapy. Prochlorperazine may inhibit phenytoin metabolism. There is a theoretical risk of hypotension being exacerbated by the epinephrine in dental local anaesthetics.

Procyclidine hydrochloride (Arpicolin, Kemadrin)

Description

An antimuscarinic drug.

Indications

Used in the management of Parkinsonism.

Effects on oral and dental structures

Xerostomia and glossitis may occur.

Effects on patient management

Xerostomia may increase caries incidence and thus a preventive regimen is important. If the xerostomia is severe, artificial saliva may be indicated. Parkinsonism can lead to management problems as the patient may have uncontrollable movement. Short appointments are recommended.

Drug interactions

Absorption of ketoconazole is decreased. Side effects increased with concurrent medication with tricyclic and monoamine oxidase inhibitor antidepressants.

Progestogen

Description

A female sex hormone.

Indications

As a constituent of hormone replacement therapy in patients with a uterus.

Effects on oral and dental structures

Progestogen can exacerbate an existing gingivitis due to a hormone-induced increase in gingival vascular permeability.

Effects on patient management
Patients on HRT are very likely to be at risk or suffering from osteoporosis. The latter may be regarded as a significant risk factor for periodontal disease.

Drug interactions
None of any dental significance (but see Contraceptive pill).

Proguanil hydrochloride (Paludrine)

Description
An anti-protozoal drug.

Indications
Used in the prophylaxis of malaria.

Effects on oral and dental structures
Stomatitis and oral ulceration may occur.

Effects on patient management
None specific.

Drug interactions
This drug enhances the anticoagulant effect of warfarin.

Proguanil hydrochloride with Atovaquone (Malorone)

Description
An anti-protozoal drug.

Indications
Used in the treatment of malaria.

Effects on oral and dental structures
Altered taste, candidal stomatitis, and oral ulceration may occur.

Effects on patient management
Opportunistic infection such as candida should be suspected and treated early. The drug can cause anaemia and leucopenia which will interfere with general anaesthesia, sedation, and postoperative healing.

Drug interactions
Tetracycline reduces plasma levels of atovaquone which may lead to failure in therapy. This drug combination enhances the anticoagulant effect of warfarin.

Promazine hydrochloride

Description
A phenothiazine medication.

Indications
Used in the short term treatment of agitation and restlessness.

Effects on oral and dental structures
Xerostomia and uncontrollable oro-facial muscle activity (tardive dyskenesia) may be produced. The oral mucosa may be discoloured. This drug may increase the incidence of candidiasis. Lichenoid reactions and Stevens–Johnson syndrome may occur.

Effects on patient management
As this drug is only used short term xerostomia should not produce significant problems, however a preventive regimen may be considered. Uncontrollable muscle movement of jaws and tongue as well as the underlying psychotic condition may interfere with management, as satisfactory co-operation may not be achieved readily. There may be problems with denture retention and certain stages of denture construction (e.g. jaw registration) can be difficult. Postural hypotension often occurs with this drug, therefore rapid changes in patient position should be avoided. This drug can produce leucocytosis, agranulocytosis and anaemia which may interfere with postoperative healing.

Drug interactions
There is increased sedation when used in combination with CNS depressant drugs such as alcohol, opioid analgesics and sedatives. Combined therapy with tricyclic antidepressants increases the chances of cardiac arrhythmias and exacerbates antimuscarinic effects such as xerostomia. The photosensitive effect of tetracycline is increased during combined therapy. There is a theoretical risk of hypotension being exacerbated by the epinephrine in dental local anaesthetics.

Promethazine hydrochloride (Phenergan)

Description
An antihistamine.

Indications
Used in the management of minor allergic reactions, sedation, insomnia, and nausea.

Presentations
 (i) 10 mg and 25 mg tablets.
 (ii) An elixir containing 5 mg/5 mL.
 (iii) A 1 mL ampoule containing 25 mg for injection.

Dose

(i) For allergy

Adult: 25 mg at night orally increased to 25 mg twice daily.
Child: 2–5 years 5–15 mg daily in 1–2 doses.
Child: 5–10 years 10–25 mg daily in 1–2 doses.

(ii) For sedation

Child: 2–5 years 15–20 mg.
Child: 5–10 years 20–25 mg.

(iii) For nausea

Adult: 25 mg.
Child: 2–5 years 5 mg.
Child: 5–10 years 10 mg.

Contraindications

Children under 2 years of age.
Severe liver disease.
Glaucoma.
Porphyria.

Precautions

Liver disease.
Heart disease.
Prostatic hypertrophy and urinary retention.

Unwanted effects

Xerostomia.
Headache.
Visual disturbances.
Nasal stuffiness.
Tinnitus.
Hypotension.

Drug interactions

Alcohol, antidepressant medication (monoamine oxidase inhibitors and tricyclics), hypnotic/anxiolytic drugs, and opioid analgesics all increase the sedative effects of promethazine.

Promethazine teoclate (Avomine)

Description

An antihistamine.

Indications

Used in the management of motion sickness, vertigo, labyrinthine disorders, and nausea.

Effects on oral and dental structures

This drug can produce xerostomia.

Effects on patient management

If use is prolonged xerostomia may increase caries incidence and thus a preventive regimen is important. If the xerostomia is severe, artificial saliva may be indicated.

Drug interactions

Alcohol, antidepressant medication (monoamine oxidase inhibitors and tricyclics), hypnotic/anxiolytic drugs, and opioid analgesics all increase the sedative effects of promethazine.

Propafenone hydrochloride (Arythmol)

Description

An antidysrhythmic drug.

Indications

Ventricular arrhythmias.

Effects on oral and dental structures

Xerostomia occurs due to antimuscarinic actions – leading to increased risk of root caries, candidal infection, and poor denture retention. Bitter taste and altered taste sensation can be produced.

Effect on patient management

Postural hypotension may occur and the patient may feel dizzy when the dental chair is restored to upright after they have been treated in the supine position.

Drug interactions

None of any dental significance.

Propanolol (Inderal)

Description

A non-selective beta adrenoceptor blocking drug.

Indications

Hypertension, angina, arrhythmia, prophylaxis after myocardial infarction, anxiety, phaeochromocytoma, and migraine prophylaxis.

Effects on oral and dental structures

Propanolol can cause xerostomia, lichenoid eruptions, inhibition of calculus of formation, and altered sensations (numbness) of the face. The dry mouth and the actions of propanolol on saliva will make the dentate patient more susceptible to dental caries, especially root caries.

Effects on patient management

Postural hypotension may occur and patient may feel dizzy when the dental chair is restored to upright after they have been treated in the supine position. If the xerostomia is severe, dentate patients should receive topical fluoride and be offered an artificial saliva.

Drug interactions

NSAIDs such as ibuprofen may antagonize hypotensive effect; possible interaction between epinephrine and propanolol which may cause a slight increase in blood pressure. Do not exceed more than 3 cartridges of epinephrine containing local anaesthetic solution per adult patient.

Propantheline bromide (Pro-banthine)

Description

An antimuscarinic drug.

Indications

Used for symptomatic relief in gastrointestinal disorders such as dyspepsia, diverticular disease, and irritable bowel syndrome. Also used as a treatment for gustatory sweating.

Effects on oral and dental structures

This drug may cause a xerostomia.

Effects on patient management

If use is prolonged xerostomia may increase caries incidence and thus a preventive regimen is important. If the xerostomia is severe, artificial saliva may be indicated. Patients may not be comfortable in fully supine condition due to underlying gastrointestinal disorder.

Drug interactions

Absorption of ketoconazole is decreased. Propantheline delays the absorption of paracetamol although peak levels remain unchanged, thus the onset of pain relief may be delayed. Side effects increased with concurrent medication with tricyclic and monoamine oxidase inhibitor antidepressants.

Propiverine hydrochloride (Detrunorm)

Description

An antimuscarinic drug.

Indications

Urinary frequency, urgency and incontinence, neurogenic bladder instability, and nocturnal enuresis.

Effects on oral and dental structures

Dry mouth is one of the main unwanted effects of propiverine hydro-chloride. This will increase the risk of dental caries (especially root caries), impede denture retention and the patient will be more prone to candidal infections. If the xerostomia is severe, dentate patients should receive topical fluoride and be offered an artificial saliva. A rare unwanted effect of propiverine hydrochloride is angioedema which can affect the floor of the mouth, tongue, and lips.

Effects on patient management

Patients on propiverine hydrochloride may become disorientated and suffer from blurred vision.

Drug interactions

None of any dental significance.

Propofol (Diprivan)

Description

A general anaesthetic agent.

Indications

Although the main use is to induce general anaesthesia it is also employed as an intravenous infusion for conscious sedation in dentistry.

Effects on oral and dental structures

Propofol can produce xerostomia and altered taste.

Effects on patient management

Used to produce sedation in dentistry.

Drug interactions

Propofol increases the effects of other central nervous system depres-sants. Cocaine (even after topical application) and propofol in com-bination may produce seizures.

Propylthiouracil

Description

An anti-thyroid drug.

Indications

Hyperthyroidism.

Effects on oral and dental structures

Propylthiouracil has been cited as a cause of taste disturbance. It has also been reported as a cause of agranulocytosis which may result in mouth ulcers, an exacerbation of periodontal disease and an increased propensity to gingival bleeding.

Effects on patient management
Propylthiouracil-induced thrombocytopenia will cause impaired haemostasis after a dental surgical procedure. If the platelet count is low (<100,000) then the socket should be packed and sutured. Persistent bleeding may require a platelet transfusion.

Drug interactions
None of any dental significance.

Protamine zinc insulin

Description
Intermediate and long acting insulin.

Indications
Diabetes mellitus.

Effects on oral and dental structures
Soluble insulin can cause pain and swelling of the salivary glands.

Effects on patient management
The main concern with treating diabetic patients on protamine zinc insulin suspension is to avoid hypoglycaemia. Thus it is important to ensure that patients have taken their normal food and insulin prior to their dental appointment. Wherever possible treat diabetic patients in the first half of the morning and ensure that any treatment does not preclude them from eating. If an insulin-dependent diabetic requires a general anaesthetic, the patient should be referred to hospital.

Drug interactions
Aspirin and the NSAIDs can cause hypoglycaemia which could be a problem in a poorly-controlled insulin dependent diabetic. These analgesics should be used with caution in such patients. Systemic corticosteroids will antagonize the hypoglycaemic properties of insulin. If these drugs are required in an insulin dependent diabetic, then consult the patient's physician before prescribing.

Protriptyline hydrochloride (Concordin)

Description
A tricyclic antidepressant.

Indications
Used in the management of depressive illness.

Effects on oral and dental structures
Xerostomia, taste disturbance, and stomatitis may occur.

Effects on patient management
Xerostomia may increase caries incidence and thus a preventive regimen is important. If the xerostomia is severe, artificial saliva may be indicated. Postural hypotension may occur with this drug, therefore rapid changes in patient position should be avoided. This drug may cause thrombocytopenia, agranulocytosis, and leucopenia. Thrombocytopenia may cause postoperative bleeding. If the platelet count is low (<100,000) then the socket should be packed and sutured. Persistent bleeding may require platelet transfusion. Agranulocytosis and leucopenia may affect healing adversely.

Drug interactions
Increased sedation occurs with alcohol and sedative drugs such as benzodiazepines. This drug may antagonize the action of anticonvulsants such as carbamazepine and phenytoin. This drug increases the pressor effects of epinephrine. Nevertheless, the use of epinephrine-containing local anaesthetics is not contraindicated; however, epinephrine dose limitation is recommended. Normal anticoagulant control by warfarin may be upset, both increases and decreases in INR have been noted during combined therapy with tricyclic antidepressants. Combined therapy with other antidepressants should be avoided and if prescribing another class of antidepressant a period of one to two weeks should elapse between changeover. Antimuscarinic effects such as xerostomia are increased when used in combination with other anticholinergic drugs such as antipsychotics.

Pseudoephedrine hydrochloride (Galpseud, Sudafed)

Description
An adrenoceptor stimulant.

Indications
Used in the treatment of reversible airway obstruction and the management of nasal congestion.

Effects on oral and dental structures
This drug may produce xerostomia.

Effects on patient management
Patients may not be comfortable in the supine position if they have respiratory problems. As the drug is only used short term xerostomia should not produce significant problems however a preventive regimen may be considered. The use of a rubber dam in patients with

obstructive airway disease may further embarrass the airway. If a rubber dam is essential then supplemental oxygen via a nasal cannula may be required.

Drug interactions

The adrenergic effects of epinephrine in dental local anaesthetics will be enhanced by pseudoephedrine, so dose reduction should be considered. A hypertensive crisis can occur with concurrent use of monoamine oxidase inhibitors. There is an increased chance of dysrhythmia with halogenated general anaesthetic agents.

Pyramethamine (Daraprim)

Description

An antiprotozoal drug.

Indications

Used as an adjunct in the treatment and prophylaxis of malaria and in the management of toxoplasmosis.

Effects on oral and dental structures

Glossitis and xerostomia may be produced. Cervical lymphadenopathy may occur.

Effects on patient management

Xerostomia may increase caries incidence and thus a preventive regimen is important. If the xerostomia is severe, artificial saliva may be indicated. When used long term the drug can cause anaemia, aganulocytosis, leucocytosis, and thrombocytopenia. Anaemia may result in poor healing. Any anaemia will need correction prior to elective general anaesthesia and sedation. Agranulocytosis and leucopenia will affect healing adversely and if severe prophylactic antibiotics should be prescribed to cover surgical procedures. Thrombocytopenia may cause postoperative bleeding. If the platelet count is low (<100,000) then the socket should be packed and sutured. Persistent bleeding may require platelet transfusion.

Drug interactions

There is an increased anti-folate effect with phenytoin and co-trimoxazole which may potentiate haematological problems.

Pyramethamine with Dapsone (Maloprim)

Description

An antiprotozoal drug.

Indications

Used in the prophylaxis of malaria.

Effects on oral and dental structures

This drug combination may cause glossitis, xerostomia, syndrome, fixed drug eruptions, and cervical lymphadenopathy.

Effects on patient management

Xerostomia may increase caries incidence and thus a preventive regimen is important. If the xerostomia is severe, artificial saliva may be indicated. When used long term the drug can cause anaemia, aganulocytosis, leucocytosis, and thrombocytopenia. Anaemia may result in poor healing. Any anaemia will need correction prior to elective general anaesthesia and sedation. Agranulocytosis and leucopenia will affect healing adversely and if severe prophylactic antibiotics should be prescribed to cover surgical procedures. Thrombocytopenia may cause postoperative bleeding. If the platelet count is low (<100,000) then the socket should be packed and sutured. Persistent bleeding may require platelet transfusion.

Drug interactions

There is an increased anti-folate effect with phenytoin and co-trimoxazole which may potentiate haematological problems.

Pyramethamine with Sulfadoxine (Fansidar)

Description

An antiprotozoal drug.

Indications

Used as an adjunct in the treatment of malaria.

Effects on oral and dental structures

Stomatitis, glossitis, xerostomia, Stevens–Johnson syndrome, candidiasis, cervical lymphadenopathy, and salivary gland adenitis can occur.

Effects on patient management

Xerostomia may increase caries incidence and thus a preventive regimen is important. If the xerostomia is severe, artificial saliva may be indicated. When used long term this drug combination can cause anaemia, aganulocytosis, leucocytosis, and thrombocytopenia. Anaemia may result in poor healing. Any anaemia will need correction prior to elective general anaesthesia and sedation. Agranulocytosis and leucopenia will affect healing adversely and if severe prophylactic antibiotics should be prescribed to cover surgical procedures. Thrombocytopenia may cause postoperative bleeding. If the platelet count is low (<100,000) then the socket should be packed and sutured. Persistent bleeding may require platelet transfusion.

Drug interactions

There is an increased chance of methaemoglobinaemia when used in combination with prilocaine, including topical use of the anaesthetic.

The effects of the anticoagulants warfarin and nicoumalone are enhanced during combined therapy. The beneficial effects of tricyclic antidepressants may be counteracted. The plasma concentration of phenytoin is increased and there is an increased anti-folate effect with phenytoin which may potentiate haematological problems.

Pyrazinamide (Zinamide)

Description
A bactericidal antitubercular drug.

Indications
Used in combination with other drugs in the treatment of tuberculosis.

Effects on oral and dental structures
None specific.

Effects on patient management
Only emergency dental treatment should be performed during active tuberculosis and care must be exercised to eliminate spread of tuberculosis between the patient and dental personnel, e.g. masks and glasses should be worn and where possible treatment should be performed under a rubber dam to reduce aerosol spread.

Drug interactions
None of importance in dentistry.

Quetiapine (Seroquel)

Description
An atypical antipsychotic drug.

Indications
Used in the treatment of schizophrenia.

Effects on oral and dental structures
Xerostomia, taste alteration, and uncontrollable oro-facial muscle activity (tardive dyskenesia) may be produced.

Effects on patient management
Xerostomia may increase caries incidence and thus a preventive regimen is important. If the xerostomia is severe, artificial saliva may be indicated. Uncontrollable muscle movement of jaws and tongue as well as the underlying psychotic condition may interfere with management, as satisfactory co-operation may not be achieved readily. There may be problems with denture retention and certain stages of denture construction (e.g. jaw registration) can be difficult. Postural hypotension often occurs with this drug, therefore rapid

changes in patient position should be avoided. Long term use may produce blood dyscrasias which can interfere with postoperative healing. If white cell counts are low prophylactic antibiotics should be considered prior to surgery.

Drug interactions
There is increased sedation when used in combination with CNS depressant drugs such as alcohol, opioid analgesics, and sedatives. Combined therapy with tricyclic antidepressants increases the chances of cardiac arrhythmias and exacerbates antimuscarinic effects such as xerostomia.

Quinagolide (Norprolac)

Description
A dopamine receptor stimulant.

Indications
Galactorrhoea, cyclical benign breast disease, and for the treatment of prolactinomas.

Effects on oral and dental structures
Quinagolide does cause xerostomia which increases the risk of dental caries, candidal infections, and causes poor denture retention. The drug also cause dyskenesias which can result in involuntary movements of the lips, tongue, and jaws.

Effects on patient management
Quinagolide-induced dyskenesias can cause problems with denture retention and make certain stages of denture construction (e.g. jaw registration) difficult. Postural hypotension is a particular problem in the early stages of dosing with quinagolide. This can cause problems with operating on patients in the supine position and then restoring the dental chair to the upright position. If the xerostomia is severe, dentate patients should receive topical fluoride and be offered an artificial saliva.

Drug interactions
Erythromycin will raise the plasma concentration of quinagolide which increases the risk of adverse reactions.

Quinapril (Accupro)

Description
Quinapril is an ACE inhibitor, that is it inhibits the renal angiotensin converting enzyme which is necessary to convert angiotensin I to the more potent angiotensin II.

Indications

Mild to moderate hypertension, congestive heart failure, and post myocardial infarction where there is left ventricular dysfunction.

Effects on oral and dental structures

Quinapril causes taste disturbances, angioedema, dry mouth, glossitis, and lichenoid drug reactions. Many of these unwanted effects are dose related and compounded if there is an impairment of renal function. Quinapril-induced xerostomia increases the risk of fungal infections (candidiasis) and caries, especially root caries. Antifungal treatment should be used when appropriate and topical fluoride (e.g. Duraphat) will reduce the risk of root surface caries.

Effect on patient management

Quinapril-induced angioedema is perhaps the most significant unwanted effect that impacts upon dental management, as dental procedures can induce the angioedema. Management of quinapril-induced angioedema is problematic because the underlying mechanisms are poorly understood. Standard anti-anaphylactic treatment is of little value (epinephrine and hydrocortisone) because the angioedema is not mediated via mast cells or antibody/antigen interactions. Usually the angioedema subsides and patients on these drugs should be questioned as to whether they have experienced any problems with breathing or swallowing. This will alert the dental practitioner to the possible risk of this unwanted effect arising during dental treatment.

Quinapril is also associated with suppression of bone marrow activity, giving rise to possible neutropenia, agranulocytosis, thrombocytopenia, and aplastic anaemia. Patients on quinapril who present with excessive bleeding of their gingiva, sore throats or oral ulceration should have a full haematological investigation.

Drug interactions

Non-steroidal anti-inflammatory drugs (NSAIDs) such as ibuprofen may reduce the antihypertensive effect of quinapril.

Quinidine (Kinidin)

Description

A class Ia antidysrhythmic drug.

Indications

Suppression of supraventricular tachycardias and ventricular arrhythmias.

Effects on oral and dental structures

Rarely causes angioedema which can affect the floor of the mouth, tongue, and lips.

Effects on patient management
May produce bone marrow depression (rare) resulting in agranulo-cytosis (high risk of oral ulceration and periodontal breakdown) and thrombo-cytopenia (impaired haemostasis). If the platelet count is low (<100,000) then the socket should be packed and sutured. Persistent bleeding may require a platelet transfusion.

Drug interactions
None of any dental significance.

Quinine

Description
An antiprotozoal drug.

Indications
Used in the treatment of malaria and in the management of nocturnal leg cramps.

Effects on oral and dental structures
This drug may produce lichenoid reactions.

Effects on patient management
This drug can cause a thrombocytopenia. Thrombocytopenia may cause postoperative bleeding. If the platelet count is low (<100,000) then extraction sockets should be packed and sutured. Persistent bleeding may require platelet transfusion.

Drug interactions
Quinine may increase the anticoagulant effect of warfarin. Quinine increases the toxicity of carbamazepine and phenobarbital.

Quinupristin with Dalfopristin (Synercid)

Description
A combination of two streptogramin antibiotics.

Indications
Used to treat serious Gram-positive infections when no alternative is available.

Effects on oral and dental structures
This drug combination can produce stomatitis and oral candidiasis.

Effects on patient management
See drug interaction with midazolam below. This drug combination may cause thrombocytopenia, leucopenia, and anaemia. Thrombocytopenia may cause postoperative bleeding. If the platelet count is low (<100,000) then extraction sockets should be packed and sutured.

Persistent bleeding may require platelet transfusion. Leucopenia and anaemia may result in poor healing. Any anaemia will need correction prior to elective general anaesthesia and sedation.

Drug interactions
Quinupristin with dalfopristin increases the plasma concentration of midazolam and this can lead to profound sedation at normal doses.

Rabeprazole sodium (Pariet)

Description
A proton-pump inhibitor.

Indications
Used in the management of gastrointestinal ulceration and oesophagitis.

Effects on oral and dental structures
Xerostomia, taste disturbance, and stomatitis may be produced. Stevens–Johnson syndrome may occur. The underlying condition of reflux can lead to erosion of the teeth, especially the palatal surfaces.

Effects on patient management
Xerostomia may increase caries incidence and thus a preventive regimen is important. If the xerostomia is severe, artificial saliva may be indicated. Non-steroidal anti-inflammatory drugs should be avoided due to gastrointestinal irritation. Similarly, high dose systemic steroids should not be prescribed in patients with gastrointestinal ulceration. Patients may be uncomfortable in the fully supine position as a result of their underlying gastrointestinal disorder.

Drug interactions
The absorption of the antifungals ketoconazole and itraconazole is reduced.

Raltitrexed (Tomudex)

Description
An antimetabolic agent.

Indications
For palliative treatment in patients with advanced colorectal cancer.

Effects on oral and dental structures
Raltitrexed causes bone marrow suppression with an accompanying thrombocytopenia and agranulocytosis. Bone marrow suppression can lead to troublesome oral ulceration, exacerbation of an existing periodontal condition and rapid spread of any residual (e.g. periapical) infections.

Effects on patient management

The effect of raltitrexed on the bone marrow is transient and routine dental treatment is best avoided until the white blood cells and platelet counts start to recover. If emergency dental treatment such as an extraction is required then antibiotic cover may be necessary depending on the degree of myelosuppression. If the platelet count is low (<100,000) then the socket should be packed and sutured. Persistent bleeding may require a platelet transfusion.

Patients on chemotherapeutic agents such as raltitrexed often neglect their oral hygiene and thus there could be an increase in both caries and periodontal disease. If time permits, patients about to go on chemotherapy should have a dental check up and any potential areas of infection should be treated. Similarly, to reduce the mucosal irritation (sensitivity) that often accompanies chemotherapy, it is advisable to remove any ill-fitting dentures and smooth over rough cusps or restorations.

Drug interactions

None of any dental significance.

Ramipril (Tritace)

Description

Ramipril is an ACE inhibitor, that is it inhibits the renal angiotensin converting enzyme which is necessary to convert angiotensin I to the more potent angiotensin II.

Indications

Mild to moderate hypertension, congestive heart failure, and post myocardial infarction where there is left ventricular dysfunction.

Effects on oral and dental structures

Ramipril causes taste disturbances, angioedema, dry mouth, glossitis, and lichenoid drug reactions. Many of these unwanted effects are dose related and compounded if there is an impairment of renal function. Ramipril-induced xerostomia increases the risk of fungal infections (candidiasis) and caries, especially root caries. Antifungal treatment should be used when appropriate and topical fluoride (e.g. Duraphat) will reduce the risk of root surface caries.

Effects on patient management

Ramipril-induced angioedema is perhaps the most significant unwanted effect that impacts upon dental management, as dental procedures can induce the angioedema. Management of ramipril-induced angioedema is problematic because the underlying mechanisms are poorly understood. Standard anti-anaphylactic treatment is of little value (epinephrine and hydrocortisone) because the angioedema is not mediated via mast cells or antibody/antigen interactions. Usually the angioedema subsides and patients on these drugs should be questioned as to whether they have experienced any problems with breathing or swallowing. This will alert the dental practitioner to the possible risk of this unwanted effect arising during dental treatment.

Ramipril is also associated with suppression of bone marrow activity giving rise to possible neutropenia, agranulocytosis, thrombocytopenia, and aplastic anaemia. Patients on ramipril who present with excessive bleeding of their gingiva, sore throats or oral ulceration should have a full haematological investigation.

Drug interactions
Non-steroidal anti-inflammatory drugs (NSAIDs) such as ibuprofen may reduce the antihypertensive effect of ramipril.

Ranitidine (Zantac)

Description
A histamine H_2-receptor antagonist.

Indications
Used in the treatment of gastrointestinal ulceration and reflux.

Effects on oral and dental structures
This drug occasionally causes erythema multiforme. The underlying condition of reflux can lead to erosion of the teeth, especially the palatal surfaces. H_2-receptor antagonists may cause pain and swelling of the salivary glands.

Effects on patient management
Non-steroidal anti-inflammatory drugs should be avoided due to gastrointestinal irritation. Similarly, high dose systemic steroids should not be prescribed in patients with gastrointestinal ulceration. The patient may prefer to avoid the supine position due to their underlying gastrointestinal problem. High doses of the long-acting local anaesthetic bupivacaine should be avoided (see below). This drug occasionally causes a pancytopenia which can affect postoperative healing and haemorrhage control.

Drug interactions
Ranitidine may decrease the absorption of the antifungals itraconazole and ketoconazole. It may also increase the plasma levels of the long-acting local anaesthetic bupivacaine.

Ranitidine bismuth citrate (Pylorid)

Description
A histamine H_2-receptor antagonist and bismuth chelate combination.

Indications
Used in the treatment of gastrointestinal ulceration and reflux.

Effects on oral and dental structures
This drug can cause dark staining of the tongue and taste disturbance. It occasionally causes erythema multiforme. The underlying condition of reflux can lead to erosion of the teeth, especially the palatal surfaces. H_2-receptor antagonists may cause pain and swelling of the salivary glands.

Effects on patient management
Non-steroidal anti-inflammatory drugs should be avoided due to gastrointestinal irritation. Similarly, high dose systemic steroids should not be prescribed in patients with gastrointestinal ulceration. The patient may prefer to avoid the supine position due to their underlying gastrointestinal problem. High doses of the long-acting local anaesthetic bupivacaine should be avoided (see below). This drug occasionally causes a pancytopenia which can affect postoperative healing and haemorrhage control.

Drug interactions
Ranitidine may decrease the absorption of the antifungals itraconazole and ketoconazole. It also may increase the plasma levels of the long-acting local anaesthetic bupivacaine. The bismuth component reduces the absorption of tetracyclines. See comments above concerning non-steroidals and steroids.

Reboxetine (Edronax)

Description
A norepinephrine reuptake inhibitor antidepressant drug.

Indications
Used in the management of depression.

Effects on oral and dental structures
This drug may cause xerostomia.

Effects on patient management
Xerostomia may increase caries incidence and thus a preventive regimen is important. If the xerostomia is severe, artificial saliva may be indicated. This drug may cause postural hypotension, thus the patient should not be changed from the supine to the standing position too rapidly.

Drug interactions

Erythromycin and other macrolide antibiotics should not be prescribed concurrently with reboxetine. Similarly, imidazole (such as ketoconazole and miconazole) and triazole (e.g. fluconazole and itraconazole) antifungal agents should be avoided during therapy with this antidepressant. Combined therapy with other antidepressants should be avoided and if prescribing another class of antidepressant a period of one to two weeks should elapse between changeover.

Repaglinide

Description
An oral antidiabetic drug that stimulates insulin release.

Indications
Diabetes mellitus.

Effects on oral and dental structures
None reported.

Effects on patient management
Although hypoglycaemia is less of a problem with the biguanides than the sulphonylureas, it is always wise to check that patients have both taken their medication and eaten prior to dental treatment. If there is any doubt, give the patient a glucose drink. As with any diabetic patient, try and treat in the first half of the morning and always ensure that any dental treatment does not prevent the patient from eating. If a patient on repaglinide requires a general anaesthetic then refer to hospital.

Drug interactions
Systemic corticosteroids antagonize the hypoglycaemic actions of repaglinide. If these drugs are required, then consult the patient's physician before prescribing.

Reproterol hydrochloride (Bronchodil)

Description
A beta$_2$-adrenoceptor stimulant.

Indications
Used in the management of asthma and reversible airway obstruction.

Effects on oral and dental structures
Xerostomia and taste alteration may occur.

Effects on patient management
Patients may not be comfortable in the supine position if they have respiratory problems. Aspirin-like compounds should not be prescribed as many asthmatipc patients are allergic to these analgesics. Similarly, sulphite-containing compounds (such as preservatives in epinephrine-containing local anaesthetics) can produce allergy in asthmatic patients. Xerostomia may increase caries incidence and thus a preventive regimen is important. If the xerostomia is severe, artificial saliva may be indicated. The use of a rubber dam in patients with obstructive airway disease may further embarrass the airway. If a rubber dam is essential then supplemental oxygen via a nasal cannula may be required.

Drug interactions
The hypokalaemia which may result from large doses of reproterol may be exacerbated by a reduction in potassium produced by high doses of steroids and by epinephrine in dental local anaesthetics.

Ribavarin [Tribavarin] (Rebetol, Virazole)

Description
An antiviral drug.

Indications
Used to treat respiratory syncytial virus infection and hepatitis C.

Effects on oral and dental structures
This drug can produce pharyngitis and taste disturbance.

Effects on patient management
This drug may cause thrombocytopenia, leucopenia, and anaemia. Thrombocytopenia may cause postoperative bleeding. If the platelet count is low (<100,000) then the socket should be packed and sutured. Persistent bleeding may require platelet transfusion. Leucopenia and anaemia may result in poor healing. Any anaemia will need correction prior to elective general anaesthesia and sedation.

Drug interactions
None of importance in dentistry.

Rifabutin (Mycobutin)

Description
A rifamycin antituberculous drug.

Indications
Treatment and prophylaxis of mycobacterial infections including tuberculosis.

Effects on oral and dental structures
This drug causes an orange-red discolouration of saliva and can produce taste alteration.

Effects on patient management
Only emergency dental treatment should be performed during active tuberculosis and care must be exercised to eliminate spread of tuberculosis between the patient and dental personnel, e.g. masks and glasses should be worn and where possible treatment should be performed under a rubber dam to reduce aerosol spread. This drug may cause thrombocytopenia, leucopenia, and anaemia. Thrombocytopenia may cause postoperative bleeding. If the platelet count is low (<100,000) then the socket should be packed, and sutured. Persistent bleeding may require platelet transfusion. Leucopenia and anaemia may affect healing adversely. Any anaemia will need correction prior to elective general anaesthesia and sedation.

Drug interactions
Rifamycins decrease the anticoagulant effect of warfarin and nicoumalone. The effects of phenytoin and carbamazepine are reduced during combined therapy. The antifungal fluconazole increases the toxicity of rifabutin and this may cause uveitis. Rifamycins accelerate the metabolism of diazepam and corticosteroids thus reducing the effectiveness of these drugs.

Rifampicin (Rifadin, Rimactane, Rifater, Rifinah 150, Rifinah 300, Rimactazid 150, Rimactazid 300)

Description
A rifamycin antituberculous drug.

Indications
Treatment of tuberculosis, brucellosis, Legionnaire's disease, and serious staphylococcal infections.

Effects on oral and dental structures
This drug causes stomatitis, candidiasis, thrombocytopenic purpura and an orange-red discolouration of saliva. Stevens–Johnson syndrome may occur with this drug.

Effects on patient management
Only emergency dental treatment should be performed during active tuberculosis and care must be exercised to eliminate spread of tuberculosis between the patient and dental personnel, e.g. masks and glasses should be worn and where possible treatment should be performed under a rubber dam to reduce aerosol spread. This drug

may cause thrombocytopenia, leucopenia, and anaemia. Thrombocytopenia may cause postoperative bleeding. If the platelet count is low (< 100,000) then the socket should be packed and sutured. Persistent bleeding may require platelet transfusion. Leucopenia and anaemia may affect healing adversely. Any anaemia will need correction prior to elective general anaesthesia and sedation.

Drug interactions

Rifamycins decrease the anticoagulant effect of warfarin and nicoumalone. The effects of phenytoin are reduced during combined therapy. The efficacy of the antifungals fluconazole, ketoconazole, and itraconazole is reduced by rifampicin. Similarly, the effectiveness of rifampicin is reduced by ketoconazole. Rifamycins accelerate the metabolism of diazepam and corticosteroids, thus reducing the effectiveness of these drugs.

Risperidone (Risperdal)

Description
An atypical antipsychotic drug.

Indications
Used in the treatment of schizophrenia.

Effects on oral and dental structures
Xerostomia, taste disturbance, stomatitis, and uncontrollable orofacial muscle activity (tardive dyskenesia) may be produced.

Effects on patient management
Xerostomia may increase caries incidence and thus a preventive regimen is important. If the xerostomia is severe, artificial saliva may be indicated. Uncontrollable muscle movement of jaws and tongue as well as the underlying psychotic condition may interfere with management, as satisfactory co-operation may not be achieved readily. There may be problems with denture retention and certain stages of denture construction (e.g. jaw registration) can be difficult. Postural hypotension often occurs with this drug, therefore rapid changes in patient position should be avoided. This drug may cause neutropenia and thrombocytopenia. Neutropenia will affect healing adversely, if severe prophylactic antibiotics should be prescribed to cover surgical procedures. Thrombocytopenia may cause postoperative bleeding. If the platelet count is low (< 100,000) then the socket should be packed and sutured. Persistent bleeding may require platelet transfusion.

Drug interactions
There is increased sedation when used in combination with CNS depressant drugs such as alcohol, opioid analgesics and sedatives.

Combined therapy with tricyclic antidepressants increases the chances of cardiac arrhythmias and exacerbates antimuscarinic effects such as xerostomia. Long term use of carbamazepine increases the excretion of risperidone.

Ritonavir (Norvir)

Description
A protease inhibitor antiviral drug.

Indications
Used in the management of HIV infection.

Effects on oral and dental structures
Oral ulceration, taste disturbance, xerostomia, and circumoral paraesthesia may be produced

Effects on patient management
Sedation with benzodiazepines should be avoided (see below). Dose limitation with lidocaine local anaesthetics is wise (see below). Sensitive handling of the underlying disease state is essential. Excellent preventive dentistry and regular examinations are important in patients suffering from HIV infection as dental infections are best avoided. HIV will interfere with postoperative healing and antibiotic prophylaxis prior to oral surgery may be advisable. Xerostomia may increase caries incidence and thus a preventive regimen is important. If the xerostomia is severe, artificial saliva may be indicated.

Ritonavir can produce anaemia leucopenia and an increased prothrombin time. Anaemia may result in poor healing. Any anaemia will need correction prior to elective general anaesthesia and sedation. Leucopenia will affect healing adversely and if severe prophylactic antibiotics should be prescribed to cover surgical procedures. The increased prothrombin time may cause postoperative bleeding. A preoperative INR (International normalized ratio) should be performed. If the platelet count is low (<100,000) then the socket should be packed and sutured. Persistent bleeding may require platelet transfusion.

Drug interactions
Ritonavir increases the plasma concentrations of a number of benzodiazepines, including midazolam and diazepam, and combined use should be avoided as deep sedation and respiratory depression can occur. Protease inhibitors appear to increase the plasma levels of lidocaine and increase cardiotoxicity of the latter drug. In addition the plasma concentrations of many opioid and non-steroidal anti-inflammatory drugs, macrolide antibiotics (such as erythromycin), imidazole and triazole antifungal agents, tricyclic and selective serotonin

reuptake inhibitor antidepressants, the steroids dexamethasone and prednisolone, warfarin and carbamazepine, are all increased by ritonavir. The effect of codeine may be reduced by ritinovir. Combination with metronidazole may produce a disulfiram-like reaction.

Rivastigmine (Exelon)

Description
An anticholinesterase drug.

Indications
Used in the management of Alzheimer's disease.

Effects on oral and dental structures
This drug can cause a xerostomia.

Effects on patient management
Xerostomia may increase caries incidence and thus a preventive regimen is important. If the xerostomia is severe, artificial saliva may be indicated. Non-steroidal anti-inflammatory drugs are best avoided in postoperative pain control (see drug interaction below).

Drug interactions
Gastrointestinal effects of non-steroidal anti-inflammatory drugs exacerbated.

Rizatriptan (Maxalt)

Description
A $5HT_1$ agonist.

Indications
Used in the treatment of acute migraine.

Effects on oral and dental structures
This drug may produce a xerostomia and facial oedema.

Effects on patient management
This drug is for short term use so xerostomia should not produce prolonged adverse effects. Avoid stimuli which may induce migraine, such as directly shining the dental light in the patient's eyes. The use of dark glasses may be of benefit to the patient.

Drug interactions
Combined therapy with monoamine oxidase inhibitors increases central nervous system toxicity and two weeks should elapse between use of these drugs. Other antimigraine drugs such as other $5HT_1$ agonists and ergotamine derivatives should not be administered till at least six hours after rizatriptan to avoid severe vasoconstriction.

Rofecoxib (Vioxx)

Description
A selective COX-2 inhibitor.

Indications
Pain and inflammation in osteoarthritis or rheumatoid arthritis.

Effects on oral and dental structures
Stomatitis, sinusitis, and taste disturbances can be produced.

Effects on patient management
If patient develops rofecoxib-induced stomatitis then the drug should be stopped and a full blood count carried out.

Drug interactions
Rofecoxib should not be given with other NSAIDs or aspirin since using such combinations will increase the risk of unwanted effects. The anticoagulant effects of both warfarin and heparin are enhanced by rofecoxib and could increase the risk of haemorrhage. Rofecoxib can antagonize the hypotensive effects of the ACE inhibitors (e.g. captopril, lisinopril). There is the additional increased risk of renal impairment and hyperkalaemia with these drugs and rofecoxib. Anti-diabetic drugs such as the sulphonylureas are extensively protein bound and can be displaced by rofecoxib, leading to hypoglycaemia. Rofecoxib can increase the risk of gastrointestinal haemorrhage if given to patients taking antiplatelet drugs such as clopidogrel. Rofecoxib should be avoided in patients taking beta-adrenoceptor blockers as there will be an antagonism of their hypotensive effect. Rofecoxib may exacerbate heart failure, reduce glomerular filtration rate and increase plasma concentration of digoxin. Both rofecoxib and corticosteroids (systemic) cause peptic ulceration, therefore avoid the combination. The excretion of methotrexate is reduced by rofecoxib which can lead to increased toxicity. Rofecoxib reduces the excretion of the muscle relaxant baclofen. The excretion of lithium is reduced by rofecoxib, thus increasing the risk of lithium toxicity.

Ropinirole (Requip)

Description
A dopaminergic drug.

Indications
Used in the management of Parkinsonism.

Effects on oral and dental structures
None reported.

Effects on patient management

This drug may cause postural hypotension, thus the patient should not be changed from the supine to the standing position too rapidly. Parkinsonism can lead to management problems as the patient may have uncontrollable movement. Short appointments are recommended.

Drug interactions

None of importance in dentistry.

Ropivacaine (Naropin)

Description

An amide local anaesthetic.

Indications

Used for infiltration and regional block anaesthesia in medicine but at the time of writing had only been used experimentally as a dental local anaesthetic.

Presentations

Available in ampoules at concentrations varying from 0.2 to 1%.

Dose

No more than 30 ml of the 0.75% solution in a 70 kg adult (adjust for weight in children) when used as a field block.

Contraindications

Allergy to the amide group of local anaesthetics.

Unwanted effects

Central nervous system toxicity at high dose. Less cardiotoxicity than bupivacaine.

Drug interactions

None reported.

Salbutamol (Accuhaler, Aerolin, Airomir, Asmasal, Easi-breathe, Evohaler, Nebules, Rotacaps, Ventodisks, Ventolin)

Description

A beta$_2$-adrenoceptor stimulant.

Indications

Used in the management of asthma, and obstructive airway disease.

Effects on oral and dental structures

Xerostomia, taste alteration, and discolouration of the teeth may occur.

Effects on patient management

Patients may not be comfortable in the supine position if they have respiratory problems. Aspirin-like compounds should not be prescribed as many asthmatic patients are allergic to these analgesics. Similarly, sulphite-containing compounds (such as preservatives in epinephrine-containing local anaesthetics) can produce allergy in asthmatic patients. Xerostomia may increase caries incidence and thus a preventive regimen is important. If the xerostomia is severe, artificial saliva may be indicated. The use of a rubber dam in patients with obstructive airway disease may further embarrass the airway. If a rubber dam is essential then supplemental oxygen via a nasal cannula may be required.

Drug interactions

The hypokalaemia which may result from large doses of salbutamol may be exacerbated by a reduction in potassium produced by high doses of steroids and by epinephrine in dental local anaesthetics.

Salcatonin (Calsynar)

Description

A hormone secreted by parafollicular cell of the thyroid gland.

Indications

Paget's disease of bone, hypercalcaemia.

Effects on oral and dental structures

Can cause taste disturbances.

Effects on patient management

Nothing of significance.

Drug interactions

None of any dental significance.

Saliva substitute (Glandosane, Luborant, Oralbalance, Saliva Orthana, Salivace, Salveze, Salivix)

Description

Artificial salivas containing carmellose sodium, xylitol or sorbitol, and salts. Saliva Orthana contains mucin.

Indications

Used in the symptomatic treatment of xerostomia.

Presentations

Oral sprays, gels, and lozenges.

Dose
Used as required on oral mucosa.

Contraindications
Mucin-containing products may be prohibited due to religious reasons in some patients.

Precautions
None.

Unwanted effects
None due to therapy.

Drug interactions
None of importance in dentistry.

Salmeterol (Serevent)

Description
A beta$_2$-adrenoceptor stimulant.

Indications
Used in the management of asthma and obstructive airway disease.

Effects on oral and dental structures
Xerostomia, taste alteration, and dental pain may occur.

Effects on patient management
Patients may not be comfortable in the supine position if they have respiratory problems. Aspirin-like compounds should not be prescribed as many asthmatic patients are allergic to these analgesics. Similarly, sulphite-containing compounds (such as preservatives in epinephrine-containing local anaesthetics) can produce allergy in asthmatic patients. Xerostomia may increase caries incidence and thus a preventive regimen is important. If the xerostomia is severe, artificial saliva may be indicated. The use of a rubber dam in patients with obstructive airway disease may further embarrass the airway. If a rubber dam is essential then supplemental oxygen via a nasal cannula may be required.

Drug interactions
The hypokalaemia which may result from large doses of salmeterol may be exacerbated by a reduction in potassium produced by high doses of steroids, and by epinephrine in dental local anaesthetics.

Saquinavir (Fortovase, Invirase)

Description
A protease inhibitor antiviral drug.

Indications
Used in the management of HIV infection.

Effects on oral and dental structures
Oral ulceration, stomatitis, xerostomia, taste alteration, paraesthesia and, Stevens–Johnson syndrome may be produced.

Effects on patient management
Sedation with midazolam should be avoided (see below). Dose limitation with lidocaine local anaesthetics is wise (see below). Sensitive handling of the underlying disease state is essential. Excellent preventive dentistry and regular examinations are important in patients suffering from HIV, as dental infections are best avoided. HIV will interfere with postoperative healing and antibiotic prophylaxis prior to oral surgery may be advisable. Saquinavir can produce anaemia leucopenia and thrombocytopenia. Leucopenia will affect healing adversely and if severe prophylactic antibiotics should be prescribed to cover surgical procedures. Thrombocytopenia may cause postoperative bleeding. If the platelet count is low (<100,000) then the socket should be packed and sutured. Persistent bleeding may require platelet transfusion. Xerostomia may increase caries incidence and thus a preventive regimen is important. If the xerostomia is severe, artificial saliva may be indicated.

Drug interactions
Concurrent use with midazolam produces prolonged sedation and should be avoided. Protease inhibitors appear to increase the plasma levels of lidocaine and increase cardiotoxicity of the latter drug. Carbamazepine, phenytoin, and dexamethasone reduce the plasma concentration of saquinavir. In addition protease inhibitors may increase the serum levels of carbamazepine and phenytoin. Dexamethasone decreases the plasma levels of protease inhibitors, and serum concentrations of the steroid may be increased during concurrent therapy. Saquinavir plasma levels increased by ketoconazole and possibly by other antifungal agents.

Secobarbital (Quinalbarbitone) [Tuinal]

Description
A barbiturate hypnotic.

Indications
Only used in treatment of intractable insomnia in those already taking barbiturates.

Effects on oral and dental structures
Rarely oral ulceration may be produced. Barbiturates may cause xerostomia and fixed drug eruptions.

Effects on patient management

Xerostomia may increase caries incidence and thus a preventive regimen is important. If the xerostomia is severe, artificial saliva may be indicated. The patient may be drowsy and confused. As respiratory depression is produced by this drug other drugs which produce such depression, such as sedatives, must be avoided in general practice. Long term treatment with this drug may produce anaemia, agranulocytosis and thrombocytopenia. Anaemia and agranulocytosis may result in poor healing. Any anaemia will need correction prior to elective general anaesthesia and sedation. Thrombocytopenia may cause postoperative bleeding. If the platelet count is low (<100,000) then sockets should be packed and sutured. Persistent bleeding may require platelet transfusion.

Drug interactions

All barbiturates are enzyme-inducers and thus can increase the metabolism of concurrent medication. Drugs which are metabolized more rapidly in the presence of barbiturates include warfarin, carbamazepine, corticosteroids, and tricyclic antidepressants. The effects of other CNS depressants, including alcohol, are increased in the presence of barbiturates.

Selegeline hydrochloride (Eldepryl, Zelapar)

Description

A monoamine oxidase B inhibitor.

Indications

Used in the management of Parkinsonism.

Effects on oral and dental structures

Xerostomia and stomatitis may be produced.

Effects on patient management

Xerostomia may increase caries incidence and thus a preventive regimen is important. If the xerostomia is severe, artificial saliva may be indicated. This drug may cause postural hypotension, thus the patient should not be changed from the supine to the standing position too rapidly. Parkinsonism can lead to management problems as the patient may have uncontrollable movement. Short appointments are recommended.

Drug interactions

Opioids particularly pethidine should not be prescribed as hyperpyrexia and CNS toxicity may occur. Concurrent antidepressant therapy should be avoided. Other monoamine oxidase inhibitors produce hypotension, tricyclic cause CNS toxicity, and selective serotonin reuptake inhibitors cause hypertension during concurrent use.

Senna (Manevac, Senokot)

Description
A stimulant laxative.

Indications
Used in the management of constipation.

Effects on oral and dental structures
None specific.

Effects on patient management
See drug interactions below.

Drug interactions
Prolonged use may produce a hypokalaemia and this may be exacerbated by potassium shifts due to corticosteroids and epinephrine in local anaesthetics. Avoid the use of codeine and other opioid compounds as they exacerbate constipation.

Sertindole (Serdolect)

Description
An atypical antipsychotic drug.

Indications
Used in the treatment of schizophrenia.

Effects on oral and dental structures
Xerostomia and uncontrollable oro-facial muscle activity (tardive dyskenesia) may be produced.

Effects on patient management
Xerostomia may increase caries incidence and thus a preventive regimen is important. If the xerostomia is severe, artificial saliva may be indicated. Uncontrollable muscle movement of jaws and tongue as well as the underlying psychotic condition may interfere with management, as satisfactory co-operation may not be achieved readily. There may be problems with denture retention and certain stages of denture construction (e.g. jaw registration) can be difficult. Postural hypotension often occurs with this drug, therefore rapid changes in patient position should be avoided.

Drug interactions
There is increased sedation when used in combination with CNS depressant drugs such as alcohol, opioid analgesics, and sedatives. Eythromycin and the antifungal drugs itraconazole and ketoconazole increase the toxicity of sertindole. Both carbamazepine and phenytoin increase the metabolism of sertindole. Combined therapy with

tricyclic antidepressants increases the chances of cardiac arrythmias and exacerbates antimuscarinic effects such as xerostomia.

Sertraline (Lustral)

Description
A selective serotonin reuptake inhibitor.

Indications
Used in the management of depression.

Effects on oral and dental structures
Xerostomia and taste alteration be produced. Aphthous ulceration and Stevens–Johnson syndrome may occur.

Effects on patient management
Xerostomia may increase caries incidence and thus a preventive regimen is important. If the xerostomia is severe, artificial saliva may be indicated. Sertraline may produce thrombocytopenia. Thrombo-cytopenia may cause postoperative bleeding. If the platelet count is low (<100,000) then sockets should be packed and sutured. Persis-tent bleeding may require platelet transfusion. Gingival bleeding may also be produced as a result of thrombocytopenia.

Drug interactions
Combined therapy with other antidepressants should be avoided. Treatment with selective serotonin reuptake inhibitors should not begin until two weeks following cessation of monoamine oxidase inhibitor therapy. Selective serotonin reuptake inhibitors increase the anticoagulant effect of warfarin. Selective serotonin reuptake inhibitors antagonize the anticonvulsant effects of anti-epileptic medication. Sertraline inhibits the metabolism of alprazolam but does not appear to affect other benzodiazepines.

Sildenafil (Viagra)

Indications
Erectile dysfunction.

Effects on oral and dental structures
None reported.

Effects on patient management
Nothing of significance.

Drug interactions
Erythromycin and ketoconazole both increase the plasma concentra-tion of sildenafil, thus a dose reduction of the latter is required to avoid the risk of unwanted effects.

Simvastatin (Zocor)

Description
A cholesterol lowering drug.

Indications
To reduce coronary events by lowering LDL cholesterol.

Effects on oral and dental structures
None reported.

Effects on patient management
None of any significance.

Drug interactions
None of any dental significance.

Sodium bicarbonate (Peptac)

Description
An antacid and alkalinizing agent.

Indications
Used to treat dyspepsia, in the reversal of metabolic acidosis, in the emergency management of electrolyte imbalance and cardiac arrest.

Effects on oral and dental structures
None known.

Effects on patient management
Patients may not be comfortable in the fully supine position due to gastric reflux. Any drug with which there is an interaction (such as tetracycline) should be taken a few hours in advance of antacid dose.

Drug interactions
Combined therapy causes reduced absorption of phenytoin, tetracyclines, the non-steroidal analgesic diflunisal, and the antifungal drugs ketoconazole and itraconazole. Antacids can increase the excretion of aspirin and reduce plasma concentration to non-therapeutic levels.

Sodium clodronate (Bonefos)

Description
A bisphosphonate.

Indications
Osteolytic lesions, hypercalcaemia, and bone pain associated with skeletal metastases in patients with breast cancer or multiple myeloma.

Effects on oral and dental structures
Nothing reported.

Effects on patient management
Nothing of significance.

Drug interactions
Sodium clodronate does cause renal dysfunction and this can be compounded by NSAIDs such as ibuprofen. The latter drugs should be avoided or only used for the short term if the patient's renal function is satisfactory.

Sodium cromoglicate (Aerocrom, Cromogen Easi-Breathe, Intal, Nalcrom, Rynacrom)

Description
A mast cell stabilizing drug.

Indications
Used in the management of asthma, allergic rhinitis, and food allergy.

Effects on oral and dental structures
Xerostomia, burning mouth, and taste disturbance may occur.

Effects on patient management
Xerostomia may increase caries incidence and thus a preventive regimen is important. If the xerostomia is severe, artificial saliva may be indicated. Patients may not be comfortable in the supine position if they have respiratory problems. If the patient is asthmatic aspirin-like compounds should not be prescribed. Similarly sulphite-containing compounds (such as preservatives in epinephrine-containing local anaesthetics) can produce allergy in asthmatic patients.

Drug interactions
None of importance in dentistry.

Sodium fusidate (Fucidin)

Description
A narrow spectrum antibiotic.

Indications
Used to treat infections due to penicillin-resistant staphylococci, especially osteomyelitis and staphylococcal endocarditis.

Effects on oral and dental structures
None specific.

Effects on patient management
Patients receiving this drug are probably extremely ill and only emergency dental treatment is indicated.

Drug interactions
None of importance in dentistry.

Sodium ironedetate

Description
An iron salt.

Indications
Iron deficiency anaemia.

Effects on oral and dental structures
Iron salts can cause staining of the teeth and tongue.

Effect on patient management
Nothing of significance.

Drug interactions
Iron salts chelate tetracyclines which in turn prevent their absorption. The two drugs should not be given together.

Soluble insulin (Hypurin, Humulin)

Description
A short-acting insulin.

Indications
Diabetes mellitus, diabetic ketoacidosis.

Effects on oral and dental structures
Soluble insulin can cause pain and swelling of the salivary glands.

Effects on patient management
The main concern with treating diabetic patients on insulin is to avoid hypoglycaemia. Thus it is important to ensure that patients have taken their normal food and insulin prior to their dental appointment. Wherever possible treat diabetic patients in the first half of the morning and ensure that any treatment does not preclude them from eating. If an insulin-dependent diabetic requires a general anaesthetic, then referred to hospital.

Drug interactions
Aspirin and the NSAIDs can cause hypoglycaemia which could be a problem in a poorly-controlled insulin dependent diabetic. These analgesics should be used with caution in such patients. Systemic corticosteroids will antagonize the hypoglycaemic properties of insulin. If these drugs are required in an insulin dependent diabetic, then consult the patient's physician before prescribing.

Sodium perborate (Bocasan)

Description
An oxidizing agent.

Indications
Used as an aid to oral hygiene.

Presentations
In sachets containing 68.6% sodium perborate.

Dose
Use contents of sachet diluted in 30 mL water as a rinse 3 times daily.

Contraindications
Allergy.

Precautions
None.

Unwanted effects
None.

Drug interactions
None of importance in dentistry.

Sodium picosulfate

Description
A stimulant laxative.

Indications
Used in the management of constipation.

Effects on oral and dental structures
None specific.

Effects on patient management
See drug interactions below.

Drug interactions
Prolonged use may produce a hypokalaemia and this may be exacerbated by potassium shifts due to corticosteroids and epinephrine in local anaesthetics. Avoid the use of codeine and other opioid compounds as they exacerbate constipation.

Sodium stibogluconate (Pentostam)

Description
An antiprotozoal drug.

Indications
Used in the management of Leishmaniasis.

Effects on oral and dental structures
May cause gingival bleeding.

Effects on patient management
As treatment with this drug is short term, management effects are minimal.

Drug interactions
None of importance in dentistry.

Somatropin (Genotropin, Humatrope)

Description
Synthetic human growth hormone.

Indications
Turner's syndrome, defects in growth hormone secretion.

Effects on oral and dental structures
None reported.

Effects on patient management
None of significance.

Drug interactions
None of dental significance.

Sotalol hydrochloride (Beta-cardone, Sotacor)

Description
A beta-adrenoceptor blocking drug.

Indications
Prophylaxis of paroxysmal atrial tachycardia or fibrillation, ventricular arrhythmias, prophylaxis of supraventricular arrhythmias.

Effects on oral and dental structures
Sotalol can cause xerostomia, lichenoid eruptions, inhibition of calculus of formation, and altered sensations (numbness) of the face. The dry mouth and the actions of sotalol hydrochloride on saliva will make the dentate patient more susceptible to dental caries, especially root caries.

Effects on patient management
Postural hypotension may occur and the patient may feel dizzy when the dental chair is restored to upright after they have been treated in the supine position. If the xerostomia is severe, dentate patients should receive topical fluoride and be offered an artificial saliva.

Drug interactions
NSAIDs such as ibuprofen may antagonize hypotensive effect; possible interaction between epinephrine and sotalol hydrochloride which may cause a slight increase in blood pressure. Do not exceed more than 3 cartridges of epinephrine containing local anaesthetic solution per adult patient. Sotalol can cause hypokalaemia, which can be exacerbated by systemic amphotericin and epinephrine containing local anaesthetics solutions (see dose restrictions above).

Spectinomycin (robicin)

Description
An antibiotic active against Gram-negative bacteria.

Indications
Used in the treatment of penicillin-resistant gonorrhoea.

Effects on oral and dental structures
The underlying disease of gonorrhoea may show oral mucosal signs such as ulceration and erythema.

Effects on patient management
Local treatment to oral lesions of gonorrhoea may be required. However, these resolve with the systemic medication.

Drug interactions
This drug increases the toxicity of Botulinum toxin.

Spironolactone (Adactone, Spiroctan)

Description
An aldosterone antagonist.

Indications
Oedema, ascites following liver cirrhosis, congestive heart failure, and primary hyperaldosteronism.

Effects on oral and dental structures
Taste disturbances may occur due to zinc chelation.

Effects on patient management
None.

Drug interactions
Aspirin antagonizes the diuretic actions of spironolactone.

Stanozolol (Stromba)

Description
An anabolic steroid.

Indication
Behçet's disease and hereditary angioedema.

Effects on oral and dental structures
Behçet's disease will be associated with oral ulceration and patients with a history of hereditary angioedema will be susceptible to swelling of the lips, the tongue and the floor of the mouth.

Effects on patient management
Hereditary angioedema may be precipitated by dental treatment. Thus it is important to ensure patients have taken their medication prior to any dental work.

Drug interactions
None of any dental significance.

Stavudine (Zerit)

Description
A nucleoside reverse transcriptase inhibitor.

Indications
Used in the management of HIV infection.

Effects on oral and dental structures
This drug may produce oral ulceration and paraesthesia.

Effects on patient management
Sensitive handling of the underlying disease state is essential. Excellent preventive dentistry and regular examinations are important in patients suffering from HIV, as dental infections are best avoided. HIV will interfere with postoperative healing and antibiotic prophylaxis prior to oral surgery may be advisable. This drug may produce neutropenia and thrombocytopenia. Thrombocytopenia may cause postoperative bleeding. If the platelet count is low (<100,000) then sockets should be packed and sutured. Persistent bleeding may require platelet transfusion.

Drug interactions
None of importance in dentistry.

Sterculia (Normacol)

Description
A bulk-forming laxative.

Indications
Used to treat constipation.

Effects on oral and dental structures
None specific.

Effects on patient management
See drug interactions below.

Drug interactions
Avoid the use of codeine and other opioid compounds as they exacerbate constipation.

Streptomycin

Description
An antitubercular drug.

Indications
Used in the treatment of tuberculosis and brucellosis.

Effects on oral and dental structures
Streptomycin can cause oral paraesthesia.

Effects on patient management
Only emergency dental treatment should be performed during active tuberculosis and care must be exercised to eliminate spread of tuberculosis between the patient and dental personnel, e.g. masks and glasses should be worn and where possible treatment should be performed under a rubber dam to reduce aerosol spread.

Drug interactions
There is an increased risk of nephrotoxicity and ototoxicity when used in combination with vancomycin and teicoplanin. Similarly there is an increased risk of nephrotoxicity with amphotericin.

Sucralfate (Antepsin)

Description
A complex of aluminium hydroxide and sulphated sucrose.

Indications
Used in the management of gastrointestinal ulceration.

Effects on oral and dental structures
Xerostomia and a metallic taste may be produced.

Effects on patient management
Non-steroidal anti-inflammatory drugs should be avoided due to gastrointestinal irritation. Similarly, high dose systemic steroids should not be prescribed in patients with gastrointestinal ulceration. Xerostomia may increase caries incidence and thus a preventive regimen is important. If the xerostomia is severe, artificial saliva may be indicated.

Drug interactions
The absorption of amphotericin B, ketoconazole, tetracyclines, and phenytoin is reduced. Sucralfate may also reduce the effects of warfarin. See comments on non-steroidals and steroids above.

Sulfadiazine

Description
A sulfonamide antibiotic.

Indications
Used to prevent the recurrence of rheumatic fever and to treat toxoplasmosis.

Effects on oral and dental structures
Stomatitis, glossitis, Stevens–Johnson syndrome, fixed drug eruptions, and candidiasis can occur.

Effects on patient management
The patient may have a history of rheumatic fever, and thus antibiotic prophylaxis may be required prior to bacteraemia-producing dental procedures. This drug may cause thrombocytopenia, agranulocytosis, and anaemia. Thrombocytopenia may cause postoperative bleeding. If the platelet count is low (<100,000) then the socket should be packed and sutured. Persistent bleeding may require platelet transfusion. Agranulocytosis and anaemia may result in poor healing. Any anaemia will need correction prior to elective general anaesthesia and sedation.

Drug interactions
There is an increased chance of methaemoglobinaemia when used in combination with prilocaine, including topical use of the anaesthetic. The effects of the anticoagulants warfarin and nicoumalone are enhanced during combined therapy. The plasma concentration of phenytoin may be increased.

Sulfadimidine

Description
A sulfonamide antibiotic.

Indications
Used in the treatment of urinary tract infections.

Effects on oral and dental structures
Stomatitis, glossitis, Stevens–Johnson syndrome, fixed drug eruptions, and candidiasis can occur.

Effects on patient management
This drug may cause thrombocytopenia, agranulocytosis, and anaemia. Thrombocytopenia may cause postoperative bleeding. If the platelet count is low (<100,000) then sockets should be packed and sutured. Persistent bleeding may require platelet transfusion. Agranulocytosis and anaemia may result in poor healing. Any anaemia will need correction prior to elective general anaesthesia and sedation.

Drug interactions
There is an increased chance of methaemoglobinaemia when used in combination with prilocaine, including topical use of the anaesthetic. The effects of the anticoagulants warfarin and nicoumalone are enhanced during combined therapy. The plasma concentration of phenytoin may be increased.

Sulfametopyrazine

Description
A sulfonamide antibiotic.

Indications
Used in the treatment of respiratory and urinary tract infections.

Effects on oral and dental structures
Stomatitis, glossitis, fixed drug eruptions, Stevens–Johnson syndrome, and candidiasis can occur.

Effects on patient management

This drug may cause thrombocytopenia, agranulocytosis, and anaemia. Thrombocytopenia may cause postoperative bleeding. If the platelet count is low (<100,000) then sockets should be packed and sutured. Persistent bleeding may require platelet transfusion. Agranulocytosis and anaemia may result in poor healing. Any anaemia will need correction prior to elective general anaesthesia and sedation.

Drug interactions

There is an increased chance of methaemoglobinaemia when used in combination with prilocaine, including topical use of the anaesthetic. The effects of the anticoagulants warfarin and nicoumalone are enhanced during combined therapy. The plasma concentration of phenytoin may be increased.

Sulfasalazine (Salazopyrin)

Description

An aminosalicylate.

Indications

Used to treat ulcerative colitis.

Effects on oral and dental structures

May produce stomatitis, glossitis, oral ulceration, mucosal bleeding, parotitis, lichen planus, lupus erythematosus, and Stevens–Johnson syndrome.

Effects on patient management

Non-steroidal inflammatory drugs are best avoided. In order to avoid pseudomembranous ulcerative colitis discussion with the supervising physician is advised prior to prescription of an antibiotic. The aminosalicylates can produce blood dyscrasias including anaemia, leucopenia, and thrombocytopenia. Anaemia may result in poor healing. Any anaemia will need correction prior to elective general anaesthesia and sedation. Leucopenia will affect healing adversely and if severe prophylactic antibiotics should be prescribed to cover surgical procedures. Thrombocytopenia may cause postoperative bleeding. If the platelet count is low (<100,000) then sockets should be packed and sutured. Persistent bleeding may require platelet transfusion.

Patients may be receiving steroids in addition to aminosalicylates and thus the occurrence of adrenal crisis should be borne in mind. This is due to adrenal suppression. Whilst such suppression does occur physiologically, its clinical significance does appear to be overstated. As far as dentistry is concerned, there is increasing evidence that supplementary corticosteroids are not required. This would apply to all restorative procedures, periodontal surgery and the uncompli-cated dental extraction. For more complicated dentolveolar surgery, each case must be judged on its merits. An apprehensive patient may well require cover. It is important to monitor the patient's blood pressure before, during and for 30 minutes after the procedure. If diastolic pressure drops by more than 25%, then hydrocortisone 100 mg IV should be administered and patient's blood pressure con-tinues to be monitored.

Drug interactions
See comments on non-steroidals and antibiotics above.

Sulfinpyrazone (Anturan)

Indications
Gout prophylaxis, hyperuricaemia.

Effects on oral and dental structures
Sulfinpyrazone can cause bone marrow suppression, which can cause an exacerbation of oral ulceration and an increased propensity to spontaneous gingival bleeding.

Effects on patient management
Sulfinpyrazone-induced bone marrow suppression can cause an increased risk of oral infection, especially after dental surgical proce-dures. The accompanying thrombocytopenia increases the risk of haemorrhage. If the platelet count is low (<100,000) then sockets should be packed and sutured. Persistent bleeding may require a platelet transfusion.

Drug interactions
Aspirin and other salicylates antagonize the uricosuric actions of sul-finpyrazone. Such antagonism could precipitate an attack of gout.

Sulindac (Clinoril)

Description
A peripherally acting, non-steroidal anti-inflammatory analgesic.

Indications
Pain and inflammation associated with musculoskeletal disorders, e.g. rheumatoid arthritis, osteoarthritis, and ankylosing spondylitis. Dysmenorrhoea and menorrhagia.

Effects on oral and dental structures
Patients on long-term NSAIDs such as sulindac may be afforded some degree of protection against periodontal breakdown. This arises from the drug's inhibitory action on prostaglandin synthesis.

The latter is an important inflammatory mediator in the pathogenesis of periodontal breakdown.

Effects on patient management

Rare unwanted effects of sulindac include angioedema and thrombocytopenia. The latter may cause an increased bleeding tendency following any dental surgical procedure. If the platelet count is low (<100,000) then sockets should be packed and sutured. Persistent bleeding may require a platelet transfusion.

Drug interactions

Ibuprofen, aspirin, and diflunisal should be avoided in patients taking sulindac due to an increase in unwanted effects, especially gastrointestinal ulceration, renal, and liver damage. Systemic corticosteroids increase the risk of peptic ulceration and gastrointestinal bleeding.

Sulphasalazine (Salazopyrin)

Description

An anti-inflammatory agent.

Indications

Active rheumatoid arthritis and ulcerative colitis.

Effects on oral and dental structures

Sulphasalazine can cause significant haematological problems resulting in a leucopenia and thrombocytopenia. Both effects can cause an exacerbation of periodontal disease, oral ulceration and an increased propensity to spontaneous gingival bleeding.

Effects on patient management

Sulphasalazine-induced leucopenia can cause an increased risk of oral infection, especially after dental surgical procedures. The accompanying thrombocytopenia increases the risk of haemorrhage. If the platelet count is low (<100,000) then sockets should be packed and sutured. Persistent bleeding may require a platelet transfusion.

Drug interactions

None of any dental significance.

Sulpiride (Dolmatil, Sulparex, Sulpitil)

Description

A phenothiazine antipsychotic medication.

Indications

Used in the treatment of psychoses such as schizophrenia.

Effects on oral and dental structures

Xerostomia, uncontrollable oro-facial muscle activity (tardive dyskenesia), Stevens–Johnson syndrome and lichenoid reactions may occur with this drug.

Effects on patient management

Xerostomia may increase caries incidence and thus a preventive regimen is important. If the xerostomia is severe, artificial saliva may be indicated. Uncontrollable muscle movement of jaws and tongue as well as the underlying psychotic condition may interfere with management, as satisfactory co-operation may not be achieved readily. There may be problems with denture retention and certain stages of denture construction (e.g. jaw registration) can be difficult. Postural hypotension often occurs with this drug, therefore rapid changes in patient position should be avoided. This drug can produce leucocytosis, agranulocytosis, and anaemia which may interfere with postoperative healing.

Drug interactions

There is increased sedation when used in combination with CNS depressant drugs such as alcohol, opioid analgesics, and sedatives. Combined therapy with tricyclic antidepressants increases the chances of cardiac arrhythmias and exacerbates antimuscarinic effects such as xerostomia. There is a theoretical risk of hypotension being exacerbated by the epinephrine in dental local anaesthetics.

Sumatriptan (Imigran)

Description

A $5HT_1$ agonist.

Indications

Used in the treatment of acute migraine and cluster headache.

Effects on oral and dental structures

This drug can produce discomfort of the mouth and jaws.

Effects on patient management

Avoid stimuli which may induce migraine, such as directly shining the dental light in the patient's eyes. The use of dark glasses may be of benefit to the patient.

Drug interactions

Combined therapy with monoamine oxidase inhibitors increases central nervous system toxicity and two weeks should elapse between use of these drugs. Similarly, combined therapy with selective serotonin reuptake inhibitors should be avoided. Other antimigraine drugs such as other $5HT_1$ agonists and ergotamine derivatives should not be administered till at least six hours after sumatriptan to avoid severe vasoconstriction.

Tacrolimus (Prograf)

Description
An immunosuppressant.

Indications
To prevent graft rejection in organ transplantation.

Effects on oral and dental structures
The immunosuppressant properties of tacrolimus could impact upon expression of periodontal disease (reduce breakdown), cause delayed healing, and make the patient more susceptible to opportunistic oral infections such as candida or herpetic infections. Organ transplant patients on tacrolimus are more prone to malignancy and lesions which can affect the mouth, including Kaposi's sarcoma and lip cancer. Hairy leukoplakia can also develop in these patients and again this is attributed to the immunosuppressant properties of tacrolimus.

Effects on patient management
All patients on immunosuppressant therapy should receive a regular oral screening because of the increased propensity to 'oral' and lip malignancies. Any suspicious lesion must be biopsied. Likewise signs of opportunistic oral infections must be treated promptly to avoid systemic complications. The delayed healing and increased susceptibility to infection does not warrant the use of prophylactic antibiotic cover before specific dental procedures.

Drug interactions
Ibuprofen and amphotericin increase risk of tacrolimus-induced nephrotoxicity. Antifungal agents such as fluconazole and ketoconazole increase the plasma concentrations of tacrolimus.

Tamoxifen (Nolvadex)

Description
An oestrogen-receptor antagonist.

Indications
Breast cancer, anovulatory infertility.

Effects on oral and dental structures
Can cause a thrombocytopenia which can exacerbate any existing gingival bleeding.

Effects on patient management

Tamoxifen-induced thrombocytopenia can cause problems with bleeding after any dental surgical procedure. If the platelet count is low (<100,000) then sockets should be packed and sutured. Persistent bleeding may require a platelet transfusion.

Drug interactions

None of any dental significance.

Teicoplanin (Targocid)

Description

A glycopeptide antibiotic.

Indications

The only indication in dentistry is for the prophylaxis of endocarditis in those having a general anaesthetic and who cannot receive amoxicillin.

Presentations

Vials for reconstitution containing 200 mg or 400 mg.

Dose

As prophylaxis for endocarditis, 400 mg given by intravenous injection at general anaesthetic induction (gentamycin must be administered in conjunction with this treatment). For children under 14 years the dose of teicoplanin is 6 mg/kg.

Contraindications

Hypersensitivity (including hypersensitivity to vancomycin).
History of deafness.
Renal disease.

Precautions

Renal disease.

Unwanted effects

Gastrointestinal upset.
Renal toxicity including kidney failure.
Tinnitus, hearing loss, and vestibular upsets.
Hypersensitivity reactions.
Haematological disorders (such as reduction in white cells and platelets) may occur after prolonged use.
Headache and dizziness.

Drug interactions

No significant interactions with single dose used in dentistry.

Telmisartan (Micardis)

Description
An angiotensin II receptor antagonist.

Indications
Used as an alternative to ACE inhibitors where the latter cannot be tolerated

Effects on oral and dental structures
Angioedema has been reported, but the incidence of this unwanted effect is much less than when compared to ACE inhibitors.

Effect on patient management
None of any significance.

Drug interactions
NSAIDs such as ibuprofen may reduce the antihypertensive action of telmisartan.

Temazepam

Description
A benzodiazepine anxiolytic drug.

Indications
Used as an oral sedative for dental treatment (also used short term to treat insomnia).

Presentations
  (i) 10 mg and 20 mg tablets.
 (ii) 10 mg, 15 mg, 20 mg and 30 mg capsules.
(iii) Oral solution containing 10 mg/5 mL.

Dose
  (i) For insomnia
        10–20 mg at bed-time (not for use in children).
 (ii) As a sedative for dental treatment
        10–40 mg one hour before treatment.

Contraindications
Severe respiratory disease.
Severe liver disease.
Myasthenia gravis.

Precautions
Respiratory disease.
Pregnancy and breastfeeding.

Drug and alcohol abuse.
Psychoses.
Porphyria.

Unwanted effects
Dependence.
Respiratory depression.

Drug interactions
As with all benzodiazepines, enhanced effects occur with combined therapy with other CNS depressants such as alcohol and opioid analgesics. Disulfiram inhibits the metabolism of temazepam. Oral contraceptives can decrease the efficacy of temazepam.

Tenoxicam (Mobiflex)

Description
A peripherally acting, non-steroidal anti-inflammatory analgesic.

Indications
Pain and inflammation associated with musculoskeletal disorders, e.g. rheumatoid arthritis, osteoarthritis, and ankylosing spondylitis. Dysmenorrhoea and menorrhagia.

Effects on oral and dental structures
Patients on long-term NSAIDs such as tenoxicam may be afforded some degree of protection against periodontal breakdown. This arises from the drug's inhibitory action on prostaglandin synthesis. The latter is an important inflammatory mediator in the pathogenesis of periodontal breakdown.

Effects on patient management
Rare unwanted effects of tenoxicam include angioedema and thrombocytopenia. The latter may cause an increased bleeding tendency following any dental surgical procedure. If the platelet count is low (<100,000) then sockets should be packed and sutured. Persistent bleeding may require a platelet transfusion.

Drug interactions
Ibuprofen, aspirin, and diflunisal should be avoided in patients taking tenoxicam due to an increase in unwanted effects, especially gastrointestinal ulceration, renal, and liver damage. Systemic corticosteroids increase the risk of peptic ulceration and gastrointestinal bleeding.

Terazosin (Hytrin)

Description
An alpha-adrenoceptor blocking drug.

Indications
Mild to moderate hypertension and benign prostate hyperplasia.

Effects on oral and dental structures
None reported.

Effects on patient management
Nothing of dental significance.

Drug interactions
NSAIDs such as ibuprofen and systemic corticosteroids may antagonize the hypotensive action of terazosin.

Terbinafine (Lamisil)

Description
An antifungal agent.

Indications
Used in the management of fungal infections of the nails and in the treatment of ringworm.

Effects on oral and dental structures
Taste disturbance and Stevens–Johnson syndrome may occur.

Effects on patient management
Terbinafine produces a neutropenia which may impair healing.

Drug interactions
None of importance in dentistry.

Terbutaline sulphate (Bricanyl, Monovent)

Description
A beta$_2$-adrenoceptor stimulant.

Indications
Used in the management of asthma and obstructive airway disease.

Effects on oral and dental structures
Xerostomia and taste alteration may occur.

Effects on patient management
Patients may not be comfortable in the supine position if they have respiratory problems. Aspirin-like compounds should not be prescribed as many asthmatic patients are allergic to these analgesics. Similarly, sulphite-containing compounds (such as preservatives in epinephrine-containing local anaesthetics) can produce allergy in asthmatic patients. Xerostomia may increase caries incidence and thus a preventive regimen is important. If the xerostomia is severe, artificial saliva may be indicated. The use of a rubber dam in patients with obstructive airway disease may further embarrass the airway. If a rubber dam is essential then supplemental oxygen via a nasal cannula may be required.

Drug interactions
The hypokalaemia which may result from large doses of terbutaline may be exacerbated by a reduction in potassium produced by high doses of steroids and by epinephrine in dental local anaesthetics.

Terfenadine (Triludan)

Description
An antihistamine.

Indications
Used in the treatment of allergies such as rhinitis and urticaria.

Effects on oral and dental structures
May produce xerostomia, but this is less common compared to older antihistamines. Stevens–Johnson syndrome may occur.

Effects on patient management
The patient may be drowsy which may interfere with co-operation. Xerostomia may increase caries incidence and thus a preventive regimen is important. If the xerostomia is severe, artificial saliva may be indicated.

Drug interactions

Eythromycin, clarithromycin, the antifungal drugs ketoconazole, miconazole, itraconazole, and fluconazole, and the antiviral agents efavirenz, indinavir, nelfinavir, ritonavir, and saquinavir can all produce dangerous arrhythmias when combined with terfenadine. Grapefruit juice must be avoided during therapy with terfenadine. Enhanced sedative effect with anxiolytic and hypnotic drugs. Tricyclic and monoamine oxidase inhibitor antidepressants increase antimuscarinic effects such as xerostomia.

Testosterone (Restandol)

Description
A male sex hormone.

Indications
Androgen deficiency in men associated with primary or secondary hypogonadism.

Effects on oral and dental structures
None reported.

Effects on patient management
Testosterone can cause significant behavioural changes, especially if misused. Patients may become aggressive, depressed or more anxious. All changes can have an impact on the delivery and acceptance of dental care.

Drug interactions
None of any dental significance.

Tetrabenazine

Description
A dopamine-depleting drug.

Indications
Used in the management of Huntington's chorea.

Effects on oral and dental structures
May cause involuntary movements of the oral and facial muscles.

Effects on patient management
Involuntary muscle movements e.g. of the tongue will interfere with operative dentistry.

Drug interactions
Combination therapy with monoamine oxidase inhibitors can cause convulsions and hypertension.

Tetracaine [Amethocaine] (Ametop)

Description
An ester local anaesthetic for topical use.

Indications
Used for topical anaesthesia of the skin prior to venepuncture.

Presentations
A 4% gel.

Dose
1.5 g applied to skin surface.

Contraindications
Allergy to ester local anaesthetics and parabens. Should not be used in infants less than one year old.

Precautions
Care must be employed in patients with liver disease, as absorption is rapid an toxicity may occur. Similarly, it should not be used on traumatized or damaged tissue or highly vascularized mucous membranes.

Unwanted effects
Allergic reactions may occur. Amethocaine is more toxic than other ester local anaesthetics because of slower metabolism and thus it is no longer used as an injectable agent.

Drug interactions
Increased systemic toxicity occurs when administered in combination with other local anaesthetics.

Tetracycline (Achromycin, Deteclo)

Description
A bacteriostatic antibiotic.

Indications
Tetracyclines are rarely indicated in the management of dental infections but are used in the treatment of periodontal disease.

Presentations
 (i) 250 mg tablets.
 (ii) 250 mg capsules.
(iii) Incorporation into slow release devices for application into periodontal pockets.

Dose

250 mg four times daily to treat infections. When used in the management of periodontal disease the duration of therapy is two weeks.

Contraindications

Pregnancy.
Breastfeeding.
Children under 12 years.
Kidney disease.
Systemic lupus erythematosus.

Precautions

Liver disease.

Unwanted effects

Staining of teeth and bones.
Lichenoid reactions.
Fixed drug eruptions.
Opportunistic fungal infections ('tetracycline sore mouth').
Hypersensitivity.
Photosensitivity.
Facial pigmentation.
Headache and visual disturbances.
Anaemia.
Hepatotoxicity.
Pancreatitis.
Gastrointestinal upset including pseudomembranous colitis.

Drug interactions

As tetracycline chelates calcium and other cations a number of drugs (and foodstuffs such as dairy products) which contain cations reduce the absorption of tetracycline. Among the drugs which reduce the absorption of tetracycline are the ACE-inhibitor quinapril, antacids, calcium, and zinc salts, ulcer-healing drugs such as sucralfate and the ion-exchange resin colestipol. Similarly tetracyclines inhibit the absorption of iron and zinc. Tetracyclines reduce the efficacy of penicillins and cephalosporins.

Tetracycline raises blood urea levels and this effect is exacerbated with combined therapy with diuretics. Tetracycline may enhance the anticoagulant effect of warfarin and the other coumarin anticoagulants. Tetracycline may interfere without the action of oral contraceptives and alternative methods of contraception should be advised during therapy. Tetracyclines have a hypoglycaemic effect and their administration to patients receiving insulin or oral hypoglycaemics should be avoided.

Tetracycline may increase the serum levels of digoxin, theophylline and the anti-malarial medication mefloquine. Tetracycline may also increase the risk of methotrexate toxicity. Combined therapy with ergotamine can produce ergotism (the most dramatic effect of ergotism is vasospasm which can cause gangrene). Patients who use a contact lens cleaner containing thiomersal have reported ocular irritation during tetracycline therapy. Cranial hypertension leading to headache and dizziness may result with the combined use of tetracycline and retinoids.

Theophylline (Lasma, Nuelin, Slo-Phyllin, Theo-Dur, Uniphyllin Continus)

Description
A bronchodilator.

Indications
Used in the management of asthma and reversible airway obstruction.

Effects on oral and dental structures
Xerostomia and taste disturbance are produced. Stevens–Johnson syndrome may occur with this drug.

Effects on patient management
Patients may not be comfortable in the supine position if they have respiratory problems. If the patient suffers from asthma then aspirin-like compounds should not be prescribed as many asthmatic patients are allergic to these analgesics. Similarly, sulphite-containing compounds (such as preservatives in epinephrine-containing local anaesthetics) can produce allergy in asthmatic patients. Xerostomia may increase caries incidence and thus a preventive regimen is important. If the xerostomia is severe, artificial saliva may be indicated. The use of a rubber dam in patients with obstructive airway disease may further embarrass the airway. If a rubber dam is essential then supplemental oxygen via a nasal cannula may be required. (See drug interactions below.)

Drug interactions
There is an increased chance of dysrhythmia with halogenated general anaesthetic agents during combined therapy. Theophylline decreases the sedative and anxiolytic effects of some benzodiazepines including diazepam. Plasma theophylline levels are reduced by carbamazepine and phenytoin. Plasma theophylline concentration is increased by ciprofloxacin, clarithromycin, erythromycin, fluconazole, and ketoconazole and tetracyclines. Theophylline decreases the plasma concentration of erythromycin. Theophylline levels may be affected by corticosteroids. Hydrocortisone and methylprednisolone have been shown to both increase and decrease theophylline levels. Concurrent therapy with quinolone antibacterials such as ciprofloxacin may lead to convulsions.

Thioridazine (Melleril)

Description
A phenothiazine antipsychotic medication.

Indications
Used in the treatment of psychoses such as schizophrenia and in short term management of severe anxiety.

Effects on oral and dental structures
Xerostomia and uncontrollable oro-facial muscle activity (tardive dyskenesia) may be produced. The oral mucosa may be discoloured. Stevens–Johnson syndrome and lichenoid reactions may be produced.

Effects on patient management
As the drug is only used short term xerostomia should not produce significant problems, however a preventive regimen may be considered. Uncontrollable muscle movement of jaws and tongue as well as the underlying psychotic condition may interfere with management, as satisfactory co-operation may not be achieved readily. There may be problems with denture retention and certain stages of denture construction (e.g. jaw registration) can be difficult. Postural hypotension often occurs with this drug, therefore rapid changes in patient position should be avoided. This drug can produce leucocytosis, agranluocytosis, and anaemia which may interfere with postoperative healing.

Drug interactions
There is increased sedation when used in combination with CNS depressant drugs such as alcohol, opioid analgesics, and sedatives. Combined therapy with tricyclic antidepressants increases the chances of cardiac arrythmias and exacerbates antimuscarinic effects such as xerostomia. The photosensitivity produced by tetracyclines is increased during combined therapy. There is a theoretical risk of hypotension being exacerbated by the epinephrine in dental local anaesthetics.

Thiotepa

Description
An alkylating agent.

Indications
Bladder cancer and certain types of malignant effusions.

Effects on oral and dental structures
Thiotepa causes bone marrow suppression with an accompanying thrombocytopenia and agranulocytosis. Bone marrow suppression

can lead to troublesome oral ulceration, exacerbation of an existing periodontal condition and rapid spread of any residual (e.g. periapical) infections.

Effects on patient management

The effect of thiotepa on the bone marrow is transient and routine dental treatment is best avoided until the white blood cells and platelet counts start to recover. If emergency dental treatment such as an extraction is required then antibiotic cover may be neccessary depending on the degree of myelosuppression. If the platelet count is low (<100,000) then sockets should be packed and sutured. Persistent bleeding may require a platelet transfusion.

Patients on chemotherapeutic agents such as thiotepa often neglect their oral hygiene and thus there could be an increase in both caries and periodontal disease. If time permits, patients about to go on chemotherapy should have a dental check up and any potential areas of infection should be treated. Similarly, to reduce the mucosal irritation (sensitivity) that often accompanies chemotherapy, it is advisable to remove any ill-fitting dentures and smooth over rough cusps or restorations.

Drug interactions

None of any dental significance.

Thymol

Description

An antiseptic agent.

Indications

Used as an aid to oral hygiene.

Presentations

 (i) Present as a 0.05% solution in combination with 10% glycerol as an oral rinse.
(ii) As a constituent of mouthwash tablets.

Dose

Mouthwash used undiluted or diluted with 3 times volume of water as a rinse.
Tablet dissolved in a tumbler of water as a rinse.

Contraindications

Allergy.

Precautions

None.

Unwanted effects
None significant.

Drug interactions
None of importance in dentistry.

Thyroxine

Description
A thyroid hormone.

Indications
Hypothyroidism.

Effects on oral and dental structures
None reported.

Effects on patient management
High or excessive doses of thyroxine can induce a thyrotoxic state. The patient will be restless, agitated and excitable. In such circumstances, dental treatment will be difficult to complete.

Drug interactions
None of any dental significance.

Tiabendazole (Mintezol)

Description
An antihelminthic drug.

Indications
Used in the management of strongyloidiasis infection.

Effects on oral and dental structures
This drug may cause Stevens–Johnson syndrome.

Effects on patient management
None specific.

Drug interactions
Corticosteroids may reduce the efficacy of tiabendazole.

Tiagebine (Gabitril)

Description
An anticonvulsant drug.

Indications
Used as an add-on drug in epilepsy.

Effects on oral and dental structures
Xerostomia, gingivitis, stomatitis, and rarely gingival overgrowth may be produced.

Effects on patient management
Xerostomia may increase caries incidence and thus a preventive regimen is important. If the xerostomia is severe, artificial saliva may be indicated. This drug can cause confusion and reduce concentration levels, thus short treatment sessions are preferred. Epileptic fits are possible especially if the patient is stressed, therefore sympathetic handling and perhaps sedation should be considered for stressful procedures. Emergency anticonvulsant medication (diazepam or midazolam) must be available.

Drug interactions
Carbamazepine reduces the effect of tiagebine.

Tiaprofenic acid (Surgam)

Description
A peripherally acting, non-steroidal anti-inflammatory analgesic.

Indications
Pain and inflammation associated with musculoskeletal disorders, e.g. rheumatoid arthritis, osteoarthritis, and ankylosing spondylitis. Dysmenorrhoea and menorrhagia.

Effects on oral and dental structures
Patients on long-term NSAIDs such as tiaprofenic acid may be afforded some degree of protection against periodontal breakdown. This arises from the drug's inhibitory action on prostaglandin synthesis. The latter is an important inflammatory mediator in the pathogenesis of periodontal breakdown.

Effects on patient management
Rare unwanted effects of tiaprofenic acid include angioedema and thrombocytopenia. The latter may cause an increased bleeding tendency following any dental surgical procedure. If the platelet count is low (<100,000) then sockets should be packed and sutured. Persistent bleeding may require a platelet transfusion.

Drug interactions

Ibuprofen, aspirin, and diflunisal should be avoided in patients taking tiaprofenic acid due to an increase in unwanted effects, especially gastrointestinal ulceration, renal, and liver damage. Systemic corticosteroids increase the risk of peptic ulceration and gastrointestinal bleeding.

Ticarcillin (Timentin [a mixture of ticarcillin and clavulanic acid])

Description
A beta-lactam antibiotic.

Indications
Used in the treatment of infections caused by *Pseudomonas aeruginosa*.

Effects on oral and dental structures
Oral candidiasis may result from prolonged use of this agent.

Effects on patient management
This drug may cause thrombocytopenia, neutropenia and anaemia. Thrombocytopenia may cause postoperative bleeding. If the platelet count is low (<100,000) then extraction sockets should be packed and sutured. Persistent bleeding may require platelet transfusion. Neutropenia and anaemia may result in poor healing. Any anaemia will need correction prior to elective general anaesthesia and sedation.

Drug interactions
Tetracyclines reduce the effectiveness of penicillins. This drug inactivates gentamicin if they are mixed together in the same infusion and this should be avoided.

Tiludronic acid (Skelid)

Description
A bisphosphonate.

Indications
Paget's disease of bone.

Effects on oral and dental structures
Nothing reported.

Effects on patient management
Nothing of significance.

Drug interactions
Tiludronic acid does cause renal dysfunction and this can be compounded by NSAIDs such as ibuprofen. The latter drugs should be

avoided or only used for the short term provided the patient's renal function is normal.

Tinidazole (Fasigyn)

Description
An antimicrobial drug.

Indications
Used to treat anaerobic and protozoal infections.

Effects on oral and dental structures
Taste disturbance and blackening of the tongue can occur.

Effects on patient management
A leucopenia may be produced after long term use and this may interfere with post-surgical healing.

Drug interactions
A disulfiram reaction occurs with alcohol.

Tinzaparin (Innohep)

Description
A low molecular weight heparin.

Indications
Initial treatment and prevention of deep vein thrombosis and pulmonary embolism. Used to prevent blood coagulation in patients on haemodialysis. Tinzaparin and other low molecular weight heparins have a longer duration of action than heparin.

Effects on oral and dental structures
No direct effect, although if patients are repeatedly heparinized, they are susceptible to osteoporosis. This latter condition may make such patients susceptible to periodontal breakdown.

Effect on patient management
Tinzaparin can only be given parentally which reduces the impact of the drug in dental practice. However dentists, especially those working in a hospital environment, will encounter patients who are heparinized on a regular basis (e.g. renal dialysis patients). Bleeding is the main problem with treating such patients. This can arise as a direct effect on the blood coagulation system or from a drug-induced immune-mediated thrombocytopenia. From the coagulation perspective, it is best to treat heparinized patients between treatments since the half-life of the drug is approximately 4 hours. If urgent treatment is required, then the anticoagulation effect of

tinzaparin can be reversed with protamine sulphate 10 mg IV. If bleeding is due to thrombocytopenia then a platelet transfusion may be required.

Drug interactions
Aspirin and parenteral NSAIDs (e.g. diclofenac and ketorolac) should be avoided in patients who are taking tinzaparin are heparinized on a regular basis. Such analgesics cause impairment of platelet aggregation which would compound a heparin-induced thrombocytopenia and likewise cause serious problems with obtaining haemostasis.

Tioguanine (Lanvis)

Description
An antimetabolic agent.

Indications
Acute leukaemias.

Effects on oral and dental structures
Tioguanine causes bone marrow suppression with an accompanying thrombocytopenia and agranulocytosis. Bone marrow suppression can lead to troublesome oral ulceration, exacerbation of an existing periodontal condition and rapid spread of any residual (e.g. periapical) infections.

Effects on patient management
The effect of tioguanine on the bone marrow is transient and routine dental treatment is best avoided until the white blood cells and platelet counts start to recover. If emergency dental treatment such as an extraction is required then antibiotic cover may be necessary depending on the degree of myelosuppression. If the platelet count is low (<100,000) then the socket should be packed and sutured. Persistent bleeding may require a platelet transfusion.

Patients on chemotherapeutic agents such as tioguanine often neglect their oral hygiene and thus there could be an increase in both caries and periodontal disease. If time permits, patients about to go on chemotherapy should have a dental check up and any potential areas of infection should be treated. Similarly, to reduce the mucosal irritation (sensitivity) that often accompanies chemotherapy, it is advisable to remove any ill-fitting dentures and smooth over rough cusps or restorations.

Drug interactions
None of any dental significance.

Tobramycin (Nebcin)

Description
An aminoglycoside antibiotic.

Indications
Used to treat serious Gram-negative infections resistant to gentamicin.

Effects on oral and dental structures
None specific.

Effects on patient management
As this drug is only administered parenterally it is unlikely to be encountered in routine dental practice. However, it may cause thrombocytopenia and agranulocytosis. Thrombocytopenia may cause postoperative bleeding. If the platelet count is low (<100,000) then extraction sockets should be packed and sutured. Persistent bleeding may require platelet transfusion. Agranulocytosis may affect healing adversely.

Drug interactions
The ototoxic effect of this drug is exacerbated by vancomycin. Miconazole may reduce the serum concentration of tobramycin. Nephrotoxicity is increased when used in combination with amphotericin B and clindamycin. The risk of hypocalcaemia produced by bisphosphonates, which are used in the management of Paget's disease of bone, is increased by tobramycin.

Tolazamide (Tolanase)

Description
A sulphonylurea oral anti-diabetic.

Indications
Diabetes mellitus.

Effects on oral and dental structures
Tolazamide has been cited as causing oral lichenoid eruptions, erythema multiforme and oro-facial neuropathy. The latter can manifest as tingling or burning in the lips and tongue. The drug is a rare cause of blood disorders and includes thrombocytopenia, agranulocytosis, and aplastic anaemia. The blood disorders could cause oral ulceration, an exacerbation of periodontal disease and spontaneous bleeding from the gingival tissues. If the platelet count is low (<100,000) then extraction sockets should be packed and sutured. Persistent bleeding may require a platelet transfusion.

Effects on patient management

The development of hypoglycaemia is the main problem associated with tolazamide. This problem is more common in the elderly. Before commencing dental treatment, it is important to check that the patients have had their normal food intake. If there is any doubt, give the patient a glucose drink. As with any diabetic patient try and treat in the first half of the morning and ensure the patient can eat after dental treatment. If a patient on tolazamide requires a general anaesthetic then refer to hospital.

Drug interactions

Aspirin and other NSAIDs enhance the hypoglycaemic actions of tolazamide. Antifungal agents such as fluconazole and miconazole increase plasma concentrations of tolazamide. Systemic corticosteroids will antagonize the hypoglycaemic properties of tolazamide. If these drugs are required, then consult the patient's physician before prescribing.

Tolbutamide

Description

A sulphonylurea oral anti-diabetic.

Indications

Diabetes mellitus.

Effects on oral and dental structures

Tolbutamide has been cited as causing oral lichenoid eruptions, erythema multiforme, and oro-facial neuropathy. The latter can manifest as tingling or burning in the lips and tongue. The drug is a rare cause of blood disorders and includes thrombocytopenia, agranulocytosis, and aplastic anaemia. The blood disorders could cause oral ulceration, an exacerbation of periodontal disease and spontaneous bleeding from the gingival tissues. If the platelet count is low (<100,000) then extraction sockets should be packed and sutured. Persistent bleeding may require a platelet transfusion.

Effects on patient management

The development of hypoglycaemia is the main problem associated with tolbutamide. This problem is more common in the elderly. Before commencing dental treatment, it is important to check that the patients have had their normal food intake. If there is any doubt, give the patient a glucose drink. As with any diabetic patient try and treat in the first half of the morning and ensure the patient can eat after dental treatment. If a patient on tolbutamide requires a general anaesthetic then refer to hospital.

Drug interactions

Aspirin and other NSAIDs enhance the hypoglycaemic actions of tolbutamide. Antifungal agents such as fluconazole and miconazole increase plasma concentrations of tolbutamide. Systemic corticosteroids will antagonize the hypoglycaemic properties of tolbutamide. If these drugs are required, then consult the patient's physician before prescribing.

Tolfenamic acid (Clotam)

Description

A non-steroidal anti-inflammatory drug.

Indications

Used in the treatment of acute migraine attacks.

Effects on oral and dental structures

This drug may cause Stevens–Johnson syndrome.

Effects on patient management

Avoid stimuli which may induce migraine, such as directly shining the dental light in the patient's eyes. The use of dark glasses may be of benefit to the patient.

Drug interactions

As this drug is only used short term, interactions commonly found with other non-steroidals are unlikely to be a concern in dentistry.

Tolterodine tartrate (Detrusitol)

Description

An antimuscarinic drug.

Indications

Urinary frequency, urgency and incontinence, neurogenic bladder instability and nocturnal enuresis.

Effects on oral and dental structures

Dry mouth is one of the main unwanted effects of tolterodine tartrate. This will increase the risk of dental caries (especially root caries), impede denture retention and the patient will be more prone to candidial infections. If the xerostomia is severe, dentate patients should receive topical fluoride and be offered an artificial saliva. A rare unwanted effect of tolterodine tartrate is angioedema which can affect the floor of the mouth, tongue, and lips.

Effects on patient management

Patients on tolterodine tartrate may become disorientated and suffer from blurred vision.

Drug interactions
None of any dental significance.

Topiramate (Topamax)

Description
An anticonvulsant drug.

Indications
Used as an add-on drug in epilepsy.

Effects on oral and dental structures
Taste disturbance, xerostomia, and rarely gingival overgrowth can occur.

Effects on patient management
Xerostomia may increase caries incidence and thus a preventive regimen is important. If the xerostomia is severe, artificial saliva may be indicated. This drug can cause confusion and reduce concentration levels, thus short treatment sessions are preferred. Epileptic fits are possible especially if the patient is stressed, therefore sympathetic handling and perhaps sedation should be considered for stressful procedures. Emergency anticonvulsant medication (diazepam or midazolam) must be available.

Drug interactions
None of importance in dentistry.

Topotecan (Hycamtin)

Description
A topoisomerase I inhibitor.

Indications
Metastatic ovarian cancer where other therapy has failed.

Effects on oral and dental structures
Topotecan causes bone marrow suppression with an accompanying thrombocytopenia and agranulocytosis. Bone marrow suppression can lead to troublesome oral ulceration, exacerbation of an existing periodontal condition and rapid spread of any residual (e.g. periapical) infections.

Effects on patient management
The effect of topotecan on the bone marrow is transient and routine dental treatment is best avoided until the white blood cells and platelet counts start to recover. If emergency dental treatment such as an extraction is required then antibiotic cover may be necessary depending on

the degree of myelosuppression. If the platelet count is low (<100,000) then extraction sockets should be packed and sutured. Persistent bleeding may require a platelet transfusion.

Patients on chemotherapeutic agents such as topotecan often neglect their oral hygiene and thus there could be an increase in both caries and periodontal disease. If time permits, patients about to go on chemotherapy should have a dental check up and any potential areas of infection should be treated. Similarly, to reduce the mucosal irritation (sensitivity) that often accompanies chemotherapy, it is advisable to remove any ill-fitting dentures and smooth over rough cusps or restorations.

Drug interactions
None of any dental significance.

Tramadol hydrochloride (Zamadol, Zydol)

Description
An opioid analgesic.

Indications
Moderate to severe pain.

Effects on oral and dental structures
Can cause xerostomia leading to an increased risk of root caries, candidial infections, and poor denture retention. If the xerostomia is severe, dentate patients should receive topical fluoride and be offered an artificial saliva.

Effects on patient management
Tramadol hydrochloride is a drug of dependence and can thus cause withdrawal symptoms if the medication is stopped abruptly. Such cessation of tramadol hydrochloride may account for unusual behavioural changes and poor compliance with dental treatment. The drug also depresses respiration and causes postural hypotension.

Drug interactions
Tramadol hydrochloride will enhance the sedative properties of midazolam and diazepam. Reduce the dose of both sedative agents.

Trandolapril (Gopten)

Description
Trandolapril is an ACE inhibitor, that is it inhibits renal angiotensin converting enzyme which is necessary to convert angiotensin I to the more potent angiotensin II.

Indications
Mild to moderate hypertension, congestive heart failure, and post myocardial infarction where there is left ventricular dysfunction.

Effects on oral and dental structures
Tandrolapril causes taste disturbances, angioedema, dry mouth, glossitis, and lichenoid drug reactions. Many of these unwanted effects are dose related and compounded if there is an impairment of renal function. Tandrolapril-induced xerostomia increases the risk of fungal infections (candidiasis) and caries, especially root caries. Antifungal treatment should be used when appropriate and topical fluoride (e.g. Duraphat) will reduce the risk of root surface caries.

Effects on patient management
Trandolapril-induced angioedema is perhaps the most significant unwanted effect that impacts upon dental managements, because dental procedures can induce the angioedema. Management of tran-dolapril-induced angioedema is problematic since the underlying mechanism is poorly understood. Standard anti-anaphylactic treatment is of little value (epinephrine and hydrocortisone) because the angioedema is not mediated via mast cells or antibody/antigen interactions. Usually the angioedema subsides and patients on these drugs should be questioned as to whether they have experienced any problems with breathing or swallowing. This will alert the dental practitioner to the possible risk of this unwanted effect arising during dental treatment.

Trandolapril is also associated with suppression of bone marrow activity giving rise to possible neutropenia, agranulocytosis, thrombocytopenia, and aplastic anaemia. Patients on trandolapril who present with excessive bleeding of their gingiva, sore throats or oral ulceration should have a full haematological investigation.

Drug interactions
Non-steroidal anti-inflammatory drugs (NSAIDs) such as ibuprofen may reduce the antihypertensive effect of tandrolapril.

Tranexamic acid (Cyklokapron)

Description
An anti-fibrinolytic drug which inhibits plasminogen activation and fibrinolysis.

Indications
To facilitate haemostasis in haemophilia, menorrhagia, and in thrombolytic overdose. Also useful in hereditary angioedema.

Effects on oral and dental structures
None reported.

Effects on patient management
None of any significance.

Drug interactions
None of any dental significance.

Tranylcypromine (Parnate)

Description
A monoamine oxidase inhibitor.

Indications
Used in the management of depression.

Effects on oral and dental structures
Xerostomia may be produced.

Effects on patient management
Xerostomia may increase caries incidence and thus a preventive regimen is important. If the xerostomia is severe, artificial saliva may be indicated. This drug may cause postural hypotension, thus the patient should not be changed from the supine to the standing position too rapidly.

Drug interactions
Combined therapy with opioid analgesics can create serious shifts in blood pressure (both elevation and depression) and thus opioids such as pethidine must be avoided for up to two weeks after monoamine oxidase inhibitor therapy. Similarly, change to another antidepressant group such as tricyclics or selective serotonin uptake inhibitors should only take place after a gap of two weeks from the end of monoamine oxidase inhibitor therapy. The anticonvulsant effects of anti-epileptic drugs is antagonized by monoamine oxidase inhibitors. Carbamazepine should not be administered within two weeks of monoamine oxidase inhibitor therapy. Hypertensive crisis can occur if administered with ephedrine. Epinephrine in dental local anaesthetics is not a concern as this is metabolized by a route independent of monoamine oxidase.

Trazodone hydrochloride (Molipaxin)

Description
An antidepressant drug related to the tricyclic group.

Indications
Used in the management of depressive illness.

Effects on oral and dental structures

Xerostomia and taste disturbance may occur but this is less trouble-some than with traditional tricyclics, occasionally stomatitis is produced.

Effects on patient management

Xerostomia may increase caries incidence and thus a preventive regimen is important. If the xerostomia is severe, artificial saliva may be indicated. Postural hypotension may occur with this drug, there-fore rapid changes in patient position should be avoided. This drug may cause thrombocytopenia, agranulocytosis and leucopenia. Thrombocytopenia may cause postoperative bleeding. If the platelet count is low (<100,000) then extraction sockets should be packed and sutured. Persistent bleeding may require platelet transfusion. Agranulocytosis and leucopenia may affect healing adversely.

Drug interactions

Increased sedation occurs with alcohol and sedative drugs such as benzodiazepines. This drug increases the pressor effects of epineph-rine. Nevertheless, the use of epinephrine-containing local anaesthet-ics is not contraindicated. However, epinephrine dose limitation is recommended. Combined therapy with other antidepressants should be avoided and if prescribing another class of antidepressant a period of one to two weeks should elapse between changeover. Anti-muscarinic effects such as xerostomia are increased when used in combination with other anticholinergic drugs such as antipsychotics. Trazodone antagonizes the anticonvulsant effects of anti-epileptic medication, conversely it has been implicated in increasing phenytoin toxicity. Trazadone may decease the anticoagulant effect of warfarin.

Treosulphan

Description

An alkylating agent.

Indications

Ovarian cancer.

Effects on oral and dental structures

Treosulphan causes bone marrow suppression with an accompany-ing thrombocytopenia and agranulocytosis. Bone marrow suppres-sion can lead to troublesome oral ulceration, exacerbation of an existing periodontal condition, and rapid spread of any residual (e.g. periapical) infections.

Effects on patient management

The effect of treosulphan on the bone marrow is transient and rou-tine dental treatment is best avoided until the white blood cells and platelet counts start to recover. If emergency dental treatment such as an extraction is required then antibiotic cover may be necessary depending on the degree of myelosuppression. If the platelet count is low (<100,000) then the socket should be packed and sutured. Persistent bleeding may require a platelet transfusion.

Patients on chemotherapeutic agents such as treosulphan often neglect their oral hygiene and thus there could be an increase in both caries and periodontal disease. If time permits, patients about to go on chemotherapy should have a dental check up and any potential areas of infection should be treated. Similarly, to reduce the mucosal irritation (sensitivity) that often accompanies chemotherapy, it is advisable to remove any ill-fitting dentures and smooth over rough cusps or restorations.

Drug interactions
None of any dental significance.

Triamcinolone (Kenalog)

Description
A corticosteroid.

Indications
Suppression of inflammation and allergic disorders. Used in the management of inflammatory bowel diseases, asthma, immunosuppression, and in various rheumatic diseases.

Effects on oral and dental structures
Although systemic corticosteroids can induce cleft lip and palate formation in mice, there is little evidence that this unwanted effect occurs in humans. The main impact of systemic corticosteroids on the mouth is to cause an increased susceptibility to opportunistic infections. These include candidiasis, and those due to herpes viruses. The anti-inflammatory and immunosuppressant properties of corticosteroids may afford the patient some degree of protection against periodontal breakdown. Paradoxically long-term systemic use can precipitate osteoporosis. The latter is now regarded as a risk factor for periodontal disease.

Effects on patient management
The main unwanted effect of corticosteroid treatment is the suppression of the adrenal cortex and the possibility of an adrenal crisis when such patients are subjected to 'stressful events'. Whilst such suppression does occur physiologically, its clinical significance does appear to be overstated. As far as dentistry is concerned, there is increasing evidence that supplementary corticosteroids are not required. This would apply to all restorative procedures, periodontal

surgery and uncomplicated dental extractions. For more complicated dentolveolar surgery, each case must be judged on its merit. An apprehensive patient may well require cover. It is important to monitor the patient's blood pressure before, during and for 30 minutes after the procedure. If diastolic pressure drops by more than 25%, then hydrocortisone 100 mg IV should be administered and the patient's blood pressure continued to be monitored.

Patients should be screened regularly for oral infections such as fungal or viral infections. When these occur, they should be treated promptly with the appropriate chemotherapeutic agent. Likewise, any patient on corticosteroids that presents with an acute dental infection should be treated urgently as such infections can readily spread.

Drug interactions
Aspirin and NSAIDs should not be prescribed to patients on long-term corticosteroids. Both drugs are ulcerogenic and hence increase the risk of gastrointestinal bleeding and ulceration. The antifungal agent amphotericin increases the risk of corticosteroid-induced hypokalaemia, whilst ketoconazole inhibits corticosteroid hepatic metabolism.

Triamterene (Dytac)

Description
A potassium-sparing diuretic.

Indications
Oedema, potassium conservation with thiazide and loop diuretics.

Effects on oral and dental structures
Xerostomia leading to an increased risk of root caries, candidial infections and poor denture retention. If the xerostomia is severe, dentate patients should receive topical fluoride and be offered an artificial saliva.

Effects on patient management
Postural hypotension may occur; this drug rarely interferes with folate metabolism causing a megaloblastic anaemia.

Drug interactions
NSAIDs can enhance triamterene-induced hyperkalaemia.

Triclofos sodium

Description
A hypnotic drug.

Indications

Sometimes used to treat insomnia in children, but these days use is limited as benzodiazepines have superseded chloral derivatives. It produces less gastric irritation than chloral hydrate, of which it is a derivative.

Effects on oral and dental structures

None known.

Effects on patient management

As this drug is used as a night time hypnotic, interference with management is minimal. However if surgery is to be performed, the interaction with warfarin mentioned below should be noted.

Drug interactions

Like other CNS depressants, triclofos interacts with alcohol and the effect may be more than additive. Some patients may experience a disulfiram (antabuse)-type reaction if alcohol is taken with chloral hydrate and this might occur with triclofos. Triclofos enhances the effects of warfarin.

Trifluoperazine (Stelazine)

Description

A phenothiazine antipsychotic medication.

Indications

Used in the treatment of psychoses such as schizophrenia and in short term management of severe agitation.

Effects on oral and dental structures

Xerostomia and uncontrollable oro-facial muscle activity (tardive dyskenesia) may be produced. The oral mucosa may be discoloured. Lichenoid reactions and Stevens–Johnson syndrome may occur.

Effects on patient management

Xerostomia may increase caries incidence and thus a preventive regimen is important. If the xerostomia is severe, artificial saliva may be indicated. Uncontrollable muscle movement of jaws and tongue as well as the underlying psychotic condition may interfere with management, as satisfactory co-operation may not be achieved readily. There may be problems with denture retention and certain stages of denture construction (e.g. jaw registration) can be difficult. Postural hypotension often occurs with this drug, therefore rapid changes in patient position should be avoided. This drug can produce leucocytosis, agranluocytosis, and anaemia which may interfere with postoperative healing.

Drug interactions

There is increased sedation when used in combination with CNS depressant drugs such as alcohol, opioid analgesics, and sedatives. Combined therapy with tricyclic antidepressants increases the chances of cardiac arrythmias and exacerbates antimuscarinic effects such as xerostomia. There is a theoretical risk of hypotension being exacerbated by the epinephrine in dental local anaesthetics.

Trihexyphenidyl hydrochloride/Benzhexol hydrochloride (Broflex)

Description

An antimuscarinic drug.

Indications

Used in the management of Parkinsonism.

Effects on oral and dental structures

Xerostomia and glossitis can occur.

Effects on patient management

Xerostomia may increase caries incidence and thus a preventive regimen is important. If the xerostomia is severe, artificial saliva may be indicated. Parkinsonism can lead to management problems as the patient may have uncontrollable movement. Short appointments are recommended.

Drug interactions

Absorption of ketoconazole is decreased. Side effects increased with concurrent medication with tricyclic and monoamine oxidase inhibitor antidepressants.

Trimeprazine tartrate/Alimemazine tartrate (Vallergan)

Description

An antihistamine.

Indications

Used in the treatment of urticaria and pruritis and as a sedative.

Effects on oral and dental structures

Can produce xerostomia.

Effects on patient management

The patient may be drowsy which may interfere with co-operation. Xerostomia may increase caries incidence and thus a preventive regimen is important. If the xerostomia is severe, artificial saliva may be indicated. This drug may cause thrombocytopenia, agranulocytosis and anaemia. Thrombocytopenia may cause postoperative bleeding. If the platelet count is low (<100,000) then extraction sockets should be packed and sutured. Persistent bleeding may require platelet transfusion. Agranulocytosis may affect healing adversely. Anaemia may result in poor healing. Any anaemia will need correction prior to elective general anaesthesia and sedation.

Drug interactions
Enhanced sedative effect with anxiolytic and hypnotic drugs and increased CNS depression with opioid analgesics. Tricyclic and monoamine oxidase inhibitor antidepressants increase antimuscarinic effects such as xerostomia.

Trimethoprim (Monotrim, Trimopan)

Description
A diaminopyrimidine antibiotic.

Indications
Used in the treatment of respiratory and urinary tract infections.

Effects on oral and dental structures
Stomatitis, glossitis, oral ulceration, Stevens–Johnson syndrome, and candidiasis can occur.

Effects on patient management
This drug may cause thrombocytopenia, agranulocytosis, and anaemia. Thrombocytopenia may cause postoperative bleeding. If the platelet count is low (<100,000) then extraction sockets should be packed and sutured. Persistent bleeding may require platelet transfusion. Agranulocytosis and anaemia may result in poor healing. Any anaemia will need correction prior to elective general anaesthesia and sedation.

Drug interactions
The plasma concentration of phenytoin is increased by trimethoprim.

Trimetrexate (Neutrexin)

Description
An antiprotozoal drug.

Indications
Used in the management of pneumocystic pneumonia, especially in AIDS patients.

Effects on oral and dental structures

Oral ulceration may occur.

Effects on patient management

The underlying chest condition will mean that local anaesthesia is the only viable form of anaesthesia. This drug can produce thrombocytopenia, anaemia, and neutropenia. Thrombocytopenia may cause postoperative bleeding. If the platelet count is low (<100,000) then extraction sockets should be packed and sutured. Persistent bleeding may require platelet transfusion. Anaemia and neutropenia will affect healing adversely and if severe prophylactic antibiotics should be prescribed to cover surgical procedures.

Drug interactions

Trimetrexate affects the plasma levels of erythromycin, ketoconazole, and fluconazole. Paracetamol influences the plasma concentration of trimetrexate.

Trimipramine (Surmontil)

Description

A tricyclic antidepressant.

Indications

Used in the management of depressive illness.

Effects on oral and dental structures

Xerostomia and taste disturbance may occur.

Effects on patient management

Xerostomia may increase caries incidence and thus a preventive regimen is important. If the xerostomia is severe, artificial saliva may be indicated. Postural hypotension may occur with this drug, therefore rapid changes in patient position should be avoided. This drug may cause thrombocytopenia, agranulocytosis, and leucopenia. Thrombocytopenia may cause postoperative bleeding. If the platelet count is low (<100,000) then extraction sockets should be packed and sutured. Persistent bleeding may require platelet transfusion. Agranulocytosis and leucopenia may affect healing adversely.

Drug interactions

Increased sedation occurs with alcohol and sedative drugs such as benzodiazepines. This drug may antagonize the action of anticonvulsants such as carbamazepine and phenytoin. This drug increases the pressor effects of epinephrine. Nevertheless, the use of epinephrine-containing local anaesthetics is not contraindicated. However, epinephrine dose limitation is recommended. Normal anticoagulant control by warfarin may be upset, both increases and decreases in

INR have been noted during combined therapy with tricyclic antidepressants. Combined therapy with other antidepressants should be avoided and if prescribing another class of antidepressant a period of one to two weeks should elapse between changeover. Antimuscarinic effects such as xerostomia are increased when used in combination with other anticholinergic drugs such as antipsychotics.

Triprolidine hydrochloride

Description
An antihistamine.

Indications
Found in cough and decongestant medications.

Effects on oral and dental structures
Can produce xerostomia and lichenoid reactions.

Effects on patient management
The patient may be drowsy which may interfere with co-operation. Xerostomia may increase caries incidence and thus a preventive regimen is important. If the xerostomia is severe, artificial saliva may be indicated. This drug may cause thrombocytopenia, agranulocytosis, and anaemia. Thrombocytopenia may cause postoperative bleeding. If the platelet count is low (<100,000) then extraction sockets should be packed and sutured. Persistent bleeding may require platelet transfusion. Agranulocytosis may affect healing adversely. Anaemia may result in poor healing. Any anaemia will need correction prior to elective general anaesthesia and sedation.

Drug interactions
Enhanced sedative effect occurs with anxiolytic and hypnotic drugs, and increased CNS depression with opioid analgesics. Tricyclic and monoamine oxidase inhibitor antidepressants increase antimuscarinic effects such as xerostomia. The photosensitive effects of tetracyclines is increased during combined therapy.

Tripotassium dicitratobismuthate (De-Noltab)

Description
A bismuth chelate.

Indications
Used in the management of duodenal and gastric ulcers.

Effects on oral and dental structures
May cause a black discolouration of the tongue and taste disturbance.

Effects on patient management
Patients may be uncomfortable in the fully supine position as a result of their underlying gastrointestinal disorder. Due to the underlying condition non-steroidal analgesics should be avoided. Similarly, high dose systemic steroids should not be prescribed in patients with gastrointestinal ulceration.

Drug interactions
This drug causes reduction of absorption of tetracyclines.

Trisodium edetate (Limclair)

Description
An intravenous chelating agent.

Indications
Hypocalcaemia, osteoporosis.

Effects on oral and dental structures
None reported.

Effects on patient management
Nothing of significance.

Drug interactions
Calcium salts chelate with tetracyclines and thus prevent absorption.

Tropisetron (Navoban)

Description
A serotonin antagonist.

Indications
Used in the treatment of nausea, especially that caused by cytotoxic chemotherapy, radiotherapy, and postoperatively.

Effects on oral and dental structures
None specific to this drug.

Effects on patient management
The patient is probably undergoing chemotherapy or radiotherapy; this will affect the timing of treatments and can interfere with surgical healing. Ideally a preventive regimen should be in place.

Drug interactions
None of importance in dentistry.

Tryptophan (Optimax)

Description
An essential amino acid.

Indications
This drug is rarely used but is occasionally employed in the management of depression which has proved intractable to other therapy.

Effects on oral and dental structures
This drug causes xerostomia.

Effects on patient management
Xerostomia may increase caries incidence and thus a preventive regimen is important. If the xerostomia is severe, artificial saliva may be indicated.

Drug interactions
Tryptophan interferes with other antidepressants, causing increased confusion and excitation.

Tulobuterol hydrochloride (Respacal)

Description
A beta$_2$-adrenoceptor stimulant.

Indications
Used in the management of asthma and reversible airway obstruction.

Effects on oral and dental structures
Xerostomia and taste alteration may occur.

Effects on patient management
Patients may not be comfortable in the supine position if they have respiratory problems. Aspirin-like compounds should not be prescribed as many asthmatic patients are allergic to these analgesics. Similarly, sulphite-containing compounds (such as preservatives in epinephrine-containing local anaesthetics) can produce allergy in asthmatic patients. Xerostomia may increase caries incidence and thus a preventive regimen is important. If the xerostomia is severe, artificial saliva may be indicated. The use of a rubber dam in patients with obstructive airway disease may further embarrass the airway. If a rubber dam is essential then supplemental oxygen via a nasal cannula may be required.

Drug interactions
The hypokalaemia which may result from large doses of tulobuterol may be exacerbated by a reduction in potassium produced by high doses of steroids and by epinephrine in dental local anaesthetics.

Ursodeoxycholic acid (Destolit, Urdox, Ursofalk, Ursogal)

Description
A bile acid.

Indications
It is used to dissolve gallstones.

Effects on oral and dental structures
Stomatitis and altered taste may be produced.

Effects on patient management
Patients may be uncomfortable in the fully supine position as a result of their underlying gastrointestinal disorder.

Drug interactions
None of importance in dentistry.

Valaciclovir (Valtrex)

Description
An antiviral drug. It is a pro-drug for aciclovir.

Indications
Used to treat herpes simplex and varicella-zoster infections.

Presentations
500 mg tablets.

Dose
Adults: for herpes zoster 1 g 3 times daily for 7 days; for herpes simplex 500 mg twice daily for 5 days.
Child: Not recommended in children.

Contraindications
Hypersensitivity, children.

Precautions
Renal disease, pregnancy and breastfeeding.

Unwanted effects
Glossitis, altered taste, gastrointestinal upset, renal failure, bone marrow depression, tremors and convulsions, rash, and urticaria.

Drug interactions
Probenicid and cimetidine increase the plasma concentration of valaciclovir.

Valproate [Sodium valproate] (Epilim, Convulex)

Description
An anticonvulsant drug.

Indications
Used in the management of epilepsy.

Effects on oral and dental structures
Prolonged bleeding and delayed healing after oral surgery, Stevens–Johnson syndrome, rarely gingival overgrowth, stomatitis, and parotid gland enlargement may occur.

Effects on patient management
Epileptic fits are possible especially if the patient is stressed, therefore sympathetic handling and perhaps sedation should be considered for stressful procedures. Emergency anticonvulsant medication (diazepam or midazolam) must be available. Postoperative haemorrhage is possible due to thrombocytopenia and an increased prothrombin time and although not usually severe, local measures such as packing sockets and suturing should be considered. Aspirin should be avoided.

Drug interactions
The toxicity of sodium valproate is increased by aspirin and possibly erythromycin and isoniazid. The effect of valproate is reduced by aciclovir. Concurrent use with carbamazepine reduces the serum level of both anticonvulsants, however the increase in carbamazepine metabolites can increase side effects. Sodium valproate may raise the serum levels of diazepam and lorazepam and possibly enhances the effects of oral anticoagulants such as warfarin. The plasma concentration of the antiviral drug zidovudine is increased.

Valsartan (Diovan)

Description
An angiotensin II receptor antagonist.

Indications
Used as an alternative to ACE inhibitors where the latter cannot be tolerated.

Effects on oral and dental structures
Angioedema has been reported, but the incidence of this unwanted effect is much less than when compared to ACE inhibitors.

Effects on patient management
None of any significance.

Drug interactions
NSAIDs such as ibuprofen may reduce the antihypertensive action of valsartan.

Vancomycin (Vancocin)

Description
A glycopeptide antibiotic.

Indications
The only indication in dentistry is for the prophylaxis of endocarditis in those having a general anaesthetic and who cannot receive amoxicillin.

Presentations
(i) 250 mg and 500 mg capsules.
(ii) Powder for reconstitution for injection in vials containing 250 mg or 500 mg.

Dose
As prophylaxis for endocarditis 1 g given by slow intravenous infusion over 100 minutes prior to the procedure (gentamycin must be administered in conjunction with this treatment at induction of general anaesthesia). For children under 10 years the dose of vancomycin is 20 mg/kg.

Contraindications
History of deafness.
Pregnancy and breastfeeding.

Precautions
Renal disease.

Unwanted effects
Renal toxicity including kidney failure.
Ototoxicity.
Neuromuscular blockade.
Hypersensitivity reactions.
Haematological disorders (such as reduction in white cells and platelets) may occur after prolonged use.
Rapid intravenous infusion can cause a number of reactions including severe hypotension leading to shock and cardiac arrest. In addition dramatic flushing may occur ('red man' syndrome).

Drug interactions
The nephrotoxic effects of vancomycin appear to be additive with the adverse renal effects produced by the aminoglycosides such as

gentamicin, amphotericin B, bacitracin, polymixin N, colistin, ketorolac, viomycin, and cisplatin. The ototoxic effect of vancomycin is exacerbated by aminoglycoside antibiotics such as gentamicin and by loop diuretics. Vancomycin produces some neuromuscular blockade and can thus enhance the action of neuromuscular blocking drugs such as vecuronium and suxamethonium. The hypotension produced by rapid intravenous infusion of vancomycin may be exacerbated by vasodilatory drugs such as the calcium-channel blocking agent nifedipine.

Vancomycin enhances the anticoagulant effect of warfarin but not to a significant degree. However monitoring of coagulation is advised if vancomycin is administered to a warfarinized patient. The reduction in white cell count produced by long term use of vancomycin is exacerbated by concurrent therapy with the HIV treatment drug zidovudine. When used to treat pseudomembranous colitis the action of vancomycin in the gut is reduced when administered concurrently with the ion-exchange resin cholestyramine. This effect is not important when the antibiotic is administered parenterally.

Vasopressin (Pitressin)

Description
A posterior pituitary hormone.

Indications
Primary diabetes insipidus, bleeding from oesophageal varices.

Effects on oral and dental structures
None reported.

Effects on patient management
None of any significance.

Drug interactions
None of any dental significance.

Venlafaxine (Efexor)

Description
An inhibitor of serotonin and norepinephrine reuptake.

Indications
Used in the management of depression.

Effects on oral and dental structures
This drug may cause xerostomia, stomatitis, and candidiasis.

Effects on patient management
Xerostomia may increase caries incidence and thus a preventive regimen is important. If the xerostomia is severe, artificial saliva may be

indicated. Local therapy for candidiasis and stomatitis may be required. This drug may cause thrombocytopenia, leucopenia, and anaemia. Thrombocytopenia may cause postoperative bleeding. If the platelet count is low (<100,000) then extraction sockets should be packed and sutured. Persistent bleeding may require platelet transfusion. Leucopenia and anaemia may result in poor healing. Any anaemia will need correction prior to elective general anaesthesia and sedation.

Drug interactions

Venlaxine may increase the anticoagulant effect of warfarin. Combined therapy with other antidepressants should be avoided and if prescribing another class of antidepressant a period of one to two weeks should elapse between changeover.

Verapamil (Cordilox, Securon)

Description
A calcium-channel blocker.

Indications
Supraventricular arrhythmias, angina prophylaxis, and hypertension.

Effects on oral and dental structures
Verapamil can cause gingival overgrowth, especially in the anterior part of the mouth. It also causes taste disturbances arising from inhibiting calcium-channel activity that is necessary for the normal function of taste and smell receptors.

Effects on patient management
None of any significance.

Drug interactions
Verapamil can inhibit the metabolism of midazolam, thus causing an increase in plasma concentration and an increased sedative action. A lower titrated dose of midazolam may be necessary for dental sedation.

Vigabatrin

Description
An anticonvulsant drug.

Indications
Used in the management of epilepsy.

Effects on oral and dental structures
None known.

Effects on patient management

Epileptic fits are possible especially if the patient is stressed, therefore sympathetic handling and perhaps sedation should be considered for stressful procedures. Emergency anticonvulsant medication (diazepam or midazolam) must be available.

Drug interactions

None of importance to dentistry.

Viloxazine hydrochloride (Vivalan)

Description

An antidepressant drug related to the tricyclic group.

Indications

Used in the management of depressive illness.

Effects on oral and dental structures

Xerostomia and taste disturbance may occur but this is less troublesome than with traditional tricyclics.

Effects on patient management

Xerostomia may increase caries incidence and thus a preventive regimen is important. If the xerostomia is severe, artificial saliva may be indicated. Postural hypotension may occur with this drug, therefore rapid changes in patient position should be avoided. This drug may cause thrombocytopenia, agranulocytosis, and leucopenia. Thrombocytopenia may cause postoperative bleeding. If the platelet count is low (<100,000) then extraction sockets should be packed and sutured. Persistent bleeding may require a platelet transfusion. Agranulocytosis and leucopenia may affect healing adversely.

Drug interactions

Increased sedation occurs with alcohol and sedative drugs such as benzodiazepines. This drug increases the pressor effects of epinephrine. Nevertheless, the use of epinephrine-containing local anaesthetics is not contraindicated; however, epinephrine dose limitation is recommended. Combined therapy with other antidepressants should be avoided and if prescribing another class of antidepressant a period of one to two weeks should elapse between changeover. Antimuscarinic effects such as xerostomia are increased when used in combination with other anticholinergic drugs such as antipsychotics. Viloxazine enhances the anticoagulant effect of coumarin anticoagulants such as warfarin. This drug increases the plasma concentrations of carbamazepine and phenytoin. Co-trimoxazole may antagonize the effect of viloxazine.

Vinblastine sulphate (Velbe)

Description
A vinca alkaloid.

Indications
Acute leukaemias, lymphomas, breast, and lung cancers.

Effects on oral and dental structures
Vinblastine sulphate causes bone marrow suppression with an accompanying thrombocytopenia and agranulocytosis. Bone marrow suppression can lead to troublesome oral ulceration, exacerbation of an existing periodontal condition, and rapid spread of any residual (e.g. periapical) infections.

Effects on patient management
The effect of vinblastine sulphate on the bone marrow is transient and routine dental treatment is best avoided until the white blood cells and platelet counts start to recover. If emergency dental treatment such as an extraction is required then antibiotic cover may be necessary depending on the degree of myelosuppression. If the platelet count is low (<100,000) then the socket should be packed and sutured. Persistent bleeding may require a platelet transfusion.

Patients on chemotherapeutic agents such as vinblastine sulphate often neglect their oral hygiene and thus there could be an increase in both caries and periodontal disease. If time permits, patients about to go on chemotherapy should have a dental check up and any potential areas of infection should be treated. Similarly, to reduce the mucosal irritation (sensitivity) that often accompanies chemotherapy, it is advisable to remove any ill-fitting dentures and smooth over rough cusps or restorations.

Drug interactions
None of any dental significance.

Vincristine sulphate (Oncovin)

Description
A vinca alkaloid.

Indications
Acute leukaemias, lymphomas, breast, and lung cancers.

Effects on oral and dental structures
Vincristine sulphate causes bone marrow suppression with an accompanying thrombocytopenia and agranulocytosis. Bone marrow suppression can lead to troublesome oral ulceration, exacerbation of an

existing periodontal condition, and rapid spread of any residual (e.g. periapical) infections.

Effects on patient management
The effect of vincristine sulphate on the bone marrow is transient and routine dental treatment is best avoided until the white blood cells and platelet counts start to recover. If emergency dental treatment such as an extraction is required then antibiotic cover may be necessary depending on the degree of myelosuppression. If the platelet count is low (<100,000) then the socket should be packed and sutured. Persistent bleeding may require a platelet transfusion.

Patients on chemotherapeutic agents such as vincristine sulphate often neglect their oral hygiene and thus there could be an increase in both caries and periodontal disease. If time permits, patients about to go on chemotherapy should have a dental check up and any potential areas of infection should be treated. Similarly, to reduce the mucosal irritation (sensitivity) that often accompanies chemotherapy, it is advisable to remove any ill-fitting dentures and smooth over rough cusps or restorations.

Drug interactions
None of any dental significance.

Vindesine sulphate (Eldisine)

Description
A vinca alkaloid.

Indications
Acute leukaemias, lymphomas, breast, and lung cancers.

Effects on oral and dental structures
Vindesine sulphate causes bone marrow suppression with an accompanying thrombocytopenia and agranulocytosis. Bone marrow suppression can lead to troublesome oral ulceration, exacerbation of an existing periodontal condition, and rapid spread of any residual (e.g. periapical) infections.

Effects on patient management
The effect of vindesine sulphate on the bone marrow is transient and routine dental treatment is best avoided until the white blood cells and platelet counts start to recover. If emergency dental treatment such as an extraction is required then antibiotic cover may be necessary depending on the degree of myelosuppression. If the platelet count is low (<100,000) then the socket should be packed and sutured. Persistent bleeding may require a platelet transfusion.

Patients on chemotherapeutic agents such as vindesine sulphate often neglect their oral hygiene and thus there could be an increase in both caries and periodontal disease. If time permits, patients about to go on chemotherapy should have a dental check up and any potential areas of infection should be treated. Similarly, to reduce the mucosal irritation (sensitivity) that often accompanies chemotherapy, it is advisable to remove any ill-fitting dentures and smooth over rough cusps or restorations.

Drug interactions
None of any dental significance.

Vinorelbine (Navelbine)

Description
A vinca alkaloid.

Indications
Acute leukaemias, lymphomas, breast, and lung cancers.

Effects on oral and dental structures
Vinorelbine causes bone marrow suppression with an accompanying thrombocytopenia and agranulocytosis. Bone marrow suppression can lead to troublesome oral ulceration, exacerbation of an existing periodontal condition, and rapid spread of any residual (e.g. periapical) infections.

Effects on patient management
The effect of vinorelbine on the bone marrow is transient and routine dental treatment is best avoided until the white blood cells and platelet counts start to recover. If emergency dental treatment such as an extraction is required then antibiotic cover may be necessary depending on the degree of myelosuppression. If the platelet count is low (<100,000) then the socket should be packed and sutured. Persistent bleeding may require a platelet transfusion.

Patients on chemotherapeutic agents such as vinorelbine often neglect their oral hygiene and thus there could be an increase in both caries and periodontal disease. If time permits, patients about to go on chemotherapy should have a dental check up and any potential areas of infection should be treated. Similarly, to reduce the mucosal irritation (sensitivity) that often accompanies chemotherapy, it is advisable to remove any ill-fitting dentures and smooth over rough cusps or restorations.

Drug interactions
None of any dental significance.

Warfarin sodium

Description
A coumarin oral anticoagulant.

Indications
Prophylaxis of embolisation in atrial fibrillation, patients which prosthetic heart valves; prophylaxis and treatment of venous thrombosis and pulmonary embolism.

Effects on oral and dental structures
Warfarin therapy has been associated with haemorrhage into the submandibular salivary glands. This can present as pain and swelling in the floor of the mouth.

Effects on patient management
The main impact on patient management is the risk of haemorrhage after any dental procedure associated with blood loss. Consultation with the patient's physician is essential if elective surgery, such as removal of an impacted third molar, is required for patients taking warfarin. This is to confirm that dosages can be altered. In most instances, the patient will be required to stop their warfarin for 48 hours prior to the planned procedure. This time period is required because the drug has a long half-life (37–38 hours) and because of the variable rate of hepatic synthesis of the clotting proteins. Prior to surgery, the patient's INR may be reassessed.

Emergency single extractions can be carried out on patients taking warfarin provided that their INR does not exceed 2–2.5 times the normal value. Sockets should be packed and sutured. If haemorrhage does occur, the anticoagulant effect can be reversed by the intravenous administration of fresh frozen plasma. In very severe cases, vitamin K (phytomenadione, 10–20 mg) should be given via an intravenous infusion.

In some situations, a physician may be reluctant to stop a patient's warfarin therapy. In such instances, the patient is admitted to hospital and their anticoagulant control switched to heparin. It may take several days to achieve the appropriate haematological profile. However, the short half-life of heparin (1–2 hours) allows for greater flexibility in controlling the patient's coagulation.

Drug interactions
Warfarin is extensively protein bound and is metabolized in the liver. Thus any drug that competes with the protein binding site or affects the drug metabolizing enzymes in the liver is going to affect warfarin blood concentrations and its anticoagulant actions. Anticoagulant effect of warfarin is increased by aspirin, diclofenac, diflunisal, flurbiprofen, ibuprofen, mefenamic acid, and by prolonged

regular use of paracetamol. Anticoagulant effect is reduced by cephalosporins, erythromycin, co-trimoxazole, and metronidazole. Broad spectrum antibiotics such as ampicillin, and tetracyclines can also alter a patient's INR. Fluconazole, ketoconazole and topical miconazole all enhance the anticoagulant effect of warfarin. Carbamazepine reduces the anticoagulant actions of warfarin.

Zafirlukast (Accolate)

Description
A leukotriene receptor antagonist.

Indications
Used in the treatment of asthma.

Effects on oral and dental structures
None specific.

Effects on patient management
Patients may not be comfortable in the supine position if they have respiratory problems. Aspirin-like compounds should not be prescribed as many asthmatic patients are allergic to these analgesics. Similarly, sulphite-containing compounds (such as preservatives in epinephrine-containing local anaesthetics) can produce allergy in asthmatic patients. Zafirlukast occasionally leads to bleeding disorders and agranulocytosis, thus postoperative bleeding and poor healing may occur.

Drug interactions
The plasma concentration of zafirlukast is increased by aspirin and reduced by erythromycin. The anticoagulant effect of warfarin is increased by zafirlukast.

Zalcitabine (Hivid)

Description
A nucleoside reverse transcriptase inhibitor.

Indications
Used in the management of HIV infection.

Effects on oral and dental structures
Oral ulceration, taste disturbance, glossitis, xerostomia, and paraesthesia may be produced.

Effects on patient management
Sensitive handling of the underlying disease state is essential. Excellent preventive dentistry and regular examinations are important in

patients suffering from HIV, as dental infections are best avoided. HIV will interfere with postoperative healing and antibiotic prophylaxis prior to oral surgery may be advisable. This drug may produce anaemia, neutropenia and thrombocytopenia. Anaemia may result in poor healing. Any anaemia will need correction prior to elective general anaesthesia and sedation. Thrombocytopenia may cause postoperative bleeding.If the platelet count is low (<100,000) then extraction sockets should be packed and sutured. Persistent bleeding may require a platelet transfusion. Xerostomia may increase caries incidence and thus a preventive regimen is important. If the xerostomia is severe, artificial saliva may be indicated.

Drug interactions
Combination with aminoglycoside antibiotics (such as gentamycin), metronidazole and amphotericin increases peripheral neuropathy. Avoid trimethoprim as this increases toxicity of zalcitabine.

Zaleplon (Sonata)

Description
A pyrazolopyrimidine hypnotic.

Indications
Used for short term treatment of insomnia.

Effects on oral and dental structures
This drug is only used short term so there are no long term effects.

Effects on patient management
Dizziness, lack of co-ordination and amnesia will make management difficult and an escort may be required.

Drug interactions
There is enhanced sedative effects with other CNS depressants, including alcohol.

Zanamivir (Relenza)

Description
An anti-influenza medication.

Indications
Used in the treatment of influenza.

Effects on oral and dental structures
None specific.

Effects on patient management

As this drug is used during the early stages of influenza the patient will be generally unwell and only essential emergency treatment should be performed.

Drug interactions

None of importance in dentistry.

Zidovudine (Retrovir)

Description

A nucleoside reverse transcriptase inhibitor.

Indications

Used in the management of HIV infection.

Effects on oral and dental structures

Taste disturbance, mucosal ulceration and pigmentation, lip and tongue swelling, and paraesthesia may be produced.

Effects on patient management

Sensitive handling of the underlying disease state is essential. Excellent preventive dentistry and regular examinations are important in patients suffering from HIV, as dental infections are best avoided. HIV will interfere with postoperative healing and antibiotic prophylaxis prior to oral surgery may be advisable. This drug may produce anaemia, leucopenia, neutropenia, and thrombocytopenia. Anaemia, leucopenia, and neutropenia may result in poor healing and antibiotic prophylaxis may be required. Any anaemia will need correction prior to elective general anaesthesia and sedation. Thrombocytopenia may cause postoperative bleeding.If the platelet count is low (<100,000) then extraction sockets should be packed and sutured. Persistent bleeding may require a platelet transfusion.

Drug interactions

Non-steroidal anti-inflammatory drugs increase the risk of haematological toxicity. Paracetamol may increase the chances of bone marrow suppression and liver toxicity. Concurrent use with the antifungals amphotericin B or fluconazole increases the risk of toxicity of the antiviral agent.

Zolmitriptan (Zomig)

Description

A $5HT_1$ agonist.

Indications

Used in the treatment of acute migraine.

Effects on oral and dental structures
This drug can produce a xerostomia.

Effects on patient management
As this drug is for short term use only, xerostomia should not create long-term management problems. Avoid stimuli which may induce migraine, such as directly shining the dental light in the patient's eyes. The use of dark glasses may be of benefit to the patient.

Drug interactions
Combined therapy with monoamine oxidase inhibitors or selective serotonin reuptake inhibitors increases central nervous system toxicity. Other antimigraine drugs such as other $5HT_1$ agonists and ergotamine derivatives should not be administered until at least six hours after zolmitriptan, to avoid severe vasoconstriction.

Zolpidem tartrate (Stilnoct)

Description
An imidazopyridine hypnotic.

Indications
Short term treatment of insomnia.

Effects on oral and dental structures
Xerostomia and taste alteration can occur.

Effects on patient management
As the drug is only used short term xerostomia should not produce significant problems, however a preventive regimen may be considered. This drug can produce dizziness, ataxia, amnesia and tremors all of which may make treatment more difficult; an escort may be required.

Drug interactions
There is an additive effect with alcohol. The benzodiazepine antagonist flumazenil reverses the action of zolpidem.

Zopiclone (Zimovane)

Description
A cyclopyrrolone hypnotic.

Indications
Used in the short term management of insomnia.

Effects on oral and dental structures
Xerostomia and taste alteration (metallic or bitter taste) can occur.

Effects on patient management
As the drug is only used short term xerostomia should not produce significant problems, however a preventive regimen may be considered. Dizziness, lack of co-ordination and amnesia will make management difficult and an escort may be required. Some patients may become aggressive.

Drug interactions
Erythromycin accelerates the absorption of zopiclone, thus speeding up the hypnotic effect.

Zotepine (Zoleptil)

Description
An atypical antipsychotic drug.

Indications
Used in the treatment of schizophrenia.

Effects on oral and dental structures
Xerostomia and uncontrollable oro-facial muscle activity (tardive dyskenesia) may be produced. Alternatively hypersalivation may occur.

Effects on patient management
Xerostomia may increase caries incidence and thus a preventive regimen is important. If the xerostomia is severe, artificial saliva may be indicated. Uncontrollable muscle movement of jaws and tongue as well as the underlying psychotic condition may interfere with management, as satisfactory co-operation may not be achieved readily. There may be problems with denture retention and certain stages of denture construction (e.g. jaw registration) can be difficult.

This drug may cause blood dyscrasias. Thrombocytopenia may cause postoperative bleeding. If the platelet count is low (<100,000) then extraction sockets should be packed and sutured. Persistent bleeding may require a platelet transfusion. Leucopenia may affect healing adversely. Anaemia may result in poor healing. Any anaemia will need correction prior to elective general anaesthesia and sedation. Postural hypotension often occurs with this drug, therefore rapid changes in patient position should be avoided.

Drug interactions
There is increased sedation when used in combination with CNS depressant drugs such as alcohol, opioid analgesics, and sedatives. Combined therapy with tricyclic antidepressants increases the chances of cardiac arrythmias and exacerbates antimuscarinic effects such as xerostomia.

Zuclopenthixol acetate (Clopixol Acuphase)

Description
A phenothiazine antipsychotic medication.

Indications
Used in the short term management of acute psychoses.

Effects on oral and dental structures
Xerostomia and uncontrollable oro-facial muscle activity (tardive dyskenesia) may be produced. Stevens–Johnson syndrome and lichenoid reactions may be produced.

Effects on patient management
As the drug is only used short term xerostomia should not produce significant problems, however a preventive regimen may be considered. Uncontrollable muscle movement of jaws and tongue as well as the underlying psychotic condition may interfere with management, as satisfactory co-operation may not be achieved readily. There may be problems with denture retention and certain stages of denture construction (e.g. jaw registration) can be difficult. Postural hypotension may occur with this drug, therefore rapid changes in patient position should be avoided. This drug can produce leucocytosis, agranluocytosis, and anaemia which may interfere with postoperative healing.

Drug interactions
There is increased sedation when used in combination with CNS depressant drugs such as alcohol, opioid analgesics, and sedatives. Combined therapy with tricyclic antidepressants increases the chances of cardiac arrythmias and exacerbates antimuscarinic effects such as xerostomia. There is a theoretical risk of hypotension being exacerbated by the epinephrine in dental local anaesthetics.

Zuclopenthixol dihydrochloride (Clopixol)

Description
A phenothiazine antipsychotic medication.

Indications
Used in the treatment of psychoses such as schizophrenia.

Effects on oral and dental structures
Xerostomia and uncontrollable oro-facial muscle activity (tardive dyskenesia) may be produced. Stevens–Johnson syndrome and lichenoid reactions may occur.

Effects on patient management

Xerostomia may increase caries incidence and thus a preventive regimen is important. If the xerostomia is severe, artificial saliva may be indicated. Uncontrollable muscle movement of jaws and tongue as well as the underlying psychotic condition may interfere with management, as satisfactory co-operation may not be achieved readily. There may be problems with denture retention and certain stages of denture construction (e.g. jaw registration) can be difficult. Postural hypotension may occur with this drug, therefore rapid changes in patient position should be avoided. This drug can produce leucocytosis, agranluocytosis, and anaemia which may interfere with postoperative healing.

Drug interactions

There is increased sedation when used in combination with CNS depressant drugs such as alcohol, opioid analgesics, and sedatives. Combined therapy with tricyclic antidepressants increases the chances of cardiac arrythmias and exacerbates antimuscarinic effects such as xerostomia. There is a theoretical risk of hypotension being exacerbated by the epinephrine in dental local anaesthetics.

Zuclopenthixol decanoate (Clopixol, Clopixol Conc.)

Description

An antipsychotic depot injection.

Indications

Used in the treatment of psychoses such as schizophrenia.

Effects on oral and dental structures

Xerostomia and uncontrollable oro-facial muscle activity (tardive dyskenesia) may be produced.

Effects on patient management

Xerostomia may increase caries incidence and thus a preventive regimen is important. If the xerostomia is severe, artificial saliva may be indicated. Uncontrollable muscle movement of jaws and tongue as well as the underlying psychotic condition may interfere with management, as satisfactory co-operation may not be achieved readily. There may be problems with denture retention and certain stages of denture construction (e.g. jaw registration) can be difficult. Postural hypotension may occur with this drug, therefore rapid changes in patient position should be avoided. This drug can produce leucocytosis, agranluocytosis, and anaemia which may interfere with postoperative healing.

Drug interactions

There is increased sedation when used in combination with CNS depressant drugs such as alcohol, opioid analgesics, and sedatives. Combined therapy with tricyclic antidepressants increases the chances of cardiac arrythmias and exacerbates antimuscarinic effects such as xerostomia. There is a theoretical risk of hypotension being exacerbated by the epinephrine in dental local anaesthetics.

Appendix

Alphabetical listing of trade names

Accolate See Zafirlukast
Accuhaler See Salbutamol
Accupro See Quinapril
Acepril See Captopril
Acetaminophen See Paracetamol
Achromycin See Tetracycline
Acupan See Nefopam hydrochloride
Adactone See Spironolactone
Adalat See Nifedipine
Adizem See Diltiazem
Adrenaline in dental local anaesthetic solutions See Epinephrine
AeroBec See Beclometasone dipropionate
Aerocrom See Sodium cromoglicate
Aerolin See Salbutamol
Airomir See Salbutamol
Akineton See Biperiden
Aldomet See Methyldopa
Algicon See Alginates
Alkeran See Melphalan
Allegron See Nortriptyline
Alphaparin See Certoparin
Alu-cap See Aluminium hydroxide
Alupent See Orciprenaline sulphate
Alvercol See Alverine citrate
Amaryl See Glimepiride
Ametop See Amethocaine
Amias See Candesartan
Amikin See Amikacin

Amoxil See Amoxicillin
Amylobarbitone See Amobarbital
Anabact See Metronidazole
Anafranil See Clomipramine hydrochloride
Ancotil See Flucytosine
Androcur See Cyproterone acetate
Anexate See Flumazenil
Angiopine See Nifedipine
Angitil See Diltiazem
Anquil See Benperidol
Antabuse See Disulfiram
Antepsin See Sucralfate
Anturan See Sulfinpyrazone
Apresoline See Hydralazine
Aprovel See Irbesartan
Aricept See Donepezil hydrochloride
Arimidex See Anastrozole
Arosmasin See Exemestan
Arpicolin See Procyclidine hydrochloride
Arythmol See Propafenone hydrochloride
Asacol See Mesalazine
Asendis See Amoxapine
AsmaBec See Beclometasone dipropionate
Asmasal See Salbutamol
Aspirin See Acetylsalicylic acid
Atarax See Hydroxyzine hydrochloride

Atrovent See Ipratropium bromide
Augmentin See Co-amoxiclav
Augmentin-Duo See Co-amoxiclav
Avloclor See Chloroquine
Avomine See Promethazine teoclate
Axid See Nizatidine
Azactam See Aztreonam
Azopt See Brinzolamide

BCNU See Carmustine
Bambec See Bambuterol
      hydrochloride
Baratol See Indoramin
Baxan See Cefadroxil
Becloforte See Beclometasone
      dipropionate
Becodisks See Beclometasone
      dipropionate
Beconase See Beclometasone
      dipropionate
Becotide See Beclometasone
      dipropionate
Benadryl allergy relief See Acrivastine
Benemid See Probenecid
Berotec See Fenoterol hydrobromide
Beta-cardone See Sotalol
      hydrochloride
Betadine See Povidone-iodine
Betaloc See Metoprolol
Betnesol See Betamethasone
Bicillin See Procaine
      penicillin/Procaine
      benzylpenicillin
Bioplex See Carbenoxolone sodium
Bioral gel See Carbenoxolone sodium
Biorphen See Orphenadrine
      hydrochloride
Bocasan See Sodium perborate
Bonefos See Sodium clodronate
Botox See Botulinum A Toxin
Bricanyl See Terbutaline sulphate
BritLofex See Lofexadine
      hydrochloride
Britaject See Apomorphine
      hydrochloride
Broflex See Benzhexol hydrochloride/
      Trihexyphenidyl hydrochloride
Bronchodil See Reproterol
      hydrochloride
Brufen See Ibuprofen
Buccastem See Prochlorperazine

Budenofalk See Budesonide
Burinex See Bumetanide
Buscopan See Hyoscine
      butylbromide
Buspar See Buspirone hydrochloride
Butacote See Phenylbutazone
Butobarbitone See Butobarbital

Cabaser See Cabergoline
Cafegot See Ergotamine tartrate
Calcitare See Calcitonin-porcine
Calcort See Deflazacort
Calicard See Diltiazem
Calpol See Paracetamol
Calsynar See Salcatonin
Camcolit See Lithium salts
Campral EC See Acamprosate
      calcium
Campto See Irinotecan
      hydrochloride
Capastat See Capreomycin
Capoten See Captopril
Cardene See Nicardipine
Cardura See Doxazosin
Catapres See Clonidine
Cefrom See Cefpirome
Cefzil See Cefprozil
Celance See Pergolide
Celebrex See Celecoxib
Celevac See Methylcellulose
Cellcept See Mycophenolate mofetil
Ceporex See Cefalexin
Cerubidin See Daunorubicin
Chirocain See Levobupivacaine
Chloral elixir See Chloral hydrate
Chloral mixture See Chloral hydrate
Chlorohex See Chlorhexidine
      gluconate
Chloromycetin See Chloramphenicol
Cidomycin See Gentamicin
Cinobac See Cinoxacin
Cipramil See Citalopram
Ciproxin See Ciprofloxacin
Citanest See Prilocaine
Claforan See Cefotaxime
Clarityn See Loratadine
Clexane See Enoxaparin
Clinoril See Sulindac
Clomid See Clomifene
Clopixol acuphase See
      Zuclopenthixol acetate

Dyspamet See Cimetidine
Dysport See Botulinum A Toxin
Dytac See Triamterene

Easi-breathe See Salbutamol
Edronax See Reboxetine
Efcortesol See Hydrocortisone
Efexor See Venlafaxine
Efudix See Fluorouracil
Eldepryl See Selegeline hydrochloride
Eldisine See Vindesine sulphate
Eloxatin See Oxaliplatin
Elyzol Flagyl See Metronidazole
Emcor See Bisoprolol
Emeside See Ethosuximide
Emflex See Acemetacin
Endoxana See Cyclophosphamide
Entocort See Budesonide
Epanutin See Phenytoin sodium
Epilim See Valproate
Epinephrine in dental local anaesthetic solutions See Adrenaline
Epivir See Lamivudine
Equagesic See Meprobamate
Equasym See Methylphenidate hydrochloride
Erymax See Erythromycin
Erythrocin See Erythromycin
Erythroped See Erythromycin
Eskazole See Albendazole
Estracyt See Estramustine phosphate
Eucardic See Carvedilol
Eudemine See Diazoxide
Euglucon See Glibenclamide
Evohaler See Salbutamol
Exelon See Rivastigmine

Famvir See Famciclovir
Fansidar See Pyramethamine with Sulfadoxine
Fasigyn See Tinidazole
Faverin See Fluvoxamine maleate
Feldene See Piroxicam
Femara See Letrozole
Fenbid See Ibuprofen
Fenopron See Fenoprofen
Fentazin See Perphenazine
Feospan See Ferrous sulphate
Ferrograd See Ferrous sulphate
Fersaday See Ferrous fumarate
Fersamal See Ferrous fumarate

Fletcher's Enemette See Docusate sodium
Flixonase See Fluticasone propionate
Flixotide See Fluticasone propionate
Florinef See Fludrocortisone acetate
Floxapen See Flucloxacillin
Fluanxol See Flupentixol
Fludara See Fludarabine phosphate
Foradil See Eformoterol fumarate/Formoterol fumarate
Fortipine See Nifedipine
Fortovase See Saquinavir
Fortral See Pentazocine
Fortum See Ceftazidime
Fosamax See Alendronic acid
Foscavir See Foscarnet sodium
Fragmin See Dalteparin
Frisium See Clobazam
Froben See Flurbiprofen
Fucidin See Sodium fusidate
Fulcin See Griseofulvin
Fungilin See Amphotericin
Fungizone See Amphotericin
Furadantin See Nitrofurantoin
Furamide See Diloxanide furoate
Fybogel See Ispaghula husk
Fybogel See Mebeverine hydrochloride

Gabitril See Tiagebine
Galenphol See Pholcodine
Galpseud See Pseudoephedrine hydrochloride
Gamanil See Lofepramine
Gastrobid Continus See Metoclopramide hydrochloride
Gastrocote See Alginates
Gastrocote See Aluminium hydroxide
Gastrocote See Magnesium trisilicate
Gastromax See Metoclopramide hydrochloride
Gaviscon Maalox See Aluminium hydroxide
Gaviscon See Alginates
Gemzar See Gemcitabine
Genotropin See Somatropin
Genticin See Gentamicin
Glandosane See Saliva substitute
Glibenese See Glipizide

Glucobay See Acarbose
Glucophage See Metformin hydrochloride
Glurenorm See Gliquidone
Gopten See Trandolapril
Grisovin See Griseofulvin

Haldol decanoate See Haloperidol decanoate
Haldol See Haloperidol
Half Sinemet See Co-careldopa
HeliClear See Lansoprazole
Hemineverin See Clomethiazole
Heroin hydrochloride See Diamorphine
Hexopal See Nicotinic acid
Hiprex See Methenamine
Hivid See Zalcitabine
Honvan See Fosfestrol tetrasodium
Hormone Replacement Therapy See Oestrogen
Human Mixtard See Biphasic isophane insulin
Human Monotard See Insulin Zinc suspension
Humatrope See Somatropin
Humulin Lente See Insulin Zinc suspension
Humulin See Soluble insulin
Hycamtin See Topotecan
Hydrocortone See Hydrocortisone
Hygroton See Chlorthalidone
Hypnovel See Midazolam
Hypovase See Prazosin
Hypurin See Soluble insulin
Hytrin See Terazosin

Ikorel See Nicorandil
Ilosone See Erythromycin
Imigran See Sumatriptan
Imodium plus See Loperamide hydrochloride
Imodium See Loperamide hydrochloride
Imunovir See Inosine pranobex
Imuran See Azathioprine
Inderal See Propranolol
Indocid See Indomethacin
Innohep See Tinzaparin
Innovace See Enalapril

Insuman See Biphasic isophane insulin
Intal See Sodium cromoglicate
Invirase See Saquinavir
Ionamin See Phentermine
Isogel See Ispaghula husk
Istin See Amlodipine besylate

Kannasyn See Kanamycin
Kaolin mixture See Kaolin
Kefadim See Ceftazidime
Kefadol See Cefamandole
Keflex See Cefalexin
Kefzol See Cefazolin
Kemadrin See Procyclidine hydrochloride
Kemicetine See Chloramphenicol
Kenalog See Triamcinolone
Kinidin See Quinidine
Klaricid XL See Clarithromycin
Klaricid See Clarithromycin
Kolanticon See Dicyclomine hydrochloride/Dicycloverine hydrochloride
Konsyl See Ispaghula husk
Kytril See Granisetron

Lamictal See Lamotrigine
Lamisil See Terbinafine
Lamprene See Clofazimine
Lanoxin See Digoxin
Lanvis See Tioguanine
Largactil See Chlorpromazine hydrochloride
Lariam See Mefloquine
Lasix See Frusemide
Lasma See Theophylline
Lederfen See Fenbufen
Ledermycin See Demeclocycline hydrochloride
Lentaron See Formestane
Lentizol See Amitriptyline hydrochloride
Lescol See Fluvastatin
Leukeran See Chlorambucil
Leustat See Cladribine
Lexotan See Bromazepam
Librium See Chlordiazepoxide
Lignospan See Lidocaine/Lignocaine Dental preparations

Lignostab See Lidocaine/Lignocaine
    Dental preparations
Limclair See Trisodium edetate
Lingraine See Ergotamine tartrate
Lipitor See Atorvastatin
Lipobay See Cerivastatin
Lipostat See Parvastatin
Liskonum See Lithium salts
Litarex See Lithium salts
Lodine See Etodolac
Lomotil See Co-phenotrope
Loniten See Minoxidil
Lopressor See Metoprolol
Losec See Omeprazole
Loxapac See Loxapine
Luborant See Saliva substitute
Ludiomil See Maprotiline
    hydrochloride
Lustral See Sertraline

MST See Morphine
Maalox TC See Aluminium
    hydroxide
Macrobid See Nitrofurantoin
Macrodantin See Nitrofurantoin
Madopar See Co-beneldopa
Magnapen See Co-fluampicil
Maloprim See Pyramethamine with
    Dapsone
Malorone See Proguanil
    hydrochloride with
    Atovaquone
Manerix See Moclobemide
Manevac See Senna
Marcain See Bupivacaine
Maxalt See Rizatriptan
Maxolon See Metoclopramide
    hydrochloride
Medrone See Methylprednisolone
Mefoxin See Cefoxitin
Melleril See Thioridazine
Meptid See Meptazinol
Merbentyl See Dicyclomine
    hydrochloride/Dicycloverine
    hydrochloride
Merocet See Cetylpyridinium chloride
Meronem See Meropenem
Methadose See Methadone
    hydrochloride
Metrogel See Metronidazole
Metrolyl See Metronidazole

Metrotop See Metronidazole
Micardis See Telmisartan
Mictral See Nalidixic acid
Midrid See Isometheptene mucate
Migranal See Dihydroergotamine
    mesilate
Migril See Ergotamine tartrate
Minocin MR See Minocycline
Mintec See Peppermint oil
Mintezol See Tiabendazole
Mirapexin See Pramipexole
Mistamine See Mizolastine
Mitoxana See Ifosfamide
Mizollen See Mizolastine
Mobic See Meloxicam
Mobiflex See Tenoxicam
Modecate See Fluphenazine
    hydrochloride
Moditen See Fluphenazine
    hydrochloride
Mogadon See Nitrazepam
Molipaxin See Trazodone
    hydrochloride
Monocor See Bisoprolol
Monotrim See Trimethoprim
Monovent See Terbutaline sulphate
Motens See Lacidipine
Motilium See Domperidone
Motipress See Nortriptyline
Motival See Nortriptyline
Movicol See Macrogols
Mucogel See Aluminium hydroxide
Mycobutin See Rifabutin
Myleran See Busulphan
Myotonine See Bethanechol chloride
Mysoline See Primidone

Nalcrom See Sodium cromoglicate
Nalorex See Naltrexone
    hydrochloride
Naprosyn See Naproxen
Naramig See Naratriptan
Nardil See Phenelzine
Naropin See Ropivacaine
Narphen See Phenazocine
Natrillix See Indapamide
Navelbine See Vinorelbine
Navoban See Tropisetron
Nebcin See Tobramycin
Nebules See Fluticasone
    propionate/Salbutamol

Negram See Nalidixic acid
Neo-Mercazole See Carbimazole
Neoral See Ciclosporin
Netillin See Netilmicin
Neulactil See Pericyazine
Neurontin See Gabapentin
Neutrexin See Trimetrexate
NiQuitin CQ See Nicotine
Nicorette See Nicotine
Nicotinell See Nicotine
Niferex See Polysaccharide-iron complex
Nimotop See Nimodipine
Nivaquine See Chloroquine
Nivemycin See Neomycin sulphate
Nizoral See Ketoconazole
Nolvadex See Tamoxifen
Nootropil See Piracetam
Norgalax Micro-enema See Docusate sodium
Normacol See Sterculia
Norprolac See Quinagolide
Norvir See Ritonavir
Novantrone See Mitoxantrone
Nozinan See Levomepromazine/ Methotrimeprazine
Nozinan See Methotrimeprazine/ Levomepromazine
Nuelin See Theophylline
Nurofen See Ibuprofen
Nutrizym See Pancreatin
Nystan See Nystatin

Oncovin See Vincristine sulphate
Optimax See Tryptophan
Optimine See Azatadine maleate
OrLAAM See Levacetylmethadol hydrochloride
Oralbalance See Saliva substitute
Oraldene See Hexetidine
Oramorph See Morphine
Orap See Pimozide
Orelox See Cefpodoxime
Orgaran See Danaparoid
Orudis See Ketoprofen
Oxis See Eformoterol fumarate/Formoterol fumarate
Oxivent See Oxitropium bromide

Palfium See Dextromoramide
Palladone See Hydromorphone hydrochloride

Paludrine See Proguanil hydrochloride
Paludrine/Avoclor See Chloroquine
Panadol See Paracetamol
Pancrease See Pancreatin
Pancrex See Pancreatin
Paraplatin See Carboplatin
Pariet See Rabeprazole sodium
Parlodel See Bromocriptine
Parnate See Tranylcypromine
Penbritin See Ampicillin
Penicillin G See Benzyl penicillin
Penicillin V See Phenoxymethyl penicillin
Pentacarinat See Pentamidine isethionate
Pentasa See Mesalazine
Pentostam See Sodium stibogluconate
Pepcid See Famotidine
Peptac See Alginates
Perdix See Moexipril
Periactin See Cyproheptadine hydrochloride
Peroxyl See Hydrogen peroxide mouthwash
Persantin See Dipyridamole
Pharmorubicin See Epirubicin
Phenergan See Promethazine hydrochloride
Phyllocontin Continus See Aminophylline
Physeptone See Methadone hydrochloride
Physiotens See Moxonidine
Piportil Depot See Pipotiazine palmitate
Piriton See Chlorphenamine maleate / Chlorpheniramine maleate
Pitressin See Vasopressin
Plavix See Clopidogrel
Plendil See Felodipine
Plesmet See Ferrous glycine sulphate
Ponstan See Mefenamic acid
Pork Mixtard See Biphasic isophane insulin
Prepulsid See Cisapride
Prescal See Isradipine
Preservex See Aceclofenac
Priadel See Lithium salts
Priadel: Li-Liquid See Lithium salts

Primacor See Milrinone
Primalan See Mequitazine
Primaxin See Imipenem with cilastatin
Pripsen See Piperazine
Pro Epanutin See Fosphenytoin sodium
Pro-Viron See Mesterolone
Pro-banthine See Propantheline bromide
Prograf See Tacrolimus
Prominal See Methylphenobarbital
Pronestyl See Procainamide
Propaderm See Beclometasone dipropionate
Proscar See Finasteride
Prothiaden See Dosulepin hydrochloride/Dothiepin hydrochloride
Protium See Pantoprazole
Provigil See Modafinil
Prozac See Fluoxetine
Pulmicort See Budesonide
Pulmozyne See Dornase alpha
Puri-Nethol See Mercaptopurine
Pylorid See Ranitidine bismuth citrate
Pyrogastrone See Carbenoxolone sodium

Questran See Cholestyramine
Quinalbarbitone {[Tuinal]} See Secobarbital
Qvar See Beclometasone dipropionate

Rapitil See Nedocromil sodium
Raxar See Grepafloxacin
Rebetol See Ribavarin
Regulan See Ispaghula husk
Relenza See Zanamivir
Relifex See Nabumetone
Remnos See Nitrazepam
Requip See Ropinirole
Respacal See Tulobuterol hydrochloride
Respontin See Ipratropium bromide
Restandol See Testosterone
Retrovir See Zidovudine
Revanil See Lisuride maleaten
Rheumox See Azapropazone

Ridaura See Auranofin
Rifadin See Rifampicin
Rifater See Rifampicin
Rifinah 150 See Rifampicin
Rifinah 300 See Rifampicin
Rimacid See Indomethacin
Rimactane See Rifampicin
Rimactazid 150 See Rifampicin
Rimactazid 300 See Rifampicin
Rimapam See Diazepam
Risperdal See Risperidone
Ritalin See Methylphenidate hydrochloride
Rivotril See Clonazepam
Robicin See Spectinomycin
Rocephin See Ceftriaxone
Rohypnol See Flunitrazepam
Rotacaps See Salbutamol
Rozex See Metronidazole
Rynacrom. See Sodium cromoglicate
Rythmodan See Disopyramide

Salagen See Pilocarpine hydrochloride
Salazopyrin See Sulfasalazine
Saliva Orthana See Saliva substitute
Salivace See Saliva substitute
Salivix See Saliva substitute
Salofalk See Mesalazine
Saluric See Chlorothiazide
Salveze See Saliva substitute
Sanomigran See Pizotifen
Scandonest See Mepivacaine
Scopoderm See Hyoscine hydrobromide
Sectral See Acebutolol
Securon See Verapamil
Securopen See Azlocillin
Selexid See Pivmecillinam hydrochloride
Semprex See Acrivastine
Senokot See Senna
Septanenst See Articaine
Septrin See Co-trimoxazole
Serc See Betahistine dihydrochloride
Serdolect See Sertindole
Serenace See Haloperidol
Seretide See Fluticasone propionate
Serevent See Salmeterol
Seroquel See Quetiapine
Seroxat See Paroxetine

Sinemet CR See Co-careldopa
Sinemet plus See Co-careldopa
Sinemet See Co-careldopa
Sinequan See Doxepin
Singulair See Montelukast
Skelid See Tiludronic acid
Slo-Phyllin See Theophylline
Slozem See Diltiazem
Sno Phenicol See Chloramphenicol
Solfedipine See Nifedipine
Solian See Amisulpride
Solu-cortel See Hydrocortisone
Sonata See Zaleplon
Sotacor See Sotalol hydrochloride
Spiroctan See Spironolactone
Sporanox See Itraconazole
Staril See Fosinopril
Stelazine See Trifluoperazine
Stemetil See Prochlorperazine
Stesolid See Diazepam
Stilboestrol See Diethylstilbestrol
Stilnoct See Zolpidem tartrate
Stromba See Stanozolol
Stugeron See Cinnarizine
Sudafed See Pseudoephedrine
        hydrochloride
Sulparex See Sulpiride
Sulpitil See Sulpiride
Suprax See Cefixime
Suprecur See Buserelin
Surgam See Tiaprofenic acid
Surmontil See Trimipramine
Sustiva See Efavirenz
Symmetrel See Amantadine
        hydrochloride
Synagis See Palivizumab
Synercid See Quinupristin with
        Dalfopristin
Syscor See Nisoldipine

Tagamet See Cimetidine
Tambocor See Flecainide acetate
Tanatril See Imidapril
Targocid See Teicoplanin
Tarivid See Ofloxacin
Tavanic See Levofloxacin
Tavegil See Clemastine
Taxol See Paclitaxel
Taxotere See Docetaxel
Tazocin See Piperacillin
Tegretol retard See Carbamazepine

Tegretol See Carbamazepine
Telfast See Fexofenadine
        hydrochloride
Temgesic See Buprenorphine
Tenorminx See Atenolol
Tensipine See Nifedipine
Tensium See Diazepam
Terasyl 300 See Lymecycline
Teril CR See Carbamazepine
Terramycin See Oxytetracycline
Tertroxin See Liothyronine sodium
Teveten See Eprosartan
Theo-Dur See Theophylline
Tilade See Nedocromil sodium
Tildiem See Diltiazem
Tiloryth See Erythromycin
Timecef See Cefodizime
Timentin See Ticarcillin
Timonil retard. See Carbamazepine
Tofranil See Imipramine
        hydrochloride
Tolanase See Tolazamide
Tomudex See Raltitrexed
Topal See Alginates
Topamax See Topiramate
Trandate See Labetalol
Trasicor See Oxprenolol
        hydrochloride
Trileptal See Oxcarbazepine
Triludan See Terfenadine
Trimopan See Trimethoprim
Triptaphen See Amitriptyline
        hydrochloride
Tritace See Ramipril
Trusopt See Dorzolamide
Tryptizol See Amitriptyline
        hydrochloride

Ubretid See Distigmine bromide
Ucerax See Hydroxyzine
        hydrochloride
Ultralanum See Fluticasone
        propionate
Uniphyllin Continus See
        Theophylline
Unisomnia See Nitrazepam
Urdox See Ursodeoxycholic acid
Uriben See Nalidixic acid
Urispass 200 See Flavoxate
        hydrochloride
Ursofalk See Ursodeoxycholic acid

Ursogal See Ursodeoxycholic acid
Utinor See Norfloxacin

Valclair See Diazepam
Valium See Diazepam
Vallergan See Alimemazine tartrate/
   Trimeprazine tartrate
Valoid See Cyclizine
Valtrex See Valaciclovir
Vancocin See Vancomycin
Vascace See Cilazapril
Velbe See Vinblastine sulphate
Velosef See Cefradine
Ventide See Beclometasone
   dipropionate
Ventodisks See Salbutamol
Ventolin See Salbutamol
Vepesid See Etoposide
Vermox See Mebendazole
Viagra See Sildenafil
Viazem See Diltiazem
Vibramycin -D See Doxycycline
Vibramycin See Doxycycline
Videx See Didanosine
Vioxx See Rofecoxib
Viracept See Nelfinavir
Viramune See Nevirapine
Virazole See Ribavarin
Visclair See Mecysteine
   hydrochloride
Visken See Pindolol
Vistide See Cidofovir
Vivalan See Viloxazine
   hydrochloride
Voltarol See Diclofenac sodium

Welldorm See Chloral hydrate
Wellvone See Atovaquone

Xanax See Alprazolam
Xenical See Orlistat

Xylocaine See Lidocaine/Lignocaine
   Dental preparations
Xylotox See Lidocaine/Lignocaine
   Dental preparations

Yomesan See Niclosamide

Zaditen See Ketotifen
Zadstat See Metronidazole
Zamadol See Tramadol
   hydrochloride
Zandip See Lercanidipine
Zantac See Ranitidine
Zarontin See Ethosuximide
Zavedos See Idarubicin
   hydrochloride
Zelapar See Selegeline
   hydrochloride
Zemtard See Diltiazem
Zerit See Stavudine
Zestril See Lisinopril
Ziagen See Abacavir
Zimovane See Zopiclone
Zinacef See Cefuroxime
Zinamide See Pyrazinamide
Zinnat See Cefuroxime
Zirtek See Cetirizine
   hydrochloride
Zispin See Mirtazapine
Zithromax See Azithromycin
Zocor See Simvastatin
Zofran See Ondansetron
Zoleptil See Zotepine
Zomig See Zolmitriptan
Zoton See Lansoprazole
Zovirax See Aciclovir
Zyban See Amfebutamone
Zydol See Tramadol
   hydrochloride
Zyloric See Allopurinol
Zyprexa See Olanzapine